KUN QI INTENTIONAL MEDITATIVE MOVEMENT

SECTIONS   PAGE

INTRODUCTION   2
SECTION ONE - KUN QI THE ESSENCE   6
    I.   SUBTLE BODY SCAN TECHNIQUES   8
    II.   7 ELEMENT THEORY OF LIFE FORCE   10
    III.   SENTIENCE - ONE SENSATION MANY DIFFERING WAYS   13
    IV.   ANCIENT AFRICAN SPIRITUALITY & DIVINE SCIENCE   18
    V.   BREATH AND VISUALIZATION   20
    VI.   CREATING SACRED SPACE   24
    VII. ATTUNING TO THE 7 ELEMENTS OF NATURE   25
    VIII. KUN QI MERIDIAN MEDITATION   26
SECTION TWO - KUN QI KUNG THE MOVEMENTS
    IX.   SEQUENCE I – JOINT MOBILIZATION   30
    X.   THE ORGAN MERIDIAN SYSTEMS & QI   36
    XI.   THE BODIES CLOCK   40
    XII. 7 HUMAN EMOTIONS THAT AFFECT HEALTH   43
    XIII. SEQUENCE II – HEALING THE ORGANS WITH TAO YIN FA   45
    XIV. THE WORKINGS OF THE 7 ELEMENTS THEORY   53
    XV. THE UNIVERSAL CYCLES OF SEVEN   56
    XVI. THE WORKINGS OF THE CHAKRAS   61
    XVII. THE CHAKRA ASSOCIATION TO THE 7 ELEMENTS   71
    XVIII. THE USE OF MUDRAS   76
    XIX. CHAKRA MUDRAS FOR MEDITATIVE MOVEMENT   82
    XX. THE 8 DIRECTIONAL CIPHER OF KUN QI   86
    XXI. 8 EXTRAORDINARY MERIDIANS & PLANETARY EMISSARIES   89
    XXII. SACRED SPACE INVOCATION   91
    XXIII. SEQUENCE III - SITUATIONAL CLEARING   98
    XXIV. ADVANCED MOVEMENTS FOR THE 8 DIRECTIONAL CIPHER 99
    XXV. SEQUENCE IV – CHAKRA CLEARING USING THE 8 DIRECTIONS   102
    XXVI. VOCAL TONING FOR CHAKRA & MERIDIAN CLEARING   103
SECTION THREE - INTRODUCING TANRAN REIKI TO KUN QI KUNG
    XXVII. THE HISTORY OF TANRAN REIKI   104
    XXVIII. TANRAN REIKI SACRED SPACE INVOCATION   108
    XXIX. TANRAN REIKI ATUN-MENT PRAYER & HEALING SALUTATION   110
    XXX. SEQUENCE V – SITUATIONAL CLEARING WITH DAI KO MYO 111
    XXXI. SEQUENCE VI – TANRAN PERSONAL & UNIVERSAL HEALING   113
SYMBOL ACTIVATION, DETAILS, ATTRIBUTES & MEDITATIONS
    XXXII. DOHYAHNOH   114
    XXXIII. DAIKOMYO   117
    XXXIV. HONSHAZESHONEN   121
    XXXV. ZEEGAHNAH   124
    XXXVI. TANRAN   128
    XXXVII. CHOKUREI   132
    XXXVIII. SEIHEKI   135
    XXXIX. RAKU   137
    XL. SUMMARY   139
    XLI. APPENDIX TABLE OF CONTENT   140
    XLII. APPENDIXES   141

* Sequence formulated by Fabian Manman, Tama-do Academy
**Based on Willam Bagley's Tanran Reiki teachings

INTRODUCTION
KUN QI INTENTIONAL HEALING MOVEMENT

KUN QI is the way in which the original (indigenous) beings of Earth lived and moved in harmony with Earth's natural design and environmental rhythms. **QI (*pronounced as "Chi"*),** as a Nuwaupian word, refers to "Mother Earth's" life force from the time of the primordial waters Trillions of Earth years ago when all living matter that was formed on earth were aquatic or elemental. It has been modified by ancient Asiatic culture to mean "Life Force", "breath", "air", or "gas". Asiatic medical tradition refers to Qi as the intangible (subtle) currents of electromagnetic energy that flows around and through our bodies. These currents extend beyond the human skin forming an electromagnetic field 10-100 cm (4-39 inches) around our physical form. This field consists of the human emotions, mental states, intellect, and spiritual essence of each person. Every cell of the physical form is fed everything that is necessary to sustain bodily form and function-ability from these life forces.

This form of intentional movement has both internal and universal healing power to transmute blocked or stagnant energy within the physical and subtle bodies, into clear and free flowing, healthy life force. Kun Qi Kung combines the healing energies of Tanran Reiki, Qi Gong movements, specific breathing techniques, Mudras, Toning, and Intentional Visualization in ways that raise the vibration and molecular structure of one's physical and energetic body's by activating, re-aligning, and upgrading the cellular memory that resides within the physical components of one's DNA structure to that of the divine components that reside within the brains functional capacity.

The Complete term for **KUN QI is "KUN HU HIKA SAI QI** which means: "The Anthro/Metamorphic Personification of Creative Life Force Resonance"

- **KUN** means existence or being-ness
- **HU** means resonance of the universe
- **HIKA** is the manipulation of elements and chemicals of nature anthropomorphically.
- **SAI** means the personification of perception, shape, form and pattern.
- **QI** mean "Life Force"

The central component of the word, as it relates to Qi Kung, is **KUN QI "Being Life Force"** In this form of Qi Kung, you can not only increase and regulate your energy expenditure more intentionally but you can unblock and transmute unhealthy life force within your body on a conscious level so that you can move toward the experience of living in Divine health. Kun Qi Kung improves the circulation of your vital life force energy throughout the muscles, joints, internal organs and subtle bodies. The sentient nature of Tanran Reiki combined with Qi Kung activates cellular memory triggers of one's divine origins within the DNA. This ascended cellular memory then processes through our anatomical and energetic systems and at times registers Akashic information on a conscious level within our mind allowing us to access the inner wisdom of the spirit and soul that reside within our chakras and anatomy for guidance as to conscious changes one can make for their personal evolution.

Reiki is a Japanese word meaning "God's Wisdom, Knowledge and Life Force". It is an ancient spiritual practice whose origins date back to the Atlantian/Lemuria time period approximately 9000 B.C. During the destruction of Atlantis, it was brought into the temple systems of religion; it has no dogma, and there is nothing you must believe in order to learn and use Reiki. In fact, Reiki is not dependent on belief at all and will work whether you believe in it or not. Because Reiki comes from The Source of all Creation, many people find that using Reiki puts them more in touch with the experience of their religion rather than having only an intellectual concept of it and inspires one to live and act in a way that promotes harmony with all of Creation. We were meant to retain the knowledge of our inherent cellular/ molecular connection to the universe, and the knowledge of the galactic star formation or nation that the elements of our godhood come from. This is the Higher Knowledge of our oneness with universal life force or our own God-Life Force that resides within the dormant strands of our DNA and is being awakened for many, during this time. This is the aspect of Reiki that has been integrated into this system of Kun Qi Kung; its power to keep our physical and energetic (mental/emotional/spiritual) bodies attuned and aligned with Divine intelligence on a consciously. The term throughout the following curriculum that we will use to refer to this is Kun Qi Kung.

THERE ARE 7 COMPONENTS OF KUN QI KUNG:
1. Breath Work
2. Intentional Movement
3. Inner Visualization
4. Healing Mudra's
5. Creating Sacred Space
6. Innerstanding the Meridian/Chakra Systems
7. Tanran Reiki Symbolism & Attunements

Like the Eastern discipline of yoga, Kun Qi Kung combines breathing, inner awareness and gentle, flowing movements that create a meditative state. It also integrates the sentient healing power of Tanran Reiki. Tanran Reiki corresponds directly and integrally with the human and Universal chakra systems and appeals especially to those who tend to achieve a meditative state of mind through physical activity. It provides a means to tapping into and utilizing greater quantities of life force energy from our earthly elements and those of the universe; something which many alternative medical, martial arts, and healing arts practitioners recognize to be the essential life force within all of creation. The effectiveness of the various series of movements are not limited by ones levels of fitness externally or internally, therefore whether you're young or old, a beginner or a trained athlete, are perfectly healthy or have a life threatening dis-ease you can adapt these sequences to fit the level of physical challenge that best suits your current physical condition.

As mentioned, this Series of meditative movements and exercises open the meridian and chakra channels that increase the flow of universal life force, lymph, blood, oxygen and nutrients thru the internal systems throughout the physical and subtle bodies. Some of the physical and subtle body benefits you will experience are:

- The dissolving and detoxification of stagnant energy and cellular waste within the physical and energetic systems,
- Relaxation of the mind, nervous system and musculature
- Increase circulation of blood, lymph, nutrients, and oxygen throughout the body
- Increased lung capacity and cellular oxygenation
- Postural re-alignment and strengthening of the musculoskeletal system
- Rejuvenation of physical and mental agility
- Increased mental clarity and balance
- Emotional clearing
- Increased sense of alignment with Higher Self and Spiritual purpose
- Improved anatomical and subtle body health and alignment from the inside out through intentionality.
- Homeostasis of the body/mind/spirit
- Creates a transcendental state of thought manifestation potential

As one's capacity to increase the amount of oxygen and nutrients absorbed into the blood is obtained, one improves their ability to think more clearly, sleep better, and one's body to function more efficiently. This helps one to rid one's body of excess cellular and subtle body waste, thus, excess physical and psychosomatic weight. This is due to the fact that oxygen is the most important nutrient, besides water, that our body needs in order to live and operate properly. And by increasing the ability for energy to move within the body one raises their vibration one feels lighter and more even in their mental/emotional state. This naturally creates more energy to utilize which brings about a sense of well-being and self-control necessary to live a happy, productive and fulfilling life.

This meditative practice of focused intent is a key to learning to master the movement of your body and how to consciously generate and direct internal qi for the purpose of unblocking, dissolving, and releasing energies and thought forms that are outdated and no longer serve your personal objectives and Soul evolution.

Personally, it has become an integral part of my own self-healing and therapeutic practice. It allows me to sustain my energy for longer periods of time which has increased the longevity of my practice and the vividness of my empathic connection with everything and everyone. Through this application one naturally becomes a clearer channel for Divine Intelligence to flow through as one becomes better able to connect on a deeper more conscious level with the elements and intuitive Healing Guidance that is responsible for the transmutation of negative energies into healthy life force that transpires through this process of vibrational alchemy and visualization. The more facets of divine health you integrate into your daily lifestyle, such as incorporating an organic vegetarian or vegan diet, organic mineral and nutritional supplementation, regular daily focused movement and exercise, meditation, healing touch, creative expression, holistic medical treatment, spiritual and self-developmental studies, positive visualization and life affirmations, the better quality of life you will experience with greater opportunities to achieve personal and spiritual fulfillment.

One major benefit is that we become more in-tune with our internal physical, postural and psychological patterns that have been responsible for the stress and pain in our bodies and our lives. This practice provides you with a set of tools that will help you to consciously recognize, release, and re-align, holding patterns and/or physical and internal imbalances intentionally, while at the same time rebalancing and rejuvenating the circulation of qi, lymph, blood, oxygen, nutrients and divine consciousness throughout the body.

The combination of Intentional thinking, Deep Breathing, Mudras, visualizing and vocalizing the symbols of healing and Qi Kung movements improves long term health, one's sense of wellbeing and one's power to meet the challenges of life with grace and ease. But most of all, it's effective in revitalizing, and provides a way for one to gently energize the entire organ system, balance the chakras, experience situational resolution and re-connect to nature and one's own spiritual truth as a part of their personal evolution within this universal healing wave.

Right now you are standing on the precipice of change. And you may be feeling that it might be too much for you. But it is not. Too much. It is just the right amount to get you where you need to be. You may be feeling that the change is so big that it will swallow you up. But it will not. It is here to birth you into a new dimension of you that has yet to exist.

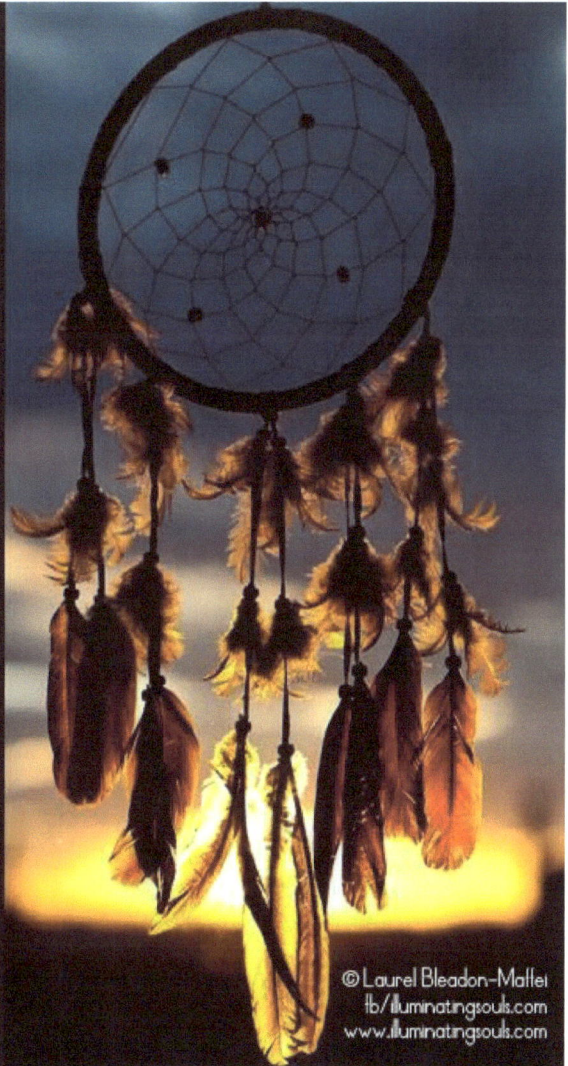

© Laurel Bleadon-Maffei
fb/illuminatingsouls.com
www.illuminatingsouls.com

KUN QI – THE ESSENCE

KUN QI is feeling, hearing, and being the breath while intentionally staying aware of activating the muscles of the body that one is using during movement at any time. This way of moving your body is based on the way in which our original ancestors moved their bodies before the constructs of city living existed. We were intuitively linked with the intelligence of the nature within all life forms and had learned to live and operate in synchronistic harmony with the environment, weather patterns, and changes caused by Mother Earth shifting her tectonic plates when needing to release her own energies. They were able to move effortlessly over land and water navigating its terrain intuitively in ways akin to the way the animal kingdom continues to migrate and hibernate in sync with seasonal changes and shifts in weather patterns. Our original psychic connection with all life forms and the knowledge of the rhythms and energetic influences of the cosmos on earth, and the properties of the plant life, allowed us to innerstand the language of nature and live in synch with its rhythms and adapt to the shifts and changes without undue stress, dis-ease or degeneration because we could read and innerstand the signs, the meanings behind their movements as a way of communication and respond to what was being communicated.

Society's man-made comfort-abilities that have been built into our modern structural environment and our food sources has created cellular degeneration, postural imbalances, un-natural muscular holding patterns, and undue stress on the internal systems creating stagnation of life force flow in the body that living in a natural environment does not. Man-made material such as vehicles of modern transportation, processed manufactured food consumption, television, microwaves, and various other devises that channel electrical waves, and chemical trails, introduce levels of toxicity that we have knowingly and for the most part, unknowingly been ingesting into our bodies. The infiltration of these material conveniences has caused a disconnection between the mind/body and nature which has had a deteriorating effect on our quality of life, our physical, mental, and spiritual function-ability and our attunement with all sentient life force. Our connection with the elements of nature needs to be re-awakened and re-established so that we can open up, attune to, and stimulate the flow of qi – "life force" between them and ourselves, throughout our meridian and chakra channels and throughout the entire body in order to reverse the aforementioned effects of modern society. This helps all aspects of one's spirit, soul, and body to synchronize rhythmically as a complete unified system raising their vibration to create a sense of well-being with the ability to handle what life presents with greater ease and to remain younger longer. As one makes it a practice to meditate on the inner workings of the body during movement one will become more deeply aware of the oneness that their mind/body and sentience were designed to operate in. With intentional awareness guiding the body you will also become more agile, able to move more effortlessly with a sense of smoothness and grace. At the same time on a subtle body level you will become more attuned to the inner wisdom from the Higher Mind which inspires harmonious intuitive insights and visions that surface within the silence rhythm of the breath during motion.

Many have adopted the belief that intellectual knowledge is the same thing as inner-standing or that the 'mind' is no more than what we consciously comprehend or recall. Yet the body and our emotions respond to stimuli without our conscious intention which proves contradictory to that belief. What lies within us is a personal link to an Infinite Source of intelligence that directs and maintains the function-ability of our bodies without our will or conscious intent. For example, the flow of adrenaline and the pace at which the heartbeat increases when confronted with fear or elation. The dropping of those same rates occurs during times of loving interaction, peaceful contemplation, or when one is engaged in those things that soul fulfilling and empowering.

How the body functions internally are also directly related to the mental/emotional state that one is in, and those things outside oneself that trigger mental/emotional responses. On a cellular level, every thought or emotionally charged memory remains lodged within our cells (clinically referred to as cellular memory). Unless the emotional charges have had an opportunity to release physically or have been confronted psycho/spiritually they become lodged within one's subconscious cellular memory and continue to cycle into ones perceptions of love, life, and relationships, unbidden and at times in an unhealthy or unproductive context. These are just a few ways in which our bodies naturally react to our mental and emotional states. When you become attuned to how your body and mind operates, you awaken to the realization of how your body responds to your mental and emotional state by producing stress, stagnation and postural holding patterns without your conscious awareness. You can then re-train your body responses by integrating various techniques such as mental body scans, focused breathing breaks and meditation in order to counter the effects of stress. You will learn how to perform Mental/Emotional body scanning exercises to identify which holding patterns of yours are self-inflicted and which ones are due to outside influence, which are behavioral, inborn, or genetic, and which of these are correctable.

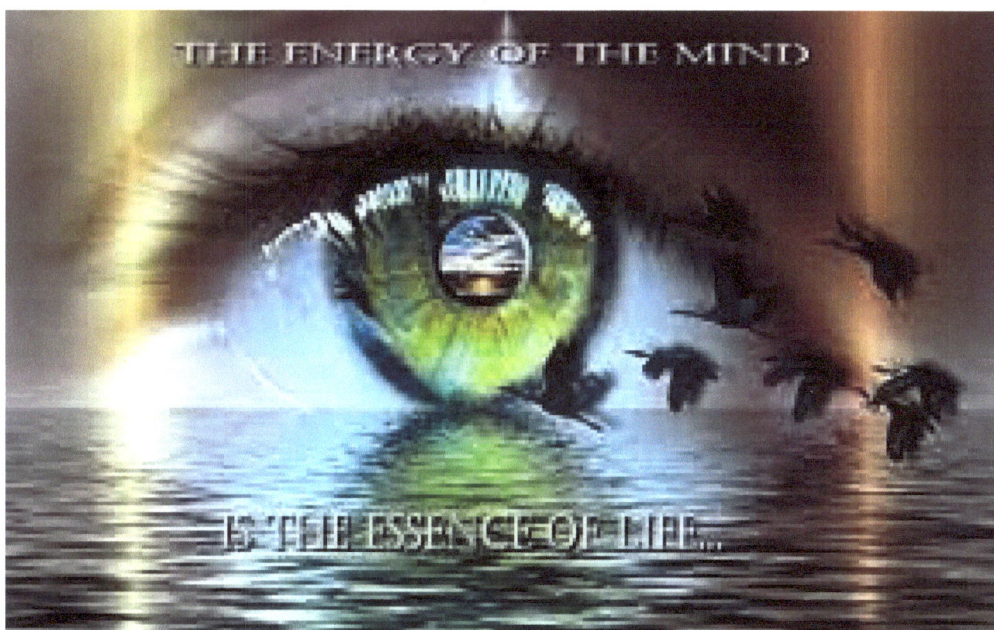

THE ENERGY OF THE MIND

IS THE ESSENCE OF LIFE...

SUBTLE BODY SCANNING TECHNIQUES

TENSION/RELAXATION SCAN

The tension/relaxation body scan is quite similar to the body scan that you will perform during your warm-up. It requires the same mental inner focus however, its purpose is to instill in you a means of quickly and automatically identifying the places in your body where you are holding tension at the time and how to automatically release the tension you are holding.

First, bring your mental attention to your shoulders. Intentionally tense or clench your head, neck, back, shoulder, and arm muscles as tight as you can as if you are bracing yourself in order to protect yourself from someone striking you. Note how that feels to do so, then using your conscious awareness intentionally relax those same muscles and allow yourself to take a few slow deep breaths focusing your mind just on your breathing and the sensation of relaxation it creates. Next move your focus down to your abdomen, glutes, and legs using your inner vision to identify and intentionally clench and tighten them for a few seconds. Now release them intentionally and take a few slow belly breaths in order to relax them even more fully just as you did with the upper body. You may repeat this a few times or choose to perform this tense/release exercise by isolating one individual muscles group or even one muscle at a time such as focusing on just the neck or just the right arm or left quad. Over time, focus on isolating, tensing, and releasing smaller and smaller areas in order to better master your ability to relax your body upon mental command instantaneously.

This exercise is designed to not only cultivate your awareness of your ability to identify and intentionally creating tension and relaxation in your body but to help you become aware of the tension patterns in your body created from performing everyday activities. This provides you with a tool to relax any area of your body at any time during any activity through the use of your mind and your breath. Once you have mastered this exercise I recommend engaging in it periodically throughout your day especially during lengthy sedentary activities such as driving, performing computer work, drumming, guitar playing, studying, etc. any activity that you are maintaining the same positioning for more than 30 minutes. As an example, while sitting at your desk typing on your computer, tense your glutes, legs, abs, upper arms, and chest while leaving your forearms, neck and lower legs relaxed. Hold the tension for 10-20 seconds then relax all your muscles paying attention to the sensation of relaxation within your body. Make sure you are breathing in a slow, deep and relaxed manner. Repeat this 2 more times. Continuing to pay attention to your breathing and the sensation of relaxation. You should feel relaxed and ready to continue to do your activities feeling calmer, looser and less mentally stressed.

Engaging is this exercise throughout your day while performing daily activities can have the benefits as working out. It increases blood flow throughout the body, firms and tones the muscles helping to improve the strength and longevity of your body and its ability to perform the activities you engage in and it is something you can do whenever and wherever it comes to mind. So, you don't necessarily need a gym membership to work your muscles.

SUBTLE BODY TRIGGER SCAN

This scanning exercise will help you to become aware of how your thoughts and emotions create postural imbalances within your body and to teach you how to become more masterful in balancing your mental/emotional state and transcending stress inducing thought patterns. Find a comfortable sitting position in either a chair or on the floor. Bring your attention to your breathing and gently slow it down breathing deeply into the diaphragm at a 3 – 6 second count during both your inhalation and exhalation. Perform this for about 60 seconds then take a moment to mentally choose either an emotion, (such as sadness or joy) or a memory of a past event that you find brings your energy down or causes it to become ignited; anything that will trigger an emotional reaction within your body. Example: envision an event such as your boss being critical about your work, or a stranger being inconsiderate, irritatingly obnoxious or confrontational publicly. Let it play out in your mind for another 60 seconds. Allow yourself to feel the emotion as though it were happening right in this moment. Once you've attuned yourself to the feeling, try to notice just what area(s) in your body are reacting to that thought and how. You may notice an increase of heat in your body, a rush of energy or blood flow, agitation inside your abdominal area, tension in the neck, your jaw may clench, you may sense butterflies in your gut or you may even notice that you physically feel like striking someone. Now, release the thought by bringing your attention back to your breath. Focus on the sound of each full inhalation and exhalation hearing the ocean in your breath for 60 seconds. As you do so, relax any areas of tension that arose by breathing into each area and letting your body melt any sense of holding with each breath.

Now, envision an event that incites joy, happiness or a peaceful feeling for 1 – 3 minutes. Again, mentally scan your body and notice the difference in your body's reaction to these types of thoughts and where you notice them taking place. Try to notice just what it is about the thought that create the physical reaction then let go of the thought while holding onto the feeling. Let the feeling grow then intentionally bring the feeling down to a more neutral state by letting it dissolve into the ocean of your breathing. By breathing through the emotion, you're able to calm the body and detach yourself physically from the thought that ignited it.

Spend some time creating emotions and diffusing them through breath work and envisioning yourself responding to all situations peacefully yet empowered by your sense of chosen action vs. reaction. Try this in real life situations and notice how your mind/body responds. You'll find that your ability to be more objectified and detached from emotionally reacting will increase. The more that you're able to become aware of what your emotional triggers are, and detach from the need to react to other peoples projected behaviors, the more you are able to master responding objectively without the feeling that you need to fix things; unless of course you do. You can then better discern what would best serve the highest good for you or for those who are being impacted by the situation and act according to what serves that purpose (which more often than not is the choice to just listen; to not respond at all. Just take the information in for future contemplation as to what it's meant to teach you about yourself and what we as a human collective, can experience).

7 ELEMENT THEORY OF LIFE FORCE

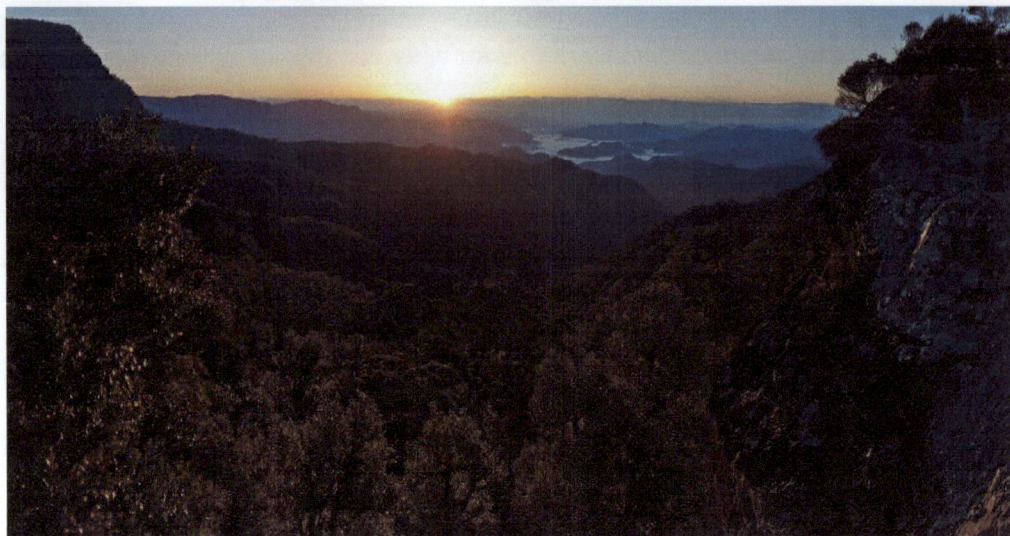

7 ELEMENTS OF NATURE
1. Air
2. Water
3. Fire
4. Mineral
5. Earth
6. Wood/Vegetation
7. Sound/Vibration

Mother Earth is a living, sentient, life giving organism of unknowable intelligence that is a part of an even larger unfathomable organism… the universe. She continues to sustain all life forms despite the destruction to her that humans cause. We, like all life forms that she sustains, are a part of an ecological organism or body that maintains itself through the oxygen/carbon exchange that allows us to live off of the air we breathe, the heat of the sun, the water we drink, the mineral and nutritional content within the food from the plant life grown within the Earths soil, and the cosmic and energetic vibrational frequencies. These 7 components of nature feed and sustain our physical and etheric bodies which create and maintain the complete composition of our molecular and energetic structures that allows us to sustain the physical package called the body that we use to express our True Selves… the spirit. When one is able to tap into all elements at once the vibrational frequency raises to such a level that one is able to transcend the limitations of mental thinking and see through the eyes of ascended consciousness the reality of the sentience, oneness and transformative life force that these elements radiate. The one location that I've found and experienced the vibrational and sacred sentient union with these elements has been at the ocean. The ocean, though not the only place where these elements meet, is the only place where the infinite vastness, magnificence, and unfathomable design of the universe displays itself in its magnitude, beauty, and profundity. It is the place where one can witness the honor and respect that these elements operate by. To me, this is the Holy Temple and the Sanctuary of Earth, where the endless waters meet the vastness of the sky and go no further, where water meets land and goes no further, where the sun and moon can reside synonymously, in the sky suspended in the ethers of space in full view, and the rock formations proceed the abundant plant life that is fed by the abundance of life force from the ocean waters, the soil and the sun. The ocean is also the location where the 7 elements of the universe can also be seen in their glory and abundance at night. Living in a time where technological and scientific evolutions have allowed us to uncover various unknown aspects of the solar system in which we dwell… the universe… the world around us… ourselves I spent some time contemplating the universe and its elements and characteristics and came to the same conclusion that The Universe also has a 7 elemental design.

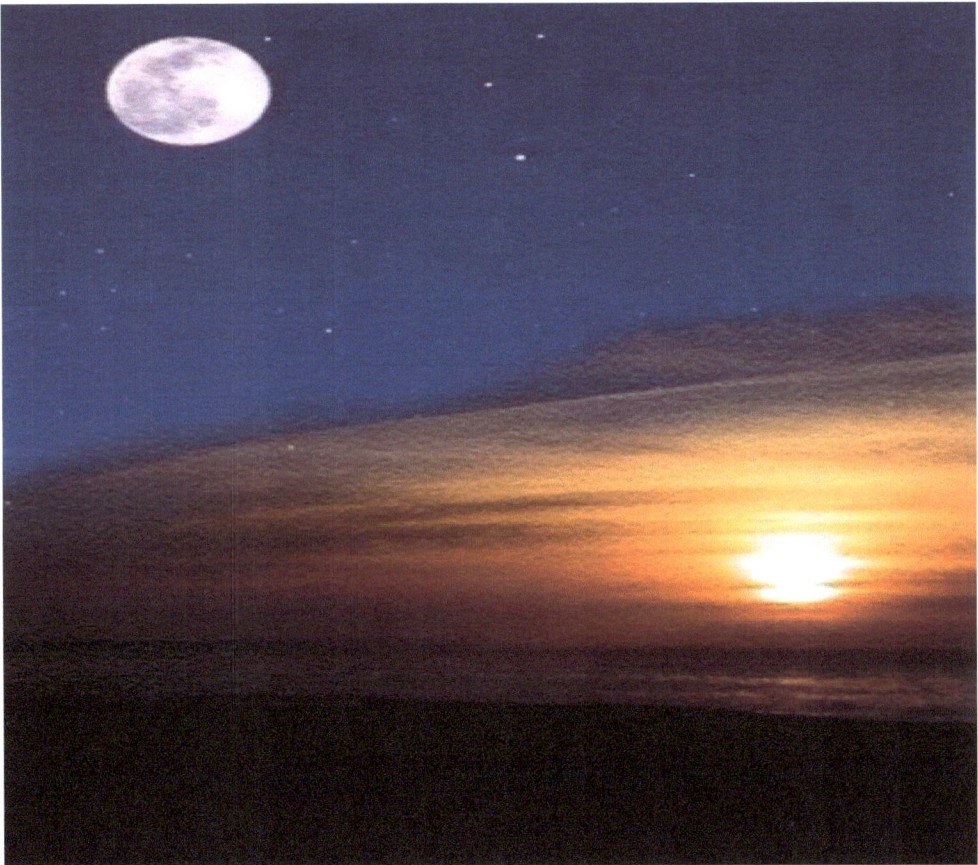

7 ELEMENTS OF THE UNIVERSE
1. Magnetism
2. Electricity
3. Light
4. Ether
5. Vibration/Sound
6. Matter
7. Intelligence

The elements of the universe provide the energetic circuitry of the soul. Though subtle, they are what allow us to consciously and unconsciously interact with all that exists within our dimensional environment. If you consider the way in which these elements function and operate, you will come to find that we reflect them in many ways.

For instance, **magnetism** is that which instinctually attracts one thing to that which reflects itself on some level of personal association. This exhibits our design from the cellular to the celestial essence of our being.

Electricity derives from the motion between two magnetized components. The communication network of our nervous system operates in the same way as electricity in that it sparks, directs, and controls the inner electrical network of the mind/body which allows us to operate the physical as well as the psychological mechanics of our being.

Light is the life force of our spirit or ka body and is maintained by the energetic frequencies that work and move through us.

The Ethers of the Universe and that of the mind are operate in the same way as the womb of a woman. They are guided by divine intelligence, which is responsible for all creative inspirations and processes whether from the Cosmic Universe or our internal Universe of the mind/body. Like a womb, the etheric space provides the incubational environment necessary for life to formulate and materialize both visually and physically. It's where the intangible transforms into the tangible giving material form and substance to all things and from where all material things are birthed. Like gaseous matter our thoughts and visualizations, though not seen through the anatomical eyes but the inner eye, are the stuff from which ALL physical matter derives.

The vibrational impact that our Spoken words coupled with our thought intentions have creates the drive and ambition that fuel the manifestation of ideas into **physical form**. This process is similar to the way in which liquid changes form but remains the same content regardless of its form. As water takes on the shape of its container yet integrates into greater quantities of itself, so do hu-man beings take on the life of their environment yet will remain ancestrally associated and intuitively connected to those of their spiritual or etheric roots. Our sensory preceptors are the mechanisms by which we are able to attune to these aspects of our outer world allowing our physical and spiritual bodies to experience our oneness with these elements. Underlying every aspect of creation is the presence of an intelligence that these elements function by that all tangible and intangible aspects of life possess at differing levels, and in differing sometimes indescribable ways.

Divine Intelligence IS at the root of all life, all that exists whether known or yet unknown and is the element that without it none of the other elements would function harmoniously as parts of a much larger Universal organism.

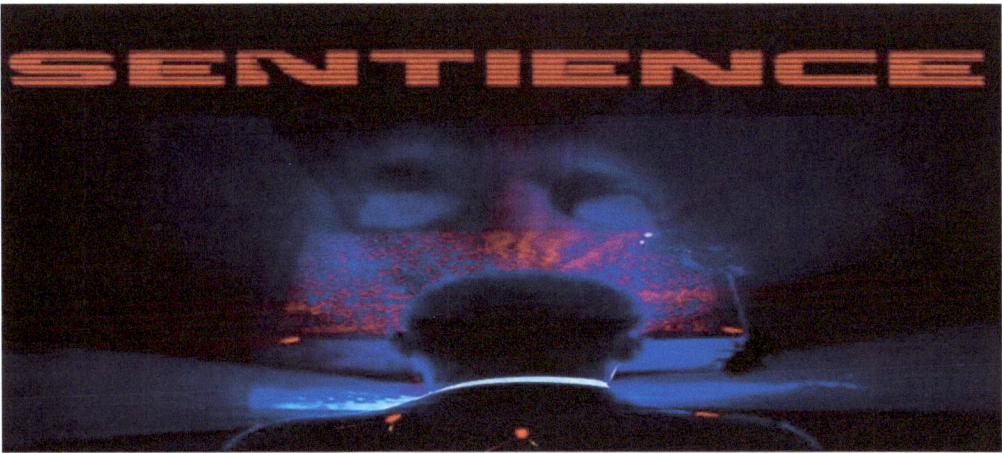

ONE SENSATION MANY DIFFERING WAYS

It has been taught that the ways in which we come to experience and interpret our environment is through our 5 physical sensory preceptors:

1. The eyes, (visual Intake)
2. The Nose, (Intake of smell)
3. The Ears (Intake by Hearing)
4. The Tongue, (Intake through taste) and
5. The Hands & Feet (Intake through touch).

However, there is one thing that I would like to bring to your awareness concerning the 5 senses and that is that all of these perceptions are encompassed within the act of touch. Thus, there is really only one physical perception happening in various physical manners. These parts of the body are designed to gather environmental information for us to innerstand and define our surroundings, and the world around us so that we can navigate its terrain. For example, when we focus the lens of our eyes on an object within our surrounding environment the light from that object penetrates through the lenses of the eyes to the membrane in the back of the eye called the Retina. The retina is in truth, a part of the brain that serves as a transducer to convert photon patterns of light made by an object into neural impulses. The way we experience sight, however, is as an image of solid material form; something we've labeled collectively in order to give the world around us meaning and thus giving life itself the same.

Though western culture has scientifically studied and used various psychic aspects of our make-up, these aspects of our personalities and human design were excluded from our educational institutions and tabooed within our religions. Newly disclosed scientific knowledge about the brain has reconfirmed the amazing powers of our psyche confirming what has been known by the ancients about the psychic sensory apparatus' that we utilize inner-dimensionally and ultra-dimensionally. These various psychic sensory apparatuses that operate within our subconscious, are part of our natural design from the beginning of man's existence.

Our inner-dimensional preceptors have 3 various ways in which our bodies navigate the space within itself and outside itself, that operate subconsciously and deals with the inner dynamics of space as well as navigating the outer dynamics of space.

Below are three internal sensory mechanism:

1. **Vestibular -** Vestibular is our sense of movement and balance
2. **Proprioception** (propulsion) - Proprioception is the signals sent by our joint receptors to tell us the position and movement of our limbs, the spatial positioning of our body within the surrounding material environment and the amount of pressure that needs to be applied to the joints in order for us to sit, walk, run, reach, grasp, throw, and hold.

3. **Interoception** (internal warning signals) - **Interoception** is the sense of our internal organs which lets us feel things like pain, nausea or butterflies in the stomach.

As human beings, we also have operating within us, various **Ultra-Dimensional Preceptors** or **Extra Sensory Preceptors,** better known as psychic abilities, which allow us to perceive and communicate with Divine Intelligence and or between minds with no physical communication or contact made.

The variety of psychic sensory mechanisms or 6th senses we possess in varying degrees are as follows:

1. **Clairvoyance,**
2. **Clairsentience,**
3. **Clairaudience,**
4. **Claircognizance,**
5. **Mental telepathy**
    a. **Latent Telepathy**
    b. **Retro-cognitive Telepathy**
    c. **Precognitive Telepathy**
    d. **Intuitive Telepathy**
    e. **Emotive Telepathy**
    f. **Super-conscious Telepathy**
    g. **Ancestral Telepathy**
    h. **Cellular Telepathy**

Clairvoyance

is the ability to visually see the spirit bodies of those who've passed on into the spirit worlds, and to read subtle body language, energy, and vibrations, and to see future events before they happen. As stated in Wikipedia, "It's the ability to gain information about an object, person, location or physical event through means other than the known human senses. It is very different from telepathy in that the information is gained directly from an external source, such as an object or celestial spirit that is present rather than being transferred from the mind of one individual to another."

Clairsentient Perception

is where one can sense people's moods, attitudes, thoughts, intentions, and feelings on a physical and/or energetic level with the ability to read between the lines and know the underlying thoughts, info or feelings that aren't being disclosed yet are the layer of truth at the root of a person's state of mind or a situation. Generally, the term refers to a person who can sense the information within the aura of other people. There are many different degrees of clairsentience ranging from the perception of existing diseases another person may have to the feeling and emotions that a person is really feeling under the surface of their expression.

Clairaudience

is the ability to hear the voices of those who reside in the spirit world or who are beyond the range of being heard by the physical ear. It refers not to actual perception of sound, but impressions made on the "inner mental ear" similar to the way many people think words without having auditory impressions. It also refers to the actual perception of sounds such as voices, tones, or noises which are not audibly apparent to other humans or commonly used recording equipment.

Claircognizance or Clear Knowing

is a form of extra-sensory perception wherein a person acquires psychic knowledge primarily by means of intrinsic knowledge. It is the ability to know something without a physical explanation why you know it, like the concept of mediums or channeling information and/or communications from entities that are beyond this dimension that are not in physical form.

Telepathy

is the ability to read the thoughts and stored information in the brain or akashic records of others. As previously mentioned, there is more than one type of telepathy. **Latent Telepathy**, formerly known as "*deferred telepathy,*" is described as being the transfer of information, through Parapsychology with an observable time-lag between transmission and receipt. **Retro-cognitive, Precognitive, and Intuitive Telepathy** is described as being the transfer of information, through Psi, about the past, future or present state of an individual's mind to another individual. **Emotive Telepathy**, also known as remote influence or emotional transfer, is the process of transferring kinesthetic or physical sensations when in altered states. **Super-conscious Telepathy** involves tapping into the collective-conscious to access the collective wisdom of the human species and its developmental experience that has been stored within the Akashic Record within the astral plane.

Ancestral Sentience and Telepathy

is the intuitional inspirations that guide our sense of group belonging and association at an inherent ancestral/bio-spiritual level as well as on a cosmic/galactic level. This level of personal association is both objective and subjective in that the sentience of our ancestral roots on a cellular memory level resides in the subjective mind. Its influence in guiding our behaviors, life perspectives, social associations and ways of generating wealth based on one's ancestral blueprint both celestially, and terrestrially. When one is able to align with their divine DNA blueprint then one will consciously seek to live according to the cosmic ways of living in harmonious existence with the environment and all life forms where malice is not the motivation behind its destructive nature.

Cellular Sentience and Telepathy

Our bodies are made up of materials that are made of both planetary and cosmic matter. The cellular composition of our bodies cells is made up from hydrogen, nitrogen, oxygen, carbon, and more. These molecular components are the same substances that many star formations, suns and planets throughout the universe also contain in varying degrees. Thus, the metaphoric reference of humans being "Children of the Stars" or "Children of God" is not just a metaphor but a literal truth on a cellular level. Since all life force and forms comes from the Divine Intelligence or The Mind of God and materializes in form we, being made in the "Image and Likeness of God" (Gen. 1:26), are made of the substance of the Universe and of the Earth and have created the material world that we live in from the infinite Divine intelligence that is accessible within our minds by acting upon our highest thoughts. This will be covered in depth later as the subject matter pertains to manifesting greater levels of health through Kun Qi Gong.

All of these senses are every bit as important and as actively used in our daily functioning and learning as our five physical senses are. As preceptors that are extra sensory or psychic in nature, they operate on an energetic subtle body level and often do not necessarily require one to be physically present to pick up. With Reiki incorporated into the meditative movement one's ultra-sensory preceptors of clairsentience and more will become either activated or deepened allowing one to consciously feel the life force and energy of all living things within one's environment and beyond. Also, one's ability to consciously receive knowledge and insights from more ascended realms and dimensions of consciousness within the universe and within oneself will also increase.

The various sequences of movements range in purpose and intent, from that of physical activation and mastery to that of conscious and subtle body awareness, integration and innerstanding of oneself and of the universal flow of life force around you and within all sentient life. Optimally, it would be best to perform these sequences in an open natural setting where all of the elements of nature are present as this allows you to connect with these elementals in a more direct way. This is not always an available option especially in urban and metropolitan areas. However, one can also create as deep of a connecting with whatever natural elements are available by performing the movements in a park, back yard, nature trails, etc. If being outdoors in the open is not an option the power of visualization and intention will serve the same purpose of attuning (Atun-ing) to the elements of life force in a conscious sentient way.

"How does this relate to meditative movement?"

The way in which this subject matter relates to meditative movement is the ancient practices based on the knowledge of the ways in which we embody and reflect the elements of life force. Through the combination of our intentions, (inner attentions) both mentally and sensory, with our breath work and movement, a way is provided for us to consciously align with, utilize and maximize the physical and psychological benefits of our physical and spiritual nature to create longevity of life. Kun Qi is also a means for one to use visualization to intentionally guide and/or follow the flow of electrical current by intentionally sending life force, (qi) to specific areas within the body and out from the body. As we focus our mental attention and inner visualization to match the rhythm of the breath we are able to literally send the vibrations of your heartfelt intentions where they need to go within the physical body and out into the world while consciously drawing in the life force frequencies of the etheric and elemental vibrations through the breath, the sensory mechanisms and through the pores of the skin.

We are also able to perceive deeper insights and innerstanding of each elemental aspect or Orisha and their functions, purposes, and abilities as they relate to life through aligning with them in meditation or contemplation which deepens our communion with the elements of earthly and cosmic life force and a deeper sentient innerstanding of the Oneness that we share with all that exists. With meditative movement one's ultra-sensory preceptors of clairsentience and more will become either activated or deepened allowing one to consciously feel the life force and energy of all living things within one's environment and beyond. Also, one's ability to consciously receive knowledge and insights from more ascended realms and dimensions of consciousness within the universe and within oneself will also increase.

The various sequences of movements range in purpose and intent, from that of physical activation and mastery to that of conscious and subtle body awareness, integration and innerstanding of oneself and of the universal flow of life force around you and within all sentient life. Optimally, it would be best to perform these sequences in an open natural setting where all of the elements of nature are present as this allows one to connect with these elementals in a more direct way. This is not always an available option especially in urban and metropolitan areas. However, one can also create as deep of a connecting with whatever natural elements are available by performing the movements in a park, back yard, nature trails, etc. If being outdoors in the open is not an option, the power of visualization and intention will serve the same purpose of attuning (Atun-ing) to the elements of life force in a conscious sentient way.

Deep breathing and rhythmic movement create a calming flow that moves one into an alpha/theta state where conscious mental awareness of one's surroundings ceases while the mind moves into a deeper state of subtle visualization and the body begins to move on its own. The use of **specific hand mudras** ignites and activates the command points of the various internal organs stimulating the flow of life force into each organ through the meridians. When combined with movement, the meridian channels are able to release tension unblocking the passageways to the organs so that the life force nutrients you ingest have a more direct effect on the inner dynamics of the body.

Vocalizing healing mantras integrates the use of sound (vibration), a shared component between the elements of the universe and those of the Earth. This creates an inner vibration that stimulates movement within the inner workings of the body that can be felt. When the tonal note of each chakra is intentionally used in combination with the corresponding mudras, visualization, circular breathing and movement, it amplifies and magnifies the clarity of one's personal resonance loosening the internal tension being generated and increasing the new life force that is being ingested throughout the subtle body. This intensifies the bodies self-healing abilities.

Visualizing symbols of healing or the elements of nature directly activates and integrates their sentient healing purpose allowing them to become a living healing frequency that radiates from within. This energy not only generates healing within oneself, it can also be sent out into the environment you are in and throughout the universe through focused intention, visualization and breath work.

Remember… we contain the likeness of The Divine Creator within us. We have the ability to actualize whatever our mind/body focuses its energies and intentions on creating. Thought intention coupled with these aforementioned frequencies will connect to and intensify all other frequencies that resonate at the same vibration. And because healing energy and intentions are of a higher and lighter vibration, they also have the ability to move through heavier negative energies transforming them or lightening them as they introduce more ascended thought forms and vibrations. Thus, meditative movement contains tools and intentions of healing that have the power to change our inner and outer experiences to provide the sense of inner peace, clarity of vision, and overall sense of wellbeing that we seek to manifest in our life experience.

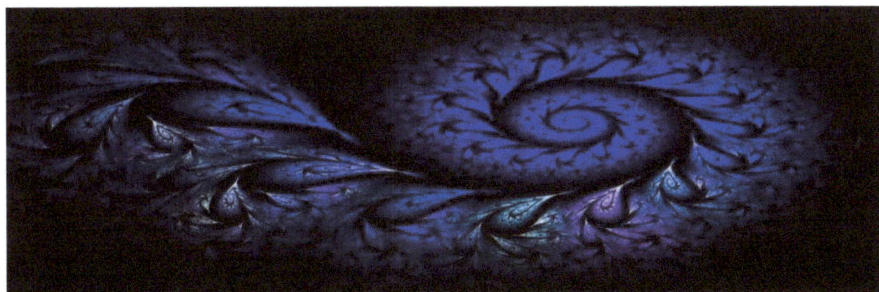

(This Visual depiction represents the Fibonacci spiral that the sequence of the golden ratio depicts mathematically. This sacred geometrical pattern exists throughout all of nature from the smallest of seashells to the largest of galaxies. Its pattern is also found in music, color, human reproduction of the family tree and more.)

17

ANCIENT AFRICAN SPIRITUALITY & DIVINE SCIENCE

In the Yoruba tradition of African spirituality, honor is given to the differing divine elemental aspects of God through what is called the Orisha; the "Ashe" within their belief system. Ashe, which is also spelled "Ase", "Axe," "Axé," "Aché," or "Ache," is the life-force that runs through all things, living and inanimate. Ashe possesses the power to create sentient life that possesses a portion of its intelligence. In this tradition, each Orisha governs various aspects of nature and reflects their various physical and metaphysical, tendencies that reside within human beings as well as all forms of life universally. Though presented as a pantheon the Orisha in truth are One Entity – Divine Intelligent Life Force Energy – that expresses different aspects of its Nature in, as, and throughout All Creation in its infinite individuated expressions.

Ashe is divine Life Force energy (Olodumare) that comes from, the Creator manifested through the sun which is associated to the Orisha Olorun. Without the sun, no life on earth would exist, just as life cannot exist without some degree of ashė. Ashe is sometimes associated with Eshu, the messenger God. For practitioners of the Yoruba/Lucumi religion, ashė represents a link to the eternal presence of God, the Orishas or elements of the Universe, and the spirit of our ancestors who have left this physical form. For those who are not familiar with this African spiritual system here is a list of the following Orisha and what they rule, regulate, or relate to within our astral/physical anatomy. I will be referring to the Elemental aspects of the Orisha every so often as they relate to various aspects of this material.

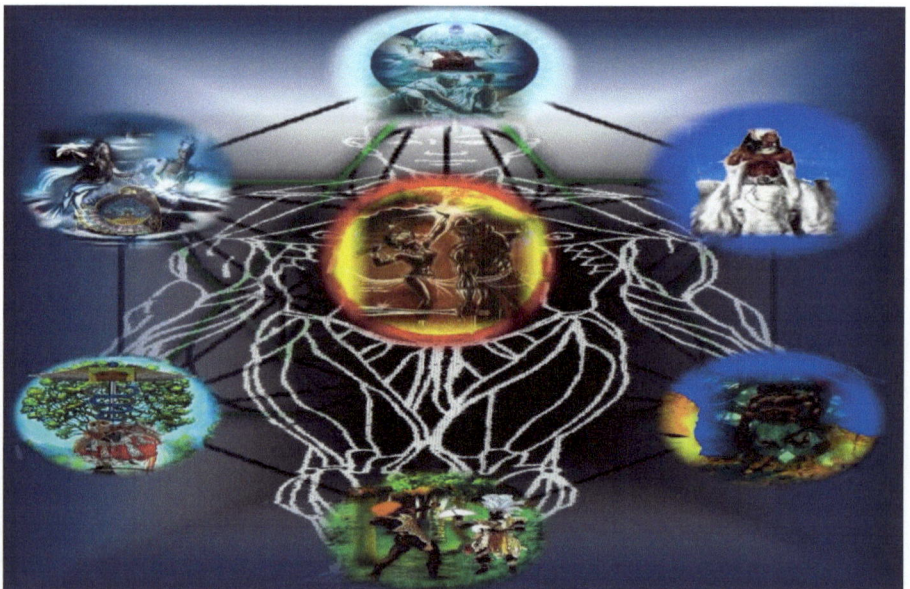

On the following page is a description of the Orisha elementals and their celestial and earthly characteristics. It describes the function abilities, and life force processes that our bodies experience as a human organism that they regulate and are responsible for.

HEAVENLY ORISHA

Olorun/Olodumare (The Sun) – Creative Life Force Intelligence of the Universe /Sentient Life Force Intelligence of Nature and All of Creation, God, The Creator of all that is

Orumila (Universal Intelligence) – The One Mind/Orisha of Divine Wisdom, Divine Intelligence, divination, our psychic gifts (Holy Spirit of God) – The Pineal Gland/The Individuated Mind - allowed to witness and comprehend the creation of the Universe by Olorun

Obatala (Air) – Father of The Orisha & Human Beings/Creator of the World of Humanity, Source of purity, wisdom, love, peace and compassion. Divine Justice, Reason and source of karmic justice,

Eleggua – Spirit/The Crossroads – Creative Thought, Spirit/Soul Intelligence, regulates the bodies operations and functions, subconscious reasoning.

Ayao (Air) – breath, the calm of the storm, source of meditative inspiration, spiritual channeling as effects of focused breathing

Oya – Whirl Winds/Tornadoes/ Transitional Change – nervous system signals (neurotransmitters), gas, facilitates connection with ancestral memory and Celestial communication with Ancestor, family genetics within our DNA.

HEAVENLY/EARTHLY ORISHA

Shango - Fire, lightning, drums – internal heat, heart rhythms, adrenals, nervous system, internal physical and subtle body rhythms,

Yemonja – Living Waters, Seas, lakes, –The Womb or incubative space within the body & mind where life is birthed from, bodily fluids, sweat, the conversion of fresh to saltwater within the body

Olokun – Deep Waters - Subconscious physical and subtle body functions and operations, psychic mechanic

EARTHLY ORISHA

Oba – Turbulent Waters – digestive imbalances, fertility and the process of insemination

Aganju – Volcanoes/fire - internal body heat, digestion, heart, skin perspiration, the elimination of bodily waste (the desert)

Ochossi – Warrior – instinct, ability for fight or flight, internal justice, breakdown of meat-based foods, the liver

Ogun – Material and technological operations and manifestation – The liver, Iron and mineral absorption and distribution of plant-based foods

Oshun – Fresh Waters – emotional healing/2nd chakra, balance, regulates the digestive and meridian channels of the organs throughout the body – distribution of blood & liquids

Babalou Aye – Orisha of healing & knowledge of all plant & mineral life force properties digestion and nutritional distribution of plant life nutrients

Erinle – Healer, Guardian of plant life, its assimilation, absorption, distribution, and elimination processes in the body along with hormonal balance.

Oko – Ruler of Harvest and fertility, consequences to actions and thought form manifestation

Osain – Rules the secret knowledge of Herbs and naturopathic medicine, the immune system and the body's ability to heal itself when supported by natural non-chemically treated nutrients

Yegua' - Orisha of cellular/physical decomposition – physical deterioration, cellular decomposition & the dying process

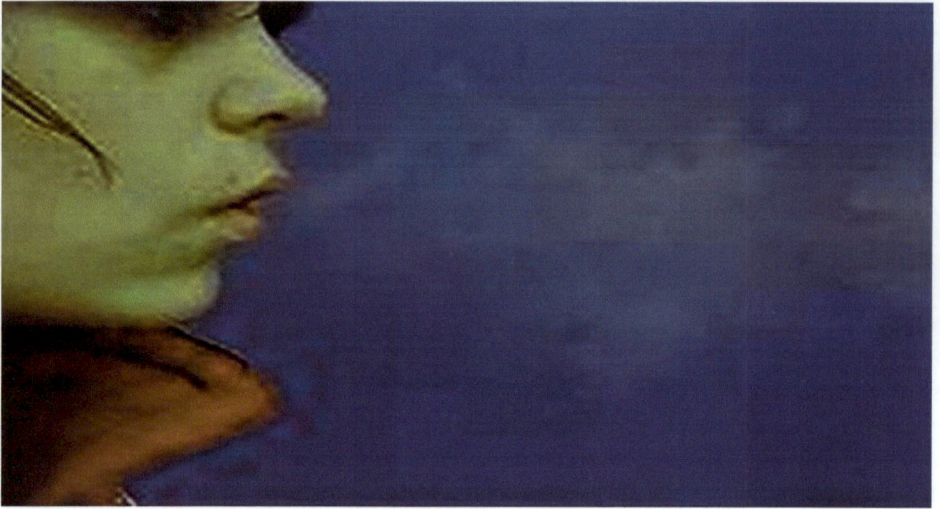

BREATH AND VISUALIZATION

Our subconscious mind controls the patterns of operation that our body follows. On a subtle body level, chronic tension patterns also have to do with activity related holding patterns, mental stress, and built-up unresolved emotional energy and forms of resistance. When we are mentally engaged in problem solving, we are subconsciously waging an internal war. Our need to force an answer to unknown factors versus trusting God, the universe, etc. to provide insights, inspirations, and wisdom through our intuitions that reveal the answers we seek - creates emotions of frustration, fear, anxiety, tension and misdirected eruptions of emotions. When we are in this state, our adrenaline increases, we breathe more shallowly for longer periods of time and we lose the connection to our awareness of our physical alignment and movements.

Breath and visualization are the key components that bring about the healing effects of Kun Qi Kung. In the tradition of Chinese medicine, we can either produce healthy or ill conditions within our physical well-being based on the way in which we breathe. Air, which main element is oxygen, is a life force containing element that each cell of our body needs in order to survive. Chronically tense muscle structures and poor postural holding patterns inhibit our capacity to take in air and expand the lungs and diaphragm fully. When we focus our awareness on our breath, we are better able to notice the patterns of tension that we hold. When we intention to turn our focus inward in order to relax we discover places in our body where we are subconsciously holding tension. The most common are the shoulders, neck and jaw. By allowing our inner sense to focus on each area of our body from head to toe, while breathing into those areas in a deep relaxed circular rhythm, we're able to feel the muscles relax as our lungs and diaphragm take in larger quantities of air and our body posture re-align itself into our spines natural curve. As this happens the body becomes lighter and we're able to breathe more fully, as well as feel a sense of weightlessness throughout the entire body.

There are two forms of breath work that are used during the meditative movement sequences and sacred space activation, circular breath work and small death breath work. Each breathing technique has a specific purpose in its application.

CIRCULAR BREATHWORK
Circular breathing is used during the body warm up exercise, joint activation sequence, and 8 directional movement sequences. With circular breathing one keeps a deep continual flow of oxygen by not holding the breath at either end of the inhalation or exhalation. In the 8 directions format of meditative movement the direction changes are performed in sync with one's inhalation and exhalation thus allowing for one to create an inner and outer rhythm that unifies conscious and ultra-conscious thought which takes you deeper into the altered states of meditation. Circular breathing will also be used during still meditation as it helps one to keep a continual flow of life force moving through the body unifying visualization with the inner terrain of the meridian and chakra channels while becoming consciously attuned to hear the body's inner wisdom communicated.

SMALL DEATH BREATHWORK
Small death-breath work is a form of deep breathing by which one holds the breath at the top of the inhalation and the bottom of the exhalation for a specific count of 4 to 8 seconds in order to bring life giving properties of the breath deeper into the inner dynamics of the mind/body thus intensifying the calming meditative healing effects of meditative movement. This form of breath work is performed during the Joint Activation warm-up, and the Tao Yin Fa sequence.

BREATH & BODY WARM-UP
Before starting the movement sequence it's important to settle into a breathing pattern that is comfortable and conducive to the rhythm of the sequence. Start with a 5 to 10-minute intentional walk or run to begin awakening and circulating Qi energy throughout your body. As time goes on, feel free to increase the duration to match your level of fitness. This helps to stimulate movement within the meridian channels increasing the amount of oxygen throughout the body and releasing toxins through the breath. It also increases your ability to consciously direct and regulate the intensity of your workout within the various healing movement sequences. As you become more adept at intentional movement you may find that you will naturally want to increase the circular count of your breathing. This is fine and can be done when you feel ready.

As you start to walk or run focus your attention on your breath. Start to regulate your breathing by inhaling and exhaling to the count of 3-6 seconds during each. If you find this difficult slow your pace to a level of intensity that's manageable so that you can maintain at least a 3 count circular rhythm. This can be done by taking shorter strides or by increasing your stride to match the rhythm. Once it starts to become comfortable and you're able to maintain this pace with ease, start to focus your attention on the muscles that are working as you're moving. By consciously engaging each muscle of the body as you move/walk/run, you help to align the spine, decrease the pressure on the joints during impact, increase the amount of oxygen getting into the lungs, muscle tissue and brain, and improve the circulation of blood, oxygen, and nutrients to the heart and throughout the body while strengthening, tightening, and firming your muscles.

Relax into your breathing, and start to allow yourself to look, with your inner vision, inside the various parts of your body. Become aware of your foot placement and how your legs and arms are moving. If your feet are rotated outward bring your foot placement forward so that your knees and toes are aligned and pointed straight ahead of you. Draw your lower abdomen in toward the spine while tightening or squeezing your glutes holding them tight and firm as you walk. By drawing your lower abdomen towards the spine and engaging your buttocks, your spine will automatically align itself and the knees will automatically soften so as not to create any jarring or strain on the joints during impact. Engaging the muscles in your glutes and quads versus using the momentum of your stride helps to shape, tone and firm your muscles from the inside out and to align the spine which takes pressure off of the knees, low back, neck and shoulders. By slightly tightening your arm, allowing them to move forward and backward in a relaxed way and intentionally engaging the muscles in your legs, glutes, abs, torso etc. you will strengthen your inner and outer body while softening your body's impact with the ground.

To become consciously in-tuned and present with your bodies rhythm and to learn how to guide it, focus your attention on intentionally using the muscles of your abs, arms, leg, and buttocks to propel you versus using the momentum of your body mass to move you forward. Focus your mind on your inner condition and allow yourself to become familiar with the physical, mental, and emotional sensations and postures that you hold. Notice where you feel tension, looseness, sluggishness, stagnation or over-stimulation, resistance, pain, discomfort and/or stress; notice how your lungs are responding to this activity. Is your breathing labored, is there any burning, is your heart feeling overtaxed or skipping, or is your heart rate beating strong and in a healthy range of the activity?

HOW TO CHECK YOUR HEART RATE: Your maximum heart rate can be determined by subtracting ½ your age from the number 210. This is your maximum heart rate. Your target heart rate should be lower, at approximately 75% of the maximum during movement. If your heart rate is over this range, slow your pace, and focus on decreasing your breath work to a lower more comfortable count. Once you have structured your movement so that your body is actively engaged in intentional propulsion and your heart rate is within healthy limits, allow your focus to go deeper by bringing your awareness to your chakras, tuning into their present state, noticing any concerns, current situations and/or issues that surface. You will be working to clear them with the Level I Situational Clearing using Dai Ko Myo or the Level III & IV Chakra Clearing Series but for now, just take note of the sensations and insights that come up for you.

Bring your attention to your root chakra. Do you feel grounded and centered in thought and at peace with your work, family, home, and current life's experiences? If so, move up to the navel chakra. If not, note what concerns or thoughts come to mind take note for later contemplation and then release them before moving to the next chakra; you will be using the information during the Situational Clearing Sequence. Moving up to the navel chakra; are there any emotional situations or feelings that come to mind? If so, note them and the questions, situations, and insights they inspire. Next bring your awareness to the Solar Plexus; your power center. Are you feeling empowered and centered in your sense of self, your boundaries, your spiritual relationship with The Creator, your Divine Self and others? If not, note where you are feeling out of tune or imbalanced, what it is that may be creating the feeling, and whatever comes to mind that challenges your sense of inner peace and oneness with The All and/or with yourself and others. Take note of what comes to the surface, allow yourself to breathe the light of the sun into your solar plexus releasing the tension, noting whatever comes to mind and move onto your heart chakra. Can you sense your love for self, your connection and oneness with life, The Creator and your Divine truth as a spiritual being? Can you envision operating with compassion towards others or are there blocks such as, judgments, anger, resentments, fears, or defenses that you are holding? Note what you feel and breath through any negativity that comes to the surface. Allow yourself to own it; view it objectively without becoming emotionally entangled in what comes up by viewing them as something that you will address and transcend through love peacefully. Next, move to the throat chakra. Does the air move freely into and out of the lungs? Do you notice any sensations of restriction, soreness, dryness or tension in the throat? Do any communication issues come to mind; things you're having trouble communicating or verbally formulating in thoughts? Notice any sensations or difficulties in speaking or living your truth that arise which reveal the blockages within your perceptions of self and others that are keeping you from expressing your needs, your desires, and from living and being comfortable in your truth. Again, take mental notes for clearing during the Situational Clearing sequence. Next bring your attention to your 1st eye and crown chakras. Are you able to remember your dreams? Are you able to envision creative and psychic insights that provide guidance to your goals or life situations? Do you feel connected and in communication receiving insights and direction from your higher self, spiritual guides, etc. note where you feel your level of connectedness to the Divine Realms as far as openness and breathe it in. Allow yourself to move through the chakras gauging your run/walk with the time necessary for you to go through all the chakras.

Once you've finished with this intentional run/walk exercise, take 2-4 minutes to cool down your body rhythms by slowing down into a walking pace until you are at a normal breathing pattern for yourself. Check your pulse to determine when you are back to your resting heart rate which can be determined by taking your pulse prior to any activity or upon waking in the morning or lying down to rest at night. Upon returning to your resting heart rate find a place that you would like to start your meditative movement exercises.

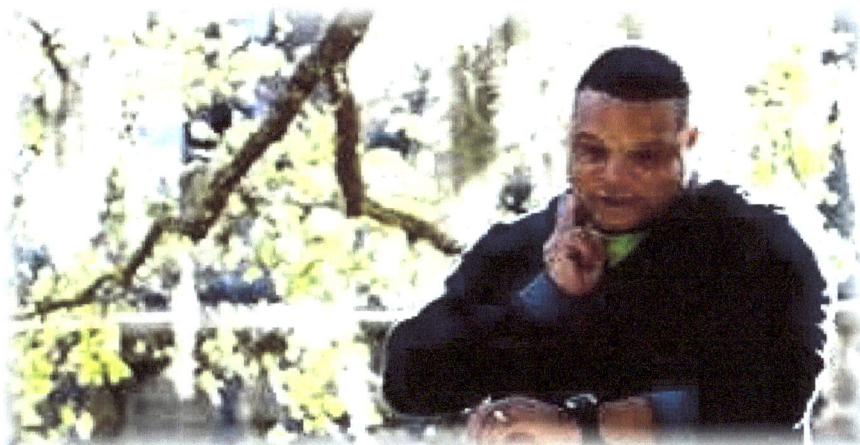

CREATING SACRED SPACE
Please note that this is not a religious ritual and performing this sacred space sequence is optional

Creating Sacred Space is a very important part of performing healing work. Attuning oneself to the sacred within all things and creating sacred space within one's environment are two of the most important aspects of personal healing and the spiritual journey towards embodiment of one's Divinity. It provides one with the ability to create energetic boundaries and vibrations that establish the essence of sacredness from the ascended realms as well as the Cosmic and Earthly Life forces in your immediate surroundings. This clears and protects you within the area you choose to work in and increases the vibration to match that of your healing intentions by welcoming in the sentient aspects of nature, as well as your spirit guides, ancestors, and totems that have chosen to be of assistance to you that you hold in a place of divine reverence and honor. The following is a short and simple sacred space invocations that are quite effective that can be used if you do not have one that you feel more comfortable with. I've also includes some more elaborate forms of creating sacred space in the appendix that are personal practices that I enjoy.

THE VIOLET FLAME SACRED SPACE INVOCATION:
This sacred space invocation is quite simple to create and can be done at any time anywhere. First take a moment to quiet and center yourself by focusing on the rhythm of your breathing. Breathe deep and to a slow count of 4 or five counts both in and out stilling your mind. If you have ways of creating protection around yourself and a space invoke them at this time, if not, envision a violet beam or flame of light surrounding you. Within this flame envision a bubble of light blue light around your body. To affirms your healing intentions welcoming higher levels of consciousness to bring greater Self- awareness and personal insights during your healing sessions by inviting your spiritual guides, ascended healing masters, ancestors, animal totems, and light beings to be present, to surround you with their Divine protection so that divine healing may take place and to guide you in your journey towards divine health.

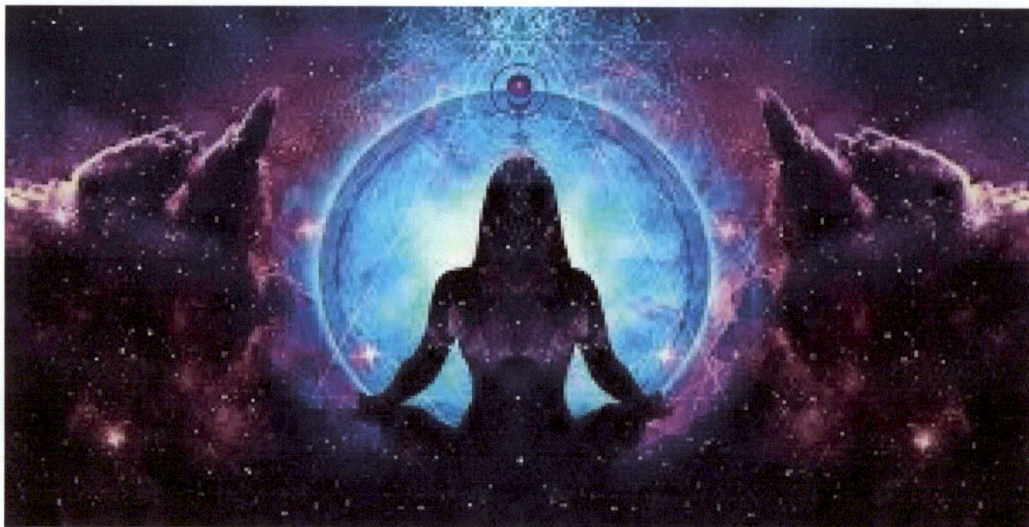

ATTUNING TO THE ELEMENTS OF NATURE

Our ability to connect to Cosmic and Earthly Life force and the ascended celestial and ancestral beings that have chosen to be of service in our personal healing and that of those that resides here on planet earth, is essential to our spiritual evolution. It is a divine birth right to live in harmony and synchronicity with our environment peacefully without being exposed to toxicity. This type of sacred attunement is a very important part of our well-being that helps to clear and purify not only oneself but the area one chooses to work in. It infuses the vibration of your Higher Self into the surrounding energetic fields vibrationally. When attuned to the life forces of the elements of nature and the spiritual beings, ancestors, and animal totems that have committed to be of assistance to us, we can shift our inner awareness and our energy fields to match that of Their vibration and intention for us. These higher intentions ride our breath as we breathe out into our environment and reverberates outward sending ripples of its energetic influence in all directions infinitely. These ripples of vibratory intention help to awaken the conscious awareness of those within its path that are even the slightest bit attuned to these life forces to be more aware of their responsibility to do their part to transmute and heal the toxic conditions that reside within this world and its Environment.

If possible, find a place outside in an open natural landscape, (Oceanside, riverside, or near a body of water is optimal) as it encompasses the 7 elements connecting you to the source and substance which your physical and Ka body derives its life force energy from. If you are not able to get to a natural landscape and must work in a walled in structure you can still connect with the elements through visualization and setting the intention within your minds desire to do so.

Stand facing the direction of the Sun, with palms together in front of your heart chakra. Begin with deep belly breathing drawing the lower abdomen in towards the spine to gently align your posture. Hold the breath at the top of the inhalation and the bottom of your exhalation for a few seconds. By doing so you will start to feel your body become somewhat lighter and your mind relax into a calmer more meditative state. As you feel yourself riding the rhythm of your breath, connect with your energy body senses and allow your energetic connection to the earth elements and the vibrations of the universe to fill your subtle sensory perception.

Envision each of the 7 elements of nature one by one focusing on each element as you open yourself up to attune with their energy as you breathe each breath. Feel the heat and warmth of the sun on your skin, listen to the rustling of the tree leaves as the wind caresses your face, notice the scent that resides within the air around you, feel the texture of the terrain under your feet envision each characteristic of each element that you that you acknowledge in its sentient function-ability. This helps you to one re-attune yourself to the elements of nature, (**sun**, **water**, **earth**, **wood**, **mineral formations**, **sound** and the **air** which moves them). You may feel a tingling or sense a slight pressure or presence around you, this is letting you know that you have connected and tuned into them.

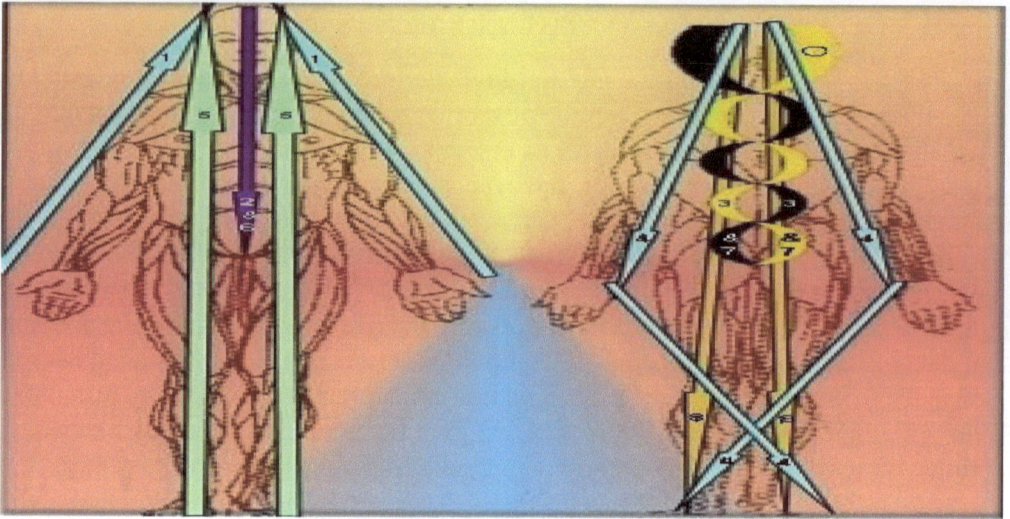

QI MERIDIAN CIRCULATION DIAGRAM

KUN QI MERIDIAN MEDITATION

The purpose of this sequence is to deepen your attunement to the energy channels within your body and for you to learn not only to feel, but to guide the movement of life force throughout your body with your mind and your breath. Feel free to refer to the charts on the previous page as a visual map of the way in which you will be guiding the flow of cosmic and earthly qi energy through your body.

To begin, stand with your knees slightly bent gently drawing the abdomen toward the spine allow it to relax and align itself naturally. If done correctly you should feel a sense of weightlessness within the core of the body starting at the pelvis and moving up along your spinal column into the shoulders, upper back and neck. Stretch your arms out in front of you at a level just below your navel with palms facing in as if you are holding a large beach ball between your arms and your body. Keep about 1" of space between the tips of your fingers in order to allow the chi force to flow freely within the lower Dan t'ian. The Dan t'ian are the "qi centers", for meditative exercise techniques in traditional Chinese medicine. This is where original qi force processes and will flow out to the hand chakra openings as well as the organ command points in the fingers. This stimulates their receptivity to cosmic and elemental life-force and creates a strong connection and even flow of energy that is drawn in, out, and throughout the body as it rides the breath. The Qi Circulation Diagram chart (shown above) is a visual depiction of the flow and order in which the meridian breath work exercise is performed.

Take a few slow relaxing breaths and focus your inner vision and sensory perceptions on connecting and aligning yourself with both the cosmic and earthly Elemental life forces (Orisha). Envision yourself being surrounded by the crystal core of the earth which is composed of Iron and Nickel (crucial in creating Earth's magnetic field). See and feel yourself standing within its gravitational pull and its library of recorded earth knowledge. This is where all the akashic records of the life experience of every entity, life form, or being that has lived on Earth have been recorded or imprinted from the beginning of earth's time to now. This same library of knowledge within the Earth's core is the marrow within the skeleton of Mother Earth. The iron within the core of Mother Earth is the source of iron that is produced within your bone marrow and flows within your bloodstream. Therefore, one has access to the history of the planet as well as that of their ancestry through the portal of their blood which operates as cellular memory within one's DNA.

Once centered within these vortexes within yourself, envision a portal of light from the galactic center of our universe encompassing you… penetrating through the crystal core that you've placed energetically around you, and absorbing into the iron within each blood cell of your body. As you inhale, envision these energies flowing into and merging within your heart chakra filling it with the life force they contain and awakening your awareness of their divine essences and their intelligence within you. As you exhale, envision their combined life force energies shooting down your spinal column and pooling within the floor of your pelvis igniting your primordial energy (also known as kundalini) that resides there. Inhale again sensing the primordial chi winding up (view black and gold spiral in previous image) through the root, navel, solar plexus, heart, throat, and stopping at a point between your 1st eye and the crown chakra. Hold the chi on either side of your head by holding your breath for a few seconds. This allows the energy to cleanse and charge the pineal and pituitary glands at the brain center. When you are ready to exhale, release the flow of qi by visualizing and feeling the life force flowing down the spinal column and radiating throughout the nervous system into every cell of your body. Repeat this sequence 2 more times as to fully align and deepen the connection. While doing so, allow yourself to become more aligned and familiar with these cosmic and earthly power centers of energy and their functions.

With your next inhalation again envision drawing the combined galactic and earth's core energies down into the heart allowing it to pool there while holding the breath. This time as you exhale envision sending the energy that you've collected within your heart out from its center into the palms and fingertips of your hands.
Upon your next inhalation feel and visualize life force energy from the surrounding vortex of cosmic and earthly elements traveling up from your fingertips through your forearms and into your elbows, shoulders, neck and head. For a few seconds, hold the qi and the breath at the point between your crown chakra and first eye that surround your pineal & pituitary glands. Now, while slowly exhaling, envision their life-force energies traveling down from the center of your head into your spinal column and descending through the chakras to pool inside the center of the pelvic floor. Again, hold the breath for a few seconds allowing the primordial energy that resides there to build.

Now, to ground and integrate the primordial energy into your body and present time experiences, inhale again sensing the Qi energy winding up through the root, navel, solar plexus, heart, throat, and 1st eye stopping there and holding the chi on either side of your crown chakra holding it there as you hold your breath. Then, upon exhalation release the flow of qi out from the top of the head down the neck into the front part of the shoulders and down the inner part of the arms into the hands and out the fingertips. At the bottom of the exhalation envision the qi energy moving across the body down into the opposite toes. Again, hold the breath a few seconds letting the energy build.

Upon inhalation, envision and feel the life force flowing up from the toes into your feet, ankles, the inner and outer legs, hips torso, shoulders, neck and head holding the breath at the top (these are the meridian channels of the stomach, spleen, liver, and gallbladder). Again, exhale all life force down the spinal column into the Dantien, hold the breath and allow it to build within the pelvic floor. This time, while inhaling, envision the qi force moving up the anterior core of the body into the acupuncture points on the inside corner ridge of the eyebrows called "drilling bamboo". Hold the qi there while holding your breath. You may feel a tingling sensation at these power points as they clear the nasal passage and charge the 1st eye chakra. As you exhale envision the combined cosmic & earthly qi energies flowing up and over the brow and crown of the head, down the back of the head through the neck and continuing down the back side of the body through the meridian channels of the bladder to the kidney point at the bottom of the feet allowing all old outdated stagnant energy that is being released to flow out of your body into the earth removing it from the entire body.

Some believe that because of the toxic abuse that Mother Earth has sustained our sending stagnant life force from our bodies back into the Earth is contributing to the toxicity of Mother Earth. Rest easy… this is not the case. The energetic toxins that you are releasing actually feed the Earth vibrationally which fuels and regenerates her power center and the carbon dioxide we exhale provides the Earth's soil and plant life with life force to thrive on.

Performing the Meridian Qi Activation Sequence at least 3 times consecutively in order to deepen your Kun Qi attunement helps to awaken and recalibrate the flow of life force through your meridian channels and your ability to connect with the sentience of these life forces within your mind multi-dimensionally. You should feel relaxed yet with a heightened sense of awareness and vibration in connection to your physical body and the elements around you.

You are now ready to start the various meditative movement sequences. Performing these exercises, opens, increases and strengthens the flow of life force to the internal organs and can help restore and regulate their function-ability to that of their natural and optimal state of operating over time with consistent practice. The meridian charts will familiarize you with the meridian channels for each organ, where they are in the body, and the directions that they flow in so that you can more effectively perform the chi activation as well as the Tao Yin Fa series of movements. The meridian charts in "Appendix A" reveal specific acupressure points for each organ and just where each organ meridian channel runs throughout the body.

Now that you've attuned to the elemental energies around you, the next step is to create sacred space that acknowledges their sentience and affirms your healing intentions by welcoming higher levels of consciousness to protect your energy fields and to bring greater Self-awareness and personal insights during your meditative movement sessions. I've included the following Dantien diagrams to visually elaborate on their locations, functions and how they operate within our physical body for your greater innerstanding.

Upper Dantian — Yintang
Middle Dantian — Tanzhong
Lower Dantian — Qihai

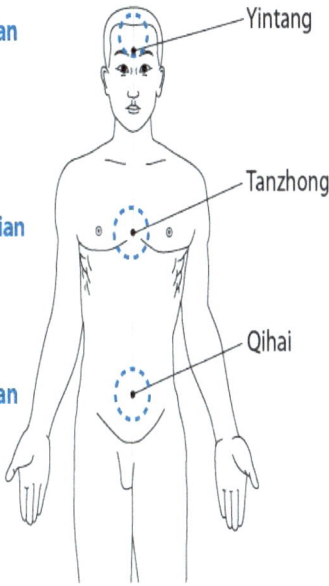

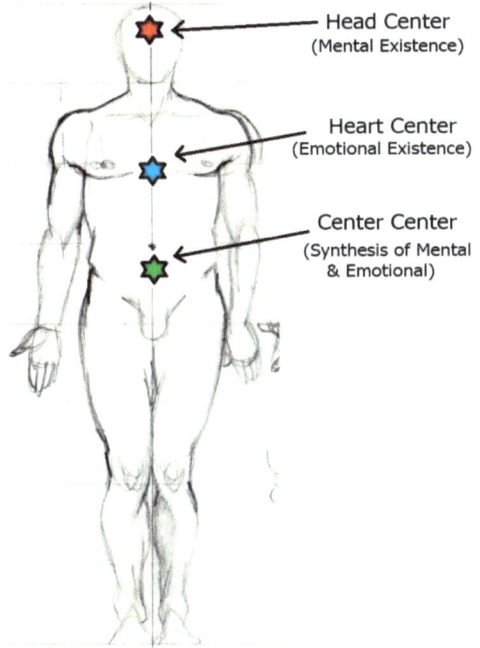

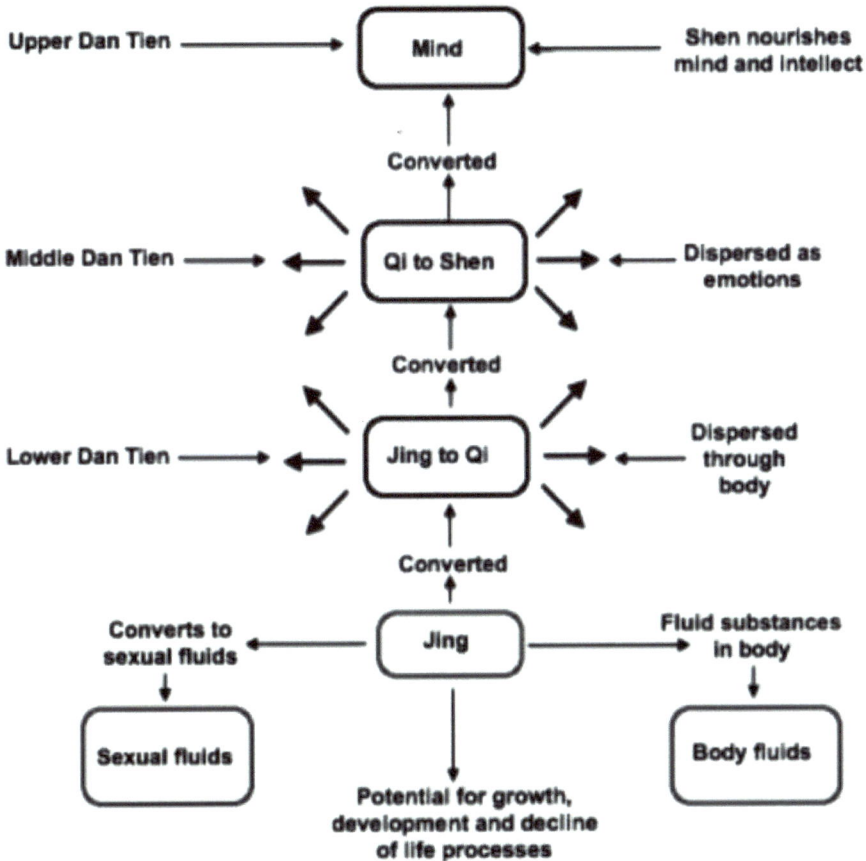

Head Center
(Mental Existence)

Heart Center
(Emotional Existence)

Center Center
(Synthesis of Mental
& Emotional)

Upper Dan Tien → Mind ← Shen nourishes mind and intellect

Converted

Middle Dan Tien → ← Qi to Shen → ← Dispersed as emotions

Converted

Lower Dan Tien → ← Jing to Qi → ← Dispersed through body

Converted

Converts to sexual fluids ← Jing → Fluid substances in body

Sexual fluids

Body fluids

Potential for growth, development and decline of life processes

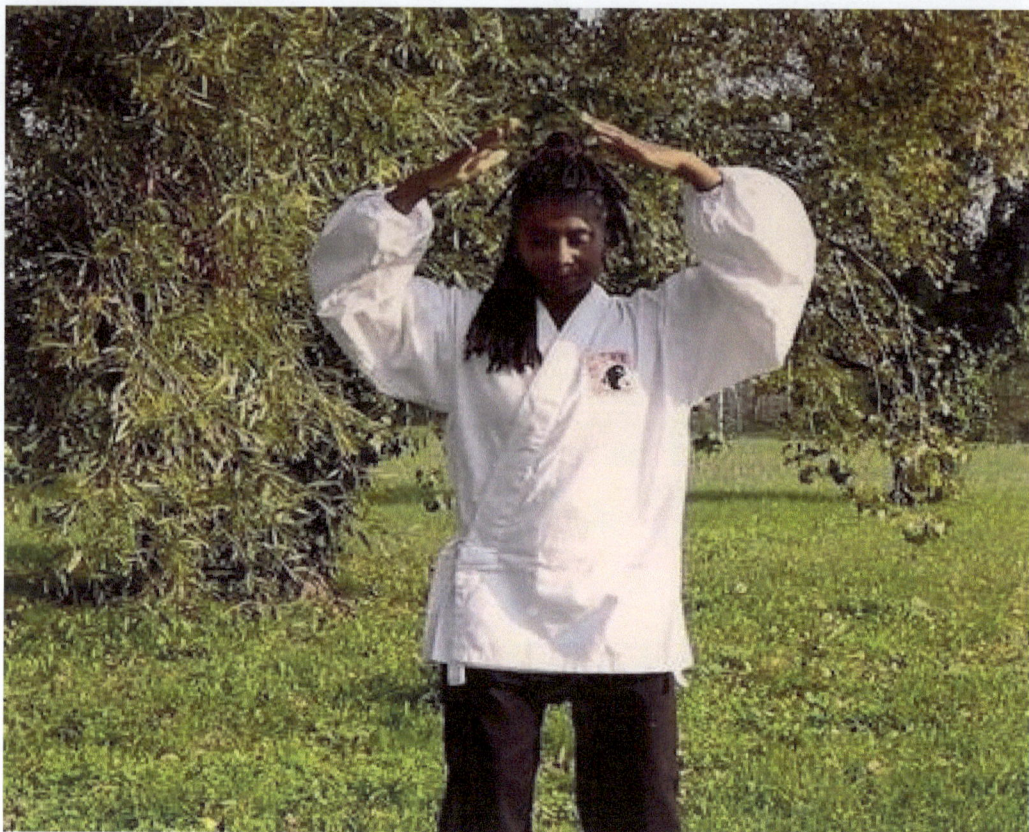

KUN CHI QI KUNG THE MOVEMENTS

SEQUENCE I - JOINT MOBILIZATION

The joint mobilization sequence is designed to activate, balance, strengthen and remove blockages from the major and sub major chakras within the joints and the meridian channels along the body by easing oneself into movement and learning how to move with intention through inner awareness. This Sequence will start at the ankles and moves up the body joint by joint opening and stimulating the synovial fluid and qi (life force) within them and within the organ channels located along the body. This sequence helps to release the buildup of nitrogen, synovial fluid and calcification in the joints and restore suppleness and central balance to the chakras within the joints and to the body.

Begin by standing with your toes facing forward and your legs shoulder width apart with knees slightly bent to allow the pelvis to align centrally. Draw the lower abdomen in toward the spine and slightly engage your buttocks. This will naturally align your entire spinal column bringing your center of gravity into its most balanced alignment. Focus your attention on listening to and becoming one with your breath and begin tuning your attention into your body. Inwardly check to see if your lower abs and glutes are engaged then allow your body and mind to relax more deeply into your breath becoming even more attuned to the feel of your body from within. At this point you are ready to start the exercise.

Follow the Joint Mobilization sequence below making sure that each movement, each rotation, each transition is performed with the muscles. Make sure that the muscles surround the joint you are moving are fully engaged and activated while the rest of your muscles are in a resting state. The inner tension allows you to properly use the power of the musculature to move the joints instead of the force of momentum through the use of the skeletal. The joint rotation count for each movement starts with 9 rotations in each direction and can be increased up to 18 counts for those who want to increase the intensity level of the exercise. The sequence is designed to be performed standing but can also be modified to a seated position for those with physical restrictions in movement or those requiring greater stability to balance.

JOINT MOBILIZATION MOVEMENTS

ANKLES - Lift the left leg up so that the knee is suspended in air at approximately 90 degrees in angle. Again, gently tighten the buttocks and the abdomen to naturally align the body inward, balancing the pelvis and spine to create stability and balance of the entire body. Bring your inner attention to the ankle joint and with intent, tighten and use the Tibial (shins) and ankle muscles. Very slowly rotate each foot medially (inward) 9 - 18 rotations and then reverse direction rotating laterally (outward) for the same count. Stretch as far in each direction as you can while circling, feeling the tension, soreness, and achiness that is generated in the musculature when you use the supporting muscles to move each foot versus momentum. Be sure to go slow paying inner attention to fully feel and identify all the muscles that it actually takes to move the foot at the ankle joint. Remember, the slower you go, the more you use your musculature to move you and the more benefits from the movement that you will achieve.

KNEES - Next move the focus of rotation up to the knee joint of the same leg. Use your quadricep muscles to propel the rotation of the knee for the same amount of rotations as you did for the ankle, medially first and then laterally. You may hear popping or crunching at the joints during rotation which is not uncommon due to nitrogen and synovial fluid buildup in the joint cavity caused by postural misalignments, not having utilized the surrounding muscles properly when moving the joint and lack of consistent stretching and strengthening of the muscles and joints. You can expect this to decrease over time as the synovial fluid starts to evenly distribute and the intentional mobility of the exercise loosens and strengthens the surrounding tendons and muscles. Once completed switch legs and repeat the ankle and knee rotations with the other leg. When finished, stand with both feet facing forward with knees slightly bent.

HIPS – Now, widen your stance to a little beyond shoulder width apart and with intent, rotate the hips in a wide circle first in one direction for 9 rotations then the other. Again, make sure to focus your inner attention on using the muscles of the hips and leg to direct the movement versus momentum. You want to synchronize your breathing to fit in alignment with the positioning of the chest and abdomen. As you bring the pelvis forward in front of you, exhale through the mouth fully. As you move the hips towards the rear, inhale deeply, fully filling up the diaphragm and lungs. Complete 9 rotations in each direction then once finished, center yourself and drop the hips by bending the knees a little more deeply. Isolate the pelvis circling the hips alone keeping everything above the waist as well as the legs stationary. This movement is exceptional for releasing energetic and vertebral blockages in the lower back region, especially within the SI joint and in the sciatic nerve area. It's a good exercise to incorporate periodically throughout your day as a treatment for low back pain and stiffness.

CHEST - The next area of rotation is the thoracic cage. While holding the hips stable isolate the chest cavity and shift it to the left. Try to keep the shoulders down focusing on using only the chest cavity in the movement. Be assured, this movement will get easier and smoother with practice. While exhaling, rotate the chest cavity posteriorly letting it sink back, fully compressing all the air out of the chest cavity and diaphragm. Then, while shifting to the right, begin to inhale as you start to rotate the chest cavity forward fully pressing it as far forward as you can. Fully expanding the lungs to maximize the oxygen intake then start to slowly exhale while rotating the chest cavity to the left then back. Rotate 9 times in each direction slowly and with intention, focusing on isolating and using the muscles to move, then reverse directions performing the same number of rotations. Once complete, center the chest and then move onto the cervical joint of the neck.

NECK – While keeping the body faced forward, tighten the musculature of the neck and turn the head fully left than right while holding tension in the neck. Visually look at each shoulder to make sure they are not curving forward on either side. Now, while isolating and holding the neck as tight as you can, use it to push/pull the head to face forward while inhaling keeping the chin close to the chest as you cross over the front of the body. Intentionally focus on using the musculature in the neck to move the head. Circle the head slowly and with intent in front of the body from right to center, exhaling, then from center to left inhaling then pull the head back as far as you can while exhaling. Take mental note of where you feel pain or pulling, tightness or discomfort. If you find points of pain or tension, apply pressure with the fingers of the opposite hand breathing deeply at tension points to relieve. Next, slowly circle your head behind the neck 6-9 times exhaling from right to center stopping to inhale at the center and exhaling toward the left. Once completed, bring head back up and rotate head to the right then to the left stretching as far as possible while still holding tension in the neck. Make sure that your shoulders are back and aligned. Bring head back to center. As you are performing these movements make sure to ride the breath inhaling during movements that open the windpipe and exhaling when the windpipe is being constricted. Note whether you feel any tightness, pain, or restriction of movement and make sure to stretch that area out a little more to release the tension. Next, we move onto the eyes.

EYES – With head facing forward, face relaxed and your tongue on the roof of the mouth, look up moving and stretching your eyeballs as far up as possible and hold them there for a few seconds. While keeping them stretched tight, roll them as far right as possible until you can see the side of the nose, and hold. Next circle them downward without moving the head, stretching them as far down as you can. Don't worry if the eyes blur or cross, this is normal. Hold the eyes there for a few seconds then roll them to the left and hold them there for a few seconds. Repeat this complete cycle up to 9 times. This helps to improve one's vision over time.

EARS & TONGUE – According to Chinese medicine, nerve endings that connect to the internal organs and various parts of the body reside on the ears and tongue. Stretching them out helps to stimulate the nerves and directs life force within the connecting organ meridians. Gently massage and pull the ears while sticking out your tongue as far as possible and in all directions stretching them both from top to bottom, left to right, and around. Open your jaw wider while sticking out your tongue. When done, move your jaw around in all directions doing the same with your lips and nose then squeeze your eyes shut and open them wide several times. This will stimulate blood and energy flow to the organs while stimulating blood flow through the tongue, eyes, and face.

SHOULDERS & ELBOWS – Next, lift the arms up to shoulder height and out to your sides extending them straight out with palms facing down toward the floor forming the letter "T" with your body. Focus and isolate the shoulder blades and shoulder joints using them to draw the shoulders up, back, down and forward circling using the muscles that connect to the shoulder blades and joints only for a count of nine. The forearms and hands should feel weightless and disengaged. Now, reverse directions circling in the opposite direction. Next, focus on circling just the arms from the shoulder joint disengaging the shoulder blades; you should feel this more in the upper arms versus the shoulders. While shoulders and arms are still held straight out from your sides, bend the arms at the elbows allowing the lower region of the arms and hands to go limp and circle the arms around the elbow joint. Perform each of these movement 6-9 times slowly in each direction making sure to focus on engaging the proper musculature and breathing deep down into the diaphram throughout the movements.

BICEPS & TRICEPS – Stretch the arm out in front of you at shoulder height with palms facing inward towards each other. Tighten the arms and press them toward each other as if squeezing a large beach ball, keeping the arms fully extended and elbows bent just enough to feel the biceps and deltoids engage. Begin pressing the arms inwards in slow pulses as if you are squeezing a beach ball several times. Exhale as you tighten and press inward, inhale as you tighten the triceps and pull outward. Do sets of 9 and then flip the palms outward facing away from the body and repeat. Next are bicep curls. Bring your arms down to your sides. Bend one forearm up to a 90-degree angle. Put the palm of the other hand squarely over the palm that is facing up press down with that hand as you curl the arm up towards the shoulder. Perform slow bicep curls using the top hand as resistance, pressing downward while you're pressing upward with the other hand. Do 9 – 18 repetitions each arm. Next, we work on the triceps. Straighten the arms on either side of you allowing them to hang by your sides. With legs shoulder width apart and knees bent, lean your upper body forward to about a 45-degree angle while at the same time making sure to keep your spine straight. Face palms towards the back of you and with arms straight, press the palms and arms back and up behind the back using the triceps to make the movements. Slowly press upward riding the breath for a count of 18. Once completed bring the arms straight back as far behind you as you can and hold them up. With elbows pointed towards the ceiling, or sky, perform Triceps extensions for a count of 18, squeezing them tightly at each full extension.

WRISTS & HANDS – With fingers extended and stretched as far out as you can, slowly circle your wrists. You should feel stretching and lengthening within the region of the forearms. While doing this movement fan the fingers as well from pointer to pinky bringing them one by one down to the palm and reversing one by one to stretch them out again. Rotate in both directions 6 – 9 times then go in the opposite direction and fan the fingers pinky to pointer fanning them down to the palm and then out again. You will really feel this in the forearms which happen to be one of the most overworked yet neglected areas of the body when it comes to intentional exercise. Next, hyperextend the fingers backwards, away from the palms stretching each finger out successively starting from the pinky until all fingers have been fully extended. You should feel a tight stretch within the hand and along the fingers. Shake hands out and bring palms and fingers together with arms extended straight out in front of the body. Flip one palm over so that the back of the right hand is cradled inside the palm of the left. While pressing the hands together, draw the hands in towards the chest and towards the right bending the elbows outward and keeping the arms shoulder height. Perform 6 – 9 times and repeat on other side then shake arms out once completed.

MERIDIAN ACTIVATION – Extend your arms out in front of your body as if you're holding onto a large beach ball. Using your left hand, make a fist and gently tap the outer side of the right arm from your wrist up to the top of the shoulder the continue tapping downward on the inner side of the arm. Switch arms and repeat on other side. Once completed, use both hands tapping down the inside of the legs down to the ankles then come up the outside of the legs to the hips. Move up to the upper back and tap along the back side of the body down to the floor.

FULL BODY SWING – Stand with legs wide holding body loosely allowing the arms to hang at your sides. Using your hips and legs to move and turn your body first towards the right and then the left like a washing machine letting the arms swing freely as you turn to each side. Perform the full body swing for a count of nine then turn your upper body so that it is facing over either leg having one facing forward and one straddled behind you in a lunge position.

LEG & HIP RELEASE – while facing in the direction chosen, do a set of 9 dips keeping the upper body upright and focusing mainly on using the back leg and quadricep muscles to do the work. Do another set of dips this time going deeper bringing your knees down to a 90-degree angle. Next, with hips facing toward the front leg, lunge your body forward leaning your upper body and hips over your front leg. Do another set of 9 lunges focusing on using your glutes and hamstrings to perform the movement by pressing with your front heal and keeping the glutes tight throughout the movement. Next, straighten the front leg in the lunge position and bend down until you feel the hamstrings stretch with hands on the floor on either side of the front foot or on your lower shin. Breathe deeply a few times allowing your body to move deeper into the stretch with each exhale. Next, move your body into a front straddle position walking your hands around to centerline of the body. Now shift your body to one side aligning it over one leg while keeping the other leg extended at an angle. Bring your body down into a side lunge position allowing the inner thighs of the opposite leg to stretch for a few seconds. You can add to the stretch by pressing the inner thigh of the knee that is bent back with your elbow. Finally, walk your hands back to the centerline while gently lifting your body by straightening the legs. Allow your chest and upper torso to drop down between your legs creating a stretch in the pelvis and low back elongating the spine. Repeat this sequence for the other side then once centered in front again, bring feet together and slowly lower yourself into a sitting lotus position with feet together in front of you.

GLUTE RELEASE – while sitting in lotus position with feet together in front of you, grab your feet with both hands, elongate the spine and gently, while exhaling, draw your chest down towards the floor stretching the lower back, hips and inner thighs. Hold this stretch momentarily, inhale deeply and as you exhale, draw yourself deeper into the stretch. You can add more intensity to the stretch by using your elbows to gently press your knees out and down as you sink your chest and upper body deeper towards the floor with each exhalation. When ready, bring your upper body upright into its proper alignment. Slide your right foot over towards your the left hip until it rests underneath or near it. Place your left foot on the other side of your right knee. If you find this position difficult, you can acchieve the same stretch by stretching your left leg straight out in front of you, then crossing the right foot over to the outer side of the left leg as close to your hip as is comfortable. Once you are in position, wrap your arms around your knee and gently draw it into your chest while elongating your spine. As you do so you will start to feel areas in the glutes that are tight or restricted. Hold each position that you experience tension in, and take 3-4 deep relaxing breaths each time moving a little bit deeper into the tension with each exhalation. When ready switch sides and repeat the same stretch with your other leg.

ABDOMINAL TONING – Now that you have fully stretched and opened up the hip area, lie down on your back and bring your legs into a position where your feet are flat on the floor hip width apart and your knees are pointed towards the ceiling. You will want to draw the lower abdominal wall in toward the spine and tuck the hips slightly in order to keeping your low back flat against the floor. Once positioned, extend your arms between your legs, and perform 9-18 sit-ups curling your upper body in as far as you can while keeping your lower back flush against the floor. When complete bring your arms to the outside of either leg for side crunches and repeat on the other side. If you're feeling up to challenging yourself you can add a set or two of lower leg raises to tighten your lower abdomen specifically.

Once completed, lie flat on your back, extend your legs out straight along the floor while bringing your arms straight up over your head and arch your back. This will help to gently release any tension or cramping in your abdominal wall. Refocus your attention on your breathing allowing your mind and body to fully relax into a peaceful yet vibrant state before returning yourself to a standing position.

THE ORGAN MERIDIANS SYSTEM & QI

QI

The science of working with Qi, (pronounced chi) or "energy" as referred to in Western culture, is at the very heart of TCM (Traditional Chinese Medicine). With thousands of years of direct observation and deep experiential knowledge of energy, this holistic medicine has a complete understanding of Qi and how it moves and functions in the body and throughout nature. TCM's deep insight and expertise on energy are what make it a profoundly accurate and effective healing system.

Qi has power and intelligence. It's true that qi is energy, but what I want to bring to your awareness is the various functions and characteristics of qi and how they operate within the body. Qi provides the power source for our body's ability to move and the intelligence of how much pressure, distance and motor skills are necessary for us to remain balanced as we do. This relates to Proprioception and vestibular function are the intelligence side of qi.

What does this mean? Have you ever wondered how the rising and ebbing tide keeps perfect pace with the lunar cycle? How a tree knows it's time to sprout leaves? How your body feels the season has changed from winter to spring and adjusts its own internal rhythms? It is Qi that allows all things to communicate with each other and change at both visible and invisible levels. It is Qi that carries infinite messages and pieces of information, connecting all things and all dimensions. Both aspects are needed: you could say that the power of Qi needs the intelligence of Qi to give it direction and focus that promotes life, change and healing. Without it there can be no growth; your body cannot exist one second without Qi. When you die your Qi leaves— it's transformed. If you view any health issue from the TCM perspective, with an understanding of the fluid and transformational qualities of Qi, it becomes clear that nothing is unmovable, unworkable, or permanent. At the level of energy, nothing is impossible to heal. It's the level where miracles can happen. However, the requirements for healing must be met and maintained.

THE BODY MERIDIANS

The network by which energy or qi flows through the body is called the meridian system. The meridians are like rivers of energy connecting everything in your body. Like a road map they're like a surplus of points woven into a vast network of invisible energy pathways connecting to each other and to every atom, cell, tendon, bone, organ, and each centimeter of skin. Meridians connect everything in your body. They link the upper portion with the lower and the surface with the interior, the subtle body with the physical body, your mind, your emotions, and your spirit—everything conscious and unconscious within you so that nothing is truly separate.

These meridians flow throughout your body and connect all invisible aspects of your being as an intercommunicating whole that connect to the Organs. There are twelve major meridians that run on each side of the body, one side mirroring the other. Each meridian corresponds to an internal organ. And each organ, with its own physiological and invisible energy functions, is not only dependent on the other organ systems but also on the greater meridian network.

The sentient intelligence of Life Force Energy, Blood, and Information flow continuously through the meridians, yet they also transmit information to and among your organs and chakras. Instantaneously they send signals to raise or lower your body temperature, signs that your body needs to release water, signals to regulate emotion, among countless other functions. They coordinate the work of the organs and keep your body balanced by regulating its functions and as long as enough Qi flows freely through your meridians and your organs work in harmony, your body can remain healthy. This means that when your body's meridian system functions well, you are well. Yet they can become clogged or even blocked due to emotional or mental stress, lack of nutritional foods, injury, lack of exercise and lack of sleep, (to name a few). When this happens, it affects the function of the corresponding organ and ultimately the whole body-mind-spirit.

Meridians are also incredibly sensitive. They can carry the effects of stimulation in the form of healing energy throughout your entire being. It is this special quality that allows the various Traditional Chinese Medicinal treatment modalities to work through the use of certain food, herbs, Qigong (an energy-building practice), acupuncture, or acupressure etc. And when the flow of energy in the meridians is stimulated, balance and health are restored.

The following charts depict the meridian channels to each of the organs within the Tao Yin Fa Sequence. These will help you to familiarize yourself with the organ meridians. They can also be used as a visualization tool should you choose to direct life force through the meridians as an optional meditation. This type of meditation works well in combination with the affirmations as the combination of these two will amplify the healing and soul evolutionary effects that one is intending to achieve.

Conception Vessel

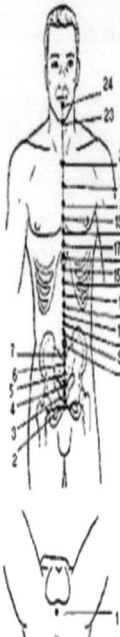

Large Intestine (LI)

Pericardium (CX P HC)

Heart (HT)

Governing Vessel

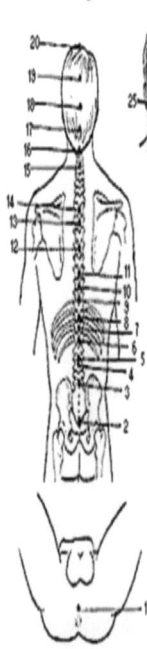

Lung (LU)

Tri-heater (TH)

Small Intestine (SI)

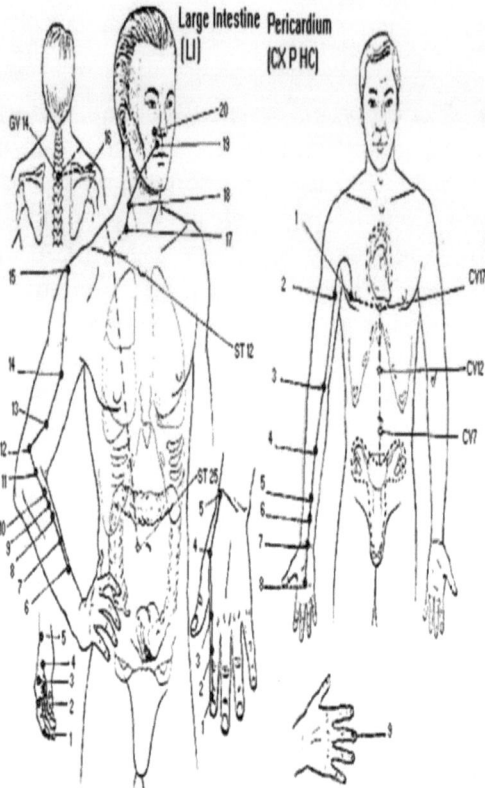

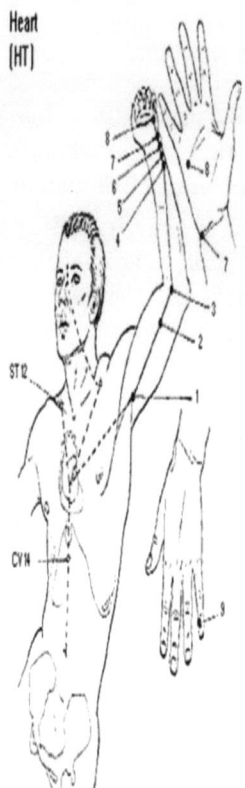

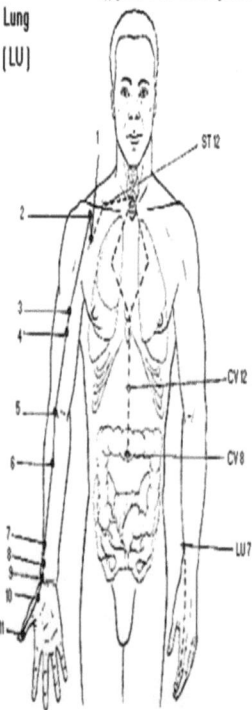

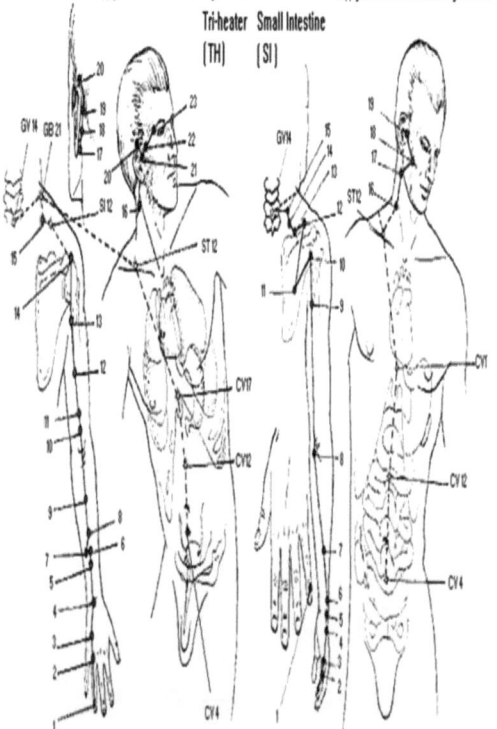

Upper Body Meridians Chart

38

Lower Body Meridians Chart

39

THE BODY'S CLOCK

In this reality, natural law operates 24/7, whether we know what these laws are or not, or whether we believe in them or not. Your body has its own built-in daily cycles of which one is the organ clock. Within Eastern medicine organ functions and operation cycles are on a 24-hour cycle with a duration of 2-hour intervals. Every two hours, a different organ energy reaches its peak of operation. This means that organ is in charge of your body's energy during that period of the day. TCM practitioners apply this knowledge when assessing your overall health picture.

Traditional Western Medicine (TWM) recognizes the rhythms of the body based on body cycle reactions to the external stimulus of sunlight and moonlight cycle which are externally driven versus internally driven. This particular science is known as the circadian rhythms which is based on the bodies sleep cycles and energetic responses effected by external lighting. The difference between the two is that the Circadian do not acknowledge the body's own function ability as a complete organism and how the body communicates and operates within itself as an organism. Another is the vast difference in styles of treatment. Traditional Western Medicine's (TWM) approach to treating imbalances of this nature is pharmaceutical drugs or at best nutritional supplementation however, both applications are administered in pill form. Traditional Chinese Medicine's (TCM) approach treating imbalances of this nature is the use of natural herbs, diet changes, Reiki, meditation and meditative movement using breathwork as a key component to bring about the rebalancing of the bodies systems.

The following diagrams present details that better explain the two viewpoint and approaches to the body's rhythms of operation. These also contains information on the bodily functions and operations that each system rules, energetically as well as physically, along with information on the internal and external operations that each approach associates to and how.

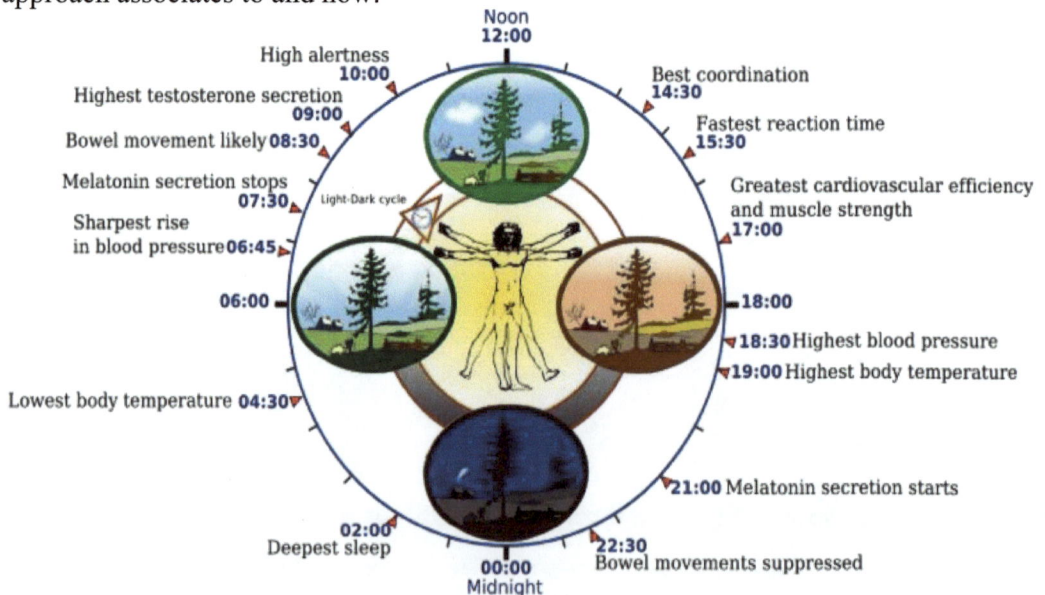

CIRCADIAN BODY CLOCK DIAGRAM

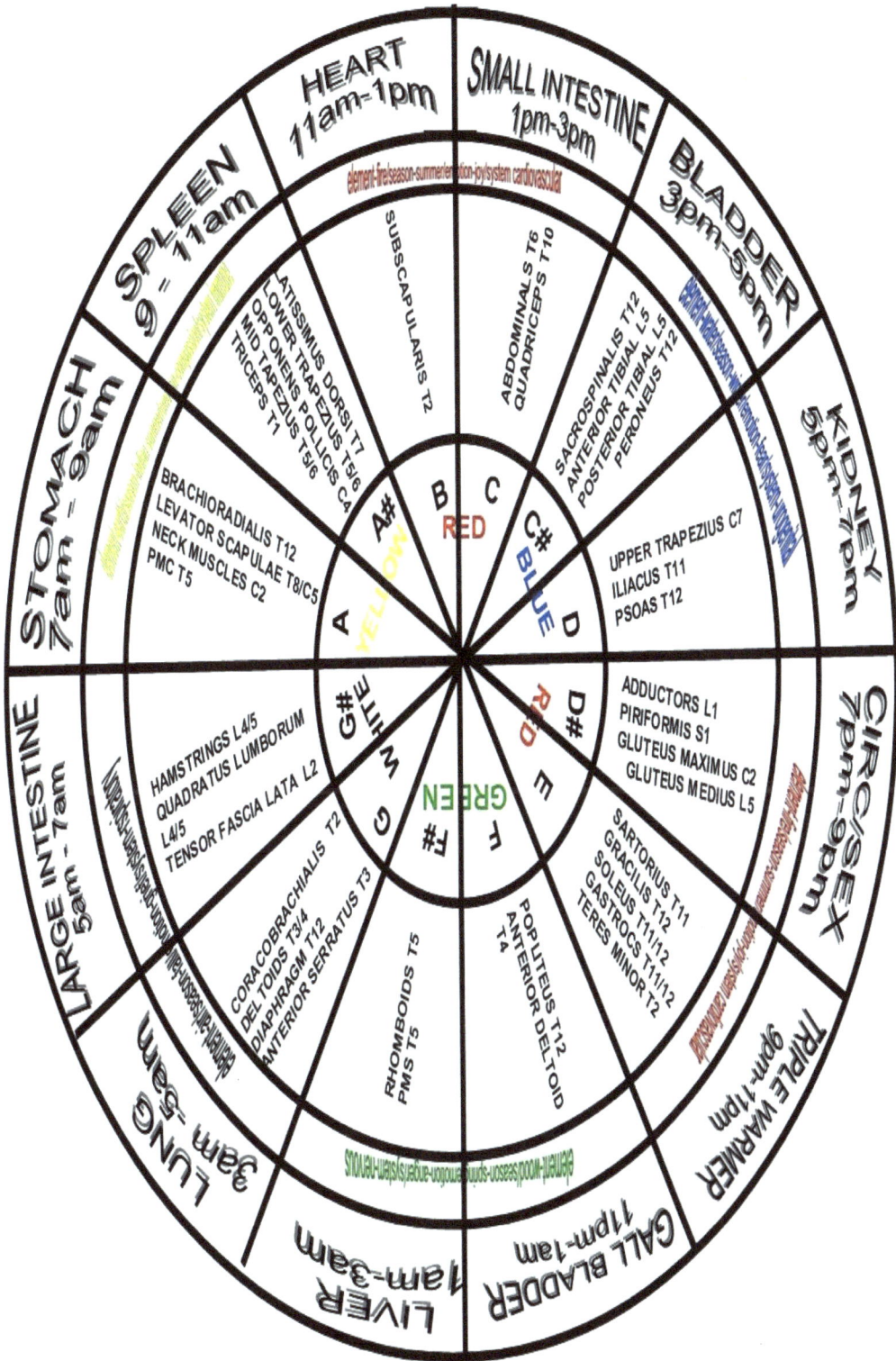

CHINESE MEDICINE ORGAN CLOCK DIAGRAM

41

TCM APPROACH TO THE CIRCADIAN BODY CLOCK

The following is an hourly breakdown combining the TWM circadian rhythms and the TCM organ clock.

3-5 am- This is the beginning of the cycle is when the **Lungs** energy are at their peak. You should be asleep during this part of the cycle. soft deep rhythmic breaths will help us sleep and process emotions. The lungs are linked with emotions such as grief.

5-7 am- The bodies Qi then moves onto be the most active within our **Large Intestine.** The body is ready to wake up and start a fresh new day! A healthy body empties it bowels soon after waking, to have a fresh start to the day, and to rid the body of waste accumulation overnight.

7-9 am- Ah yes- the **Stomach**, moving onto the beloved breakfast "the most important meal of the day". This is an ideal time to eat the biggest meal of the day as the energy of the stomach is at its highest, making the body more efficient at digestion and absorption, optimizing digestion.

9-11 am-The **Spleen** is a tricky organ system to comprehend when trying to make a correlation between Chinese medicine and western thought. It can be thought of as the spleen/pancreas, the yin earth pair to the stomachs yang energy. This is a great time of the day to get work done and exercise! The spleen helps to convert food you eat into brain food.

11-1pm- High noon bring the energy of the body to the **Heart**, the yin organ of fire. This is also when the day is at its fullest yang energy. The body is now focusing upon circulating nutrients absorbed by the food to the entirety of the system.

1-3pm- The **Small Intestine** helps to separate clear fluids from turbid and filter them to the kidneys or large intestine for waste secretion.

3-5pm- The time of the **Bladder** is often when people feel a lull in energy especially if they are not well hydrated.

5-7pm- This is when the **Kidney** energy is at its highest. The kidneys are the root of all energy in the Chinese organ system. This is a great time to eat a light and healthy meal to help replenish the bodies nutrients.

7-9pm- The time of the **Pericardium**, known as the protector of the Heart. This time frame is a wonderful time to do activities to nourish the heart such as socialize with loved ones, create art and music, or go dancing.

9-11pm-The **Triple Burner**, also known as the San Jiao, is most active at this time. It is a great time to wind down, relax and drift off to sleep. Gentle stretching, meditation, reading or cuddling can help the body quiet down. This is when melatonin secretion begins within our circadian rhythm.

11-1am- The time of the **Gallbladder-** it is said that when out of balance a person has trouble making decisions and has low self-esteem. A spike in energy can come at this time for many people, but it is best to use this time to go to bed.

1-3am- This is the time of the **Liver** and is the best time for deep sleep and dreaming. Often people with deficiencies wake during this time and experience a range of emotions.

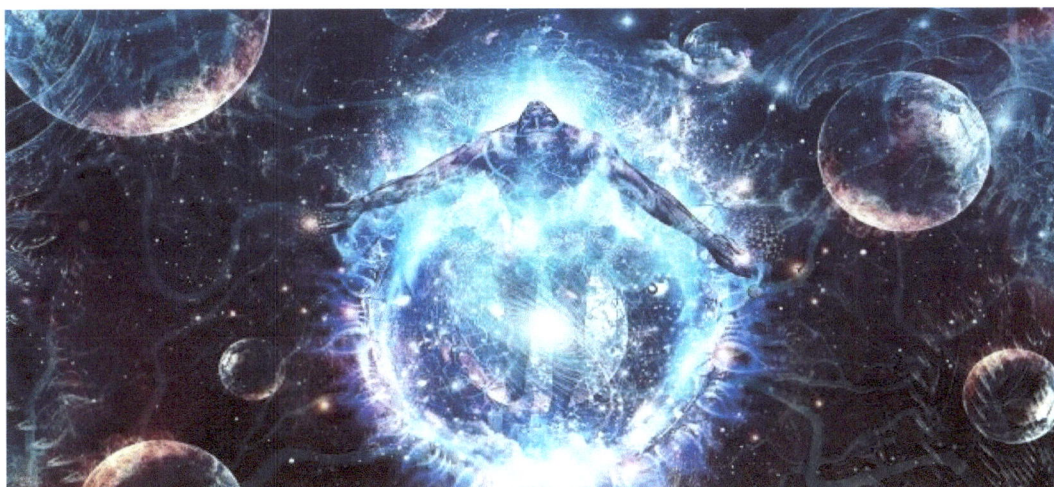

7 HUMAN EMOTIONS WHICH AFFECT HEALTH

As previously mentioned, one of the energetic subtle body functions of the organs is to regulate the emotions. Though there are 12 recognized organs within the body, I have found that there are 7 emotional roots that negatively affect the organ systems. When our organs systems are functioning properly and in homeostasis, we're able to process emotional events appropriately either through direct expression or through other forms of venting or releasing the adrenaline behind the emotion so that they do not remain in our subconscious or physical bodies. When emotions have been repressed or when our organs are not functioning properly it restricts the flow of life force through the meridian channels which not only creates dysfunction within the associated organ but affects all of the systems of our body in various ways.

1. **Anger effects on the Liver**
   - Anger makes Qi rise and symptoms will manifest in the head and neck, such as headaches, dizziness, tinnitus, neck stiffness, red blotches on the front part of the neck, a red face.
   - The term "anger" should be interpreted very broadly, to include several other related emotional states, such as resentment, repressed anger, irritability, frustration, rage, hatred, indignation, animosity or bitterness. If these emotions persist for a long time, they can affect the Liver causing stagnation of Liver-Qi or rising of Liver-Yang. *Yang is* the action potential, Qi, and heat in the body. These are the two most common Liver dis-harmonies arising out of anger.

2. **Joys effects on the Heart**
   - Joy makes the Mind peaceful and relaxed. It benefits the Nutritive and Defensive Qi and it makes Qi relax and slow down.
   - What is meant by "joy" as a cause of disease is obviously not a state of healthy contentment but one of excessive excitement and craving which can injure the Heart. This can happen when one lives in a state of continuous mental stimulation (however pleasurable) or excessive excitement. This leads to excessive stimulation of the Heart and, in time,

can lead to Heart-Fire or Heart Empty-Heat, depending on the underlying condition.

3. **Pensiveness effects on the Spleen & Heart**
   - Pensiveness makes the Heart Qi accumulate blood and causes the mind to converge: the upright Qi settles and does not move and therefore Qi stagnates."
   - Pensiveness is very similar to worry in its character and effect. It consists in brooding, constantly thinking about certain events or people (even though not worrying), sentimentally agonizing over the past and generally thinking intensely about life rather than living it. In extreme cases, pensiveness leads to obsessive thoughts. In a different sense, pensiveness also includes excessive mental work in the process of one's work or study.

4. **Worry effects on the Lungs, Spleen & Heart–**
   - Worry causes obstruction of Qi so that Qi stagnates.
   - Worry knots Qi, which means that it causes stagnation of Qi, and it affects both Lungs and Spleen: the lungs because when one is worried breathing is shallow, and the spleen because this organ is responsible for thinking and ideas. The symptoms and signs caused by worry will vary according to whether they affect the Lungs or the Spleen. If worry affects the Lungs it will cause an uncomfortable feeling of the chest, slight breathlessness, tensing of the shoulders, sometimes a dry cough, weak voice, sighing and a pale complexion.
   - If worry affects the Spleen it may cause poor appetite, gastric discomfort, some abdominal pain and distension, tiredness and a pale complexion. Worry is also the emotional counterpart of the Spleen's mental energy which is responsible for concentration and memorization. When the Spleen is healthy, we can concentrate and focus on the object of our study or work: the same type of mental energy, when disturbed by worry, leads to constantly thinking, brooding and worrying about certain events of life.
   - Finally, like all emotions, worry affects the Heart causing stagnation of Heart-Qi. This will cause palpitations, a slight feeling of tightness of the chest and insomnia.

5. **Fear effects on the Kidneys**
   - Fear diminishes one's ability to hear the voice one's heart and soul and blocks the free-flowing function of the organs and anatomy that relate to the Upper Burner (The lungs and heart). Fear causes restrictions of the intake and the circulation of air, blood and solids which blocks the flow of Qi that descends to the Lower Burner.
   - It over stimulates the adrenals which on an emotional subconscious level create feelings of distress, distrust of oneself and those around them, stagnation of one's decision making abilities as well as one's ability to distinguish when the universe is supporting them with positive opportunities to fulfill their own intentions. (Discerning the voice and/or hand of God in their life)

6. **Sadness effects on the Lungs & Heart**
   - Sadness weakens the Lungs also makes the Heart cramped and agitated, this pushes towards the lungs' lobes, the Upper Burner becomes obstructed, Nutrients and Qi that strengthens the immune system cannot circulate freely and Heat accumulates which dissolves Qi".
7. **Shock effects on the Heart**
   - Shock affects the Heart by depriving one's ability to reside in and come from their heart; the Mind overpowers one's inner senses and cannot rest, so that Qi becomes chaotic.
   - Mental shock "suspends" Qi and affects the Heart. It causes a sudden depletion of Heart-Qi, makes the Heart smaller and leads to palpitations, breathlessness and insomnia. Shock also "closes" the Heart or makes the Heart smaller. This can be observed in a bluish tinge on the forehead and a Heart pulse which is Tight and Fine.

HEALING THE ORGANS WITH TAO YIN FA

Tao Yin is a form of breathing exercises practiced by Taoists to cultivate qi or internal energy of the body based upon the principles of Traditional Chinese Medicine. The practice of **Tao Yin** was a precursor of qigong and was practiced in Chinese Taoist monasteries for health and spiritual cultivation. Tao Yin is also said to be (along with Shaolin Ch'uan) a primary formative ingredient in the well-known "soft style" Chinese martial art T'ai Chi Ch'uan. Each exercise is designed with a different goal in mind, for example: calmative effects and expanded oxygen intake, internal health and longevity.

Some of the exercises act as a means of sedating, some as a stimulant and a tonic, whilst others help in the activation, harnessing and cultivation of internal qi energy from the external Qi life force. Through the excellent health that is gained thereby, they all assist in the opening up of the whole body while enhancing the functioning of the autonomic nervous system and increasing the mental capacity of the brain. This allows for greater mind control, increased perception and intuition, the uplifting of moral standards, as well as tranquility within the mind. This in turn confers for inner homeostasis and greater happiness. As time goes by, these exercises slowly open up the control channels that feed and activate the energy within the nervous and psychic centers, enabling the individual to have a deeper understanding, and conscious awareness of the spiritual world.

The Tao Yin Fa sequence of meditative movement derives from the original practices designed by healing arts Master teacher Fabien Mannman, founder of Tama-do Academy of Sound, Color, and Movement. Its purpose is to open, clear, and rejuvenate the meridian channels, to energize the internal organs and to help keep them operating and functioning optimally as they were designed. Though not necessarily stated by Fabien, I believe that his intention was to draw life force energy (Qi) from the elements into the body more directly through this practice. In practice you will learn to directly connect to, circulate, send and receive life force from not only the Earthly Life Force Elements but also the Universal Life Force Elements through conscious awareness and intention. For those who are challenged with compromised states within the organ systems this can help to strengthen and balance one's internal state of health over time through consistent practice along with integrating other holistic practices and treatments.

Tao Yin Fa is a soft style martial arts movement that uses controlled breathing to help raise one's internal & external frequencies by re-establishing their vibrational connection to the elemental kingdoms. The added benefit with the southern styles of martial arts is that their focus on the acupuncture points to the organs along the meridians was also used as points of contact for healing the organs and subtle bodies. This form of Qi kung is best practiced in the open air where one can be surrounded by life force elements. However, it is also effective when performed within an enclosed environment with the use of visualization. What's unique about Fabian's approach within this sequence is the way in which he has designed the movements to isolate and stimulate the command points and meridian channels of each organ directly while incorporating it into a fluid movement pattern. Tao Yin Fa works on an energetic level to detoxify, rejuvenate, and strengthen the physical and subtle bodies and to energize the meridian channels helping to keep the internal organs operating and functioning optimally as they were originally designed. When an organ is experiencing a chronic condition or blockage this form of intentional movement combined with a living food diet, breath work, mudras, visualization and healing affirmations can assist in strengthening and restoring to health those organs that are out of balance or depleted in life force.

IMPORTANT NOTE FOR BOTH TAO YIN FA SEQUENCES:

Your palms and feet possess chakra openings that channel vibrational life force energy through them. Because of this, one is able to utilize them to amplify the healing aspects of ingestion and release of life force directly into and out from your own being through intention and visualization. Thus, whenever your hands are upward towards the sky or downward towards the earth, set the intention to draw in the life force elements of the Universe and those of Earth into yourself filling yourself up with their vitality.

Whichever sequence you are working with upon inhalation visualize breathing in the surrounding life force energies along with the corresponding gamma ray of the sun. Upon exhalation visualize any stagnant Qi or toxicity out either into your environment and/or into Mother Earth herself for its transmutation along with love and healing intentions.

TOA YIN FA - SEQUENCE II

LUNG/LARGE INTESTINE (LU/LI)

Create an "L" by stretching the thumb and forefinger out as far as you can while curling the remaining fingers of the hand into the palm. This opens the meridians of the Lung & Large Intestine. This movement aligns directly with the breath in that the lungs are responsible for inhaling or taking in new life force (oxygen) and the large intestine is responsible for eliminating old life force (waste) from the body. While Inhaling, extend your hand out in front of your body and move it in an upward curve until it is extended over and outward along the sagittal plane stopping at head level along the frontal plane. When you reach this point of the movement, stretch the arm as far away from the body as possible, then turn palm outward completely, flexing the wrist. In this position the life force is being optimally stimulated within the LU/LI meridian channels. Inhale deeply then hold the position and the breath while imagining the gamma-rays from the sun filling the LU/LI meridians and organs, with the color white while flooding them with life force energy. At this point, start to circle the hand downwards envision the color white taken into the organ and meridian being released into the universe while making the sound "seeeee" (like the sound of steam escaping from a pressure cooker). Repeat 6 times with each hand individually and 6 times with both hands simultaneously.

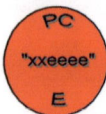

HEART/SMALL INTESTINE (HT/SI)

This mudra stimulates the Heart & Small Intestine meridians with the element of fire. Begin the movement with the arm stretched out in front of you. Create a closed circle with the thumb and forefinger while extending the other three fingers of the hand out as far as possible. On the inhale envision life force energy being drawn into the body with the hand at waist level. Move the hand back out away from the body in a figure eight movement bringing it up until it is aligned with the frontal plane of the body. At the top of the movement hold the breath while tightening the fingers and stretch the arm as far away from the body as possible. Imagine the color red filling the meridians and organs of the HT/SI with energy. As you start to bring the hand downward, envision releasing all toxicity and stagnation from the organs and meridians thru the breath into the earth while making the sound "haaaaa" in the note of C. The shift from one arm to the other is accomplished as you bring energy down from the top of the movement. In one continuous movement, transfer the energy to the left hand and continue on that side. End the movement with both hands in front of the hara (just below the navel) bringing the energy into the hara and then around and up to the top of the movement with both hands. Pause at the top to visualize the color red and then exhale as you bring the arms down with the sound "ha." Repeat 6 times with each hand individually and 6 times with both hands simultaneously.

CIRCULATORY/REPRODUCTIVE (PC/CIR)

The hand mudra for this meridian is performed by drawing the pinky and forefinger of each hand into the palm while fully extending the two middle fingers with palm open flat. THIS

MOVEMENT IS DONE WITH BOTH HANDS AT THE SAME TIME. With hand palm facing up at waist level in front of you, simultaneously draw a circle moving fingers away from the center and around. As fingers come back to the center turn the palms facing each other yet not touching and move both arms up until they are extended overhead. Once overhead fan the arms out until they are fully extended to your sides at shoulder height flexing the wrists downward so that palms are facing outward and away from the body. This movement scoops the energy up from the root to the crown chakra. Once arms are fully extended above your crown, open the arms out to your sides while still fully extended to receive cosmic energies and pause holding the breath and visualizing the color crimson filling the pericardium meridian with vital energy. Breathe out with the sound "Xeeeee" on the note E as you bring the energy down, arms out to the side. When arms are parallel to the ground turn palms downward and continue lowering towards the earth. At the level of the kidneys, gently turn the hands and bring the energy across the back to the kidneys. Caress the kidney with the back of the hands. Do not break the circular flow as you bring the hands across the sides of the body waist height and to the front. Perform this movement 18 times then move onto next movement.

URINARY BLADDER

The bladder, as well as the following meridians, travel up through the body from the feet. Invert the foot inward towards the body so that the lateral edge of the foot and toes are touching the ground in order to stimulate the bladder meridian command points. The bladder meridian also runs along the spine so remember to elongate fully to stretch the meridians. As you inhale, the hand and opposite foot, are to move synchronistically throughout the movement. Allow the foot to reach from front to back at the same time that the opposite hand reaches from being down at your side to up over your head. At the top of the arm movement open the hand wide and turn the palm so it is facing inward toward the head. Hold the breath for a moment as you visualize the color dark blue traveling up the UB meridian to the organ. Make sure to stretch and extend the body to its furthest point. Slowly bring the hand and foot back to their starting position while breathing out with the sound "shuiiiii". Repeat with the remaining hand/foot performing 6 times on each side. Turn to the front and perform just the upper body movements with both hands simultaneously 6 times before moving onto the next movement.

SPLEEN (SP)

The Spleen is stimulated by everting the foot fully outward, so the instep of the foot is facing forward. Breathe in moving the hand and opposite foot up and back synchronistically as you did in the previous movement. Move the hand up with palm away from the body while swinging the foot out and behind you in a half circle, keeping the instep of the foot facing inward. Hold the breath at the top of the movement and visualize the color yellow running through the SP meridian to the organ, then slowly breathe out with the sound "Hhhuuuuu" as you return the hand and foot to its original position. Perform 6 times then repeat with the remaining hand/foot performing 6 times on each side. Turn to the front and perform just the upper body movements with both hands simultaneously 6 times before moving onto the next movement.

KIDNEY (KI)

The next two movements are performed moving both hands simultaneously along with the left foot then repeating with the right foot. While extending the left leg out in front, flex the foot upward pressing the heel into the floor with toes are pointed up towards the sky. While keeping the foot flexed, move it in a half circle ending with the leg stretching behind you placing the foot flat on the ground. Leg should be fully extended so that the hamstrings and calves are fully stretched. Both hands should move up simultaneously with the foot movement in synchronicity with the foot movement with palms facing inward toward the head. This allows the meridian to remain stimulated throughout the movement. Hold the breath while you visualize the color dark blue running through the KI meridian to the organ, then slowly breathe out with the sound "shuiiiii" as you return the hands and foot to their original position. Perform 9 times on each side.

LIVER/GALLBLADDER (LV/GB)

This movement stretches the gall bladder meridian by pointing the tip of the big toe down towards the earth as you extend the leg out in front of you. Open both hands so the palms are facing forward in a position of receiving. The movement is again a synchronized sweeping of the foot and arms yet this time the palms are turned outward at the top of the movement stretching the arm as high as comfortable. Move the foot around in a half circle from front to back keeping the toe pointed throughout the movement. When the toe reaches the back, it should still be pointed with the same tension that you started with. At the top of the movement, hold your breath and visualize the color green bringing energy through the (LV/GB) meridians and into the organs as you turn your hands outward. Slowly breathe out with the sound "xxxuuuuu" in the note A as you return the hand and foot to its original position. Perform 9 times on each side.

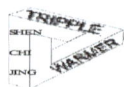
TRIPPLE WARMER

The triple warmer movement is the only movement where you will be traveling across the ground. It harmonizes the first seven movements to ground the energy and stimulate the three heaters that govern the energy of the total body. The triple warmer consists of the upper warmer = lungs & heart, mid warmer = stomach, spleen, pancreas, liver, gall bladder and lower warmer = small intestine, large intestine, kidneys and bladder. Begin this movement by touching each of the Three Heaters and then cupping the energy and bringing it into the hara or Dantien and around again to the front and up. You will have the experience of your arms encircling the energy like a cup. Here you should have finished your first step. As you shift your weight onto the foot which has taken the step, take the Grail energy in your cupped hands and cross them at the wrists with palms facing away from the body giving the energy back to the earth and the universe. This completes the movement and you have returned to the original posture and are ready to begin the movement with your other foot. Gently touch the energies of the three heaters, bring the energy back to the hara as you start a new step... and continue from here. Perform 3-4 steps of this (each foot) working in a forward movement after which you will continue moving backwards with the same movements.

TAO YIN FA AFFIRMATIONS
Affirmations can be internally or externally vocalized in conjunction with visualization while performing the corresponding movements to expand the effects of the movements into the subtle bodies consciously strengthening and increasing their healing abilities.

LUNG: "I breathe in new life visions, new ideas, new insights to self, and new experiences of unconditional love. By this I transmute all negative outdated mentalities that do not reflect my vision of living the divine life and of being in alignment with my divine truth. As I exhale, I eliminate the old outdated patterns of though, disappointments, insecurities concerning my future vision of divine health and any fear of being unconditionally loved and provided for. I breathe in self-love, the pure essence of peace, the sentient beauty of Nature's elements, and the pure essence of divine knowledge and wisdom that surround and embody me. I allow life's elements to reveal their insights to my connection with all life inhaling their life force while exhaling and eliminating any and all past pain, low self-esteem, self-doubt, self-judgments, and/or self-loathing from past lives lived as well as from ancestral memory that may reside within."

LIVER/GALL BLADDER: "I allow divine life force to filter through my, divine ideas, divine insight to Self, and healthier, happier intentions for unconditional experiences of love that sustains me through its life blood and substance feeding my thoughts, words and deeds. I allow these divine thoughts to become a part of my essence expressing its divine influences through me which inspires spiritual healing in those that I come into contact with."

STOMACH/SPLEEN: "I take in divine life force, divine ideas, divine insights to self and divine experiences of love, allowing these things to assimilate and integrate into my consciousness so that they may circulate throughout my life reproducing new healthy thought forms, experiences, and creative expressions that produce greater levels of joy and peace in my life. I allow these new insights, ideas, and experiences of love to dissolve toxic energy from past conditioning and to transmute them into that of divine health, divine wealth, and knowledge of Divine Self through divine evolution (love-u-tion)."

SMALL INTESTINE/LARGE INTESTINE: "I ingest divine life force, divine ideas, divine insights and divine visions of myself living in divine health, divine wealth, and embodiment of divine Self, the ancestors, and my celestial roots. I allow these insights to digest, assimilate within my minds meditations and permeate into my conscious way of thinking, speaking and acting so that these new insights transmute outdated patterns of self that do not reflect the image of the life I want to experience. As these meditations circulate throughout my life, they reproduce better experiences, better outcomes, and greater joy & peace in my life."

HEART/REPRODUCTIVE/CIRCULATORY SYSTEMS: "I embody unconditional love and allow divine life force, divine ideas, divine insights to Self and divine experiences of love, to break down any and all existing barriers to healing and creating healthy relationships and experiences. I release what no longer serves my divine vision of personal fulfillment of my divine desires and higher intentions. I activate & unlock my potential to live in optimal alignment with the ancestors, Divine God/Goddess/The Elementals/The

Universal Consciousness. I express a healthy attitude towards My body, my spirit, my surroundings, my family & community and my divine purpose breathing out all blockages and allow myself to flow with the blessings and infinite potential for personal and spiritual ascension that living the life I desire to live presents unhindered."

'I stand strong in my resolve to embrace the love that will generate the healing of my body, my mind, my soul, my relationships, my community and the planet."

TRIPPLE WARMER: "I am spirit housed in this body of flesh of which I choose to sustain in divine health that it may assist me in the fulfillment of my purpose, desires, and dreams. I breathe in divine life force, divine ideas, divine insights to self and divine experiences of love, while exhaling the past with each exhalation knowing that within my cellular memory resides the blueprint of my spiritual and ancestral roots. These roots guide, direct, and assimilate the wisdom from the knowledge of our past story from the beginning of time and before and inspires me to live and share the truth of our original life in order to transmute the misrepresentation and subjugation into right-us-ness and harmony of living as one with the land. And each time I embrace and breathe in this truth, I become immune to limitation, lack, fear and all forms of dis-ease instantaneously and as I exhale focused on the fulfillment of my purpose, desires, and dreams, they become manifest as my life."

URINARY BLADDER/KIDNEY: "I choose to float along the streams of divine consciousness that surround me, bathing in divine ideas, divine insights to self and divine experiences of love. I allow these things to filter through my consciousness and to flush out any and all harmful or outdated thought forms, memories, or ways of being to eliminate them from my thought of the future, my speech and my actions creating new vibrant healthy relationships and experiences of Self-fulfillment."

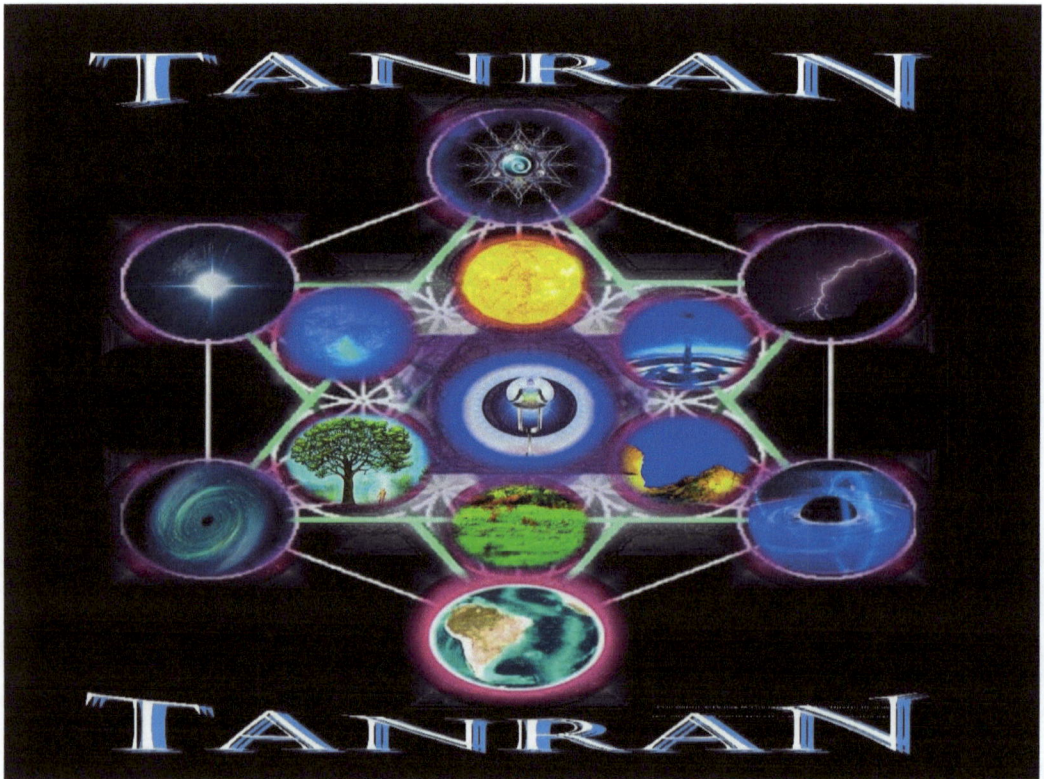

52

7 PHASE ELEMENTAL CHAKRA MERIDIAN CHART

YIN (SOLID) ORGANS

(- HT) HEART
(- PC) PERICARDIUM
(- SP) SPLEEN
(- LU) LUNGS
(- KI) KIDNEY
(- LV) LIVER
(GV) GOVERNING VESSEL

YANG (HOLLOW) ORGANS

SMALL INTESTINE(+ SI)
TRIPPLE WARMER (+ TW)
STOMACH (+ ST)
LARGE INTESTINE (+ LI)
URINARY BLADDER (+ UB)
GALL BLADDER (+ GB)
CONCEPTION VESSEL (CV)

CROWN
Color - Violet/White
Elements - Light, Vibration
Note - B/Tone - "EEE"
physicality - helps remove
obstruction allows Divine love,
wisdom, and creativity to rule
your thoughts, words, deed
Emotional impacts happiness,
intellectual development,
memory

3RD EYE
Color - Indigo
Element - Ether
Note - A/Tone "EEE"
PB - Lower Brain,
Left Eye, Pituitary Gland, Ears,
Nose, Nervous System
EMSB
Centre of creativity, intuition,
imagination, insight, devotion
to spiritual knowledge.

NAVEL
Color - Orange
Element - Water
Note - D/Tone - "O"
PB - Spleen, Gonads,
Reproductive System,
Womb, Ovaries, Testicles,
Prostate, Genitals, Bladder,
Kidneys
EMSB
Centre of feeling, emotion,
sexual desire, craving,
family life, harmony,
tolerance.

HEART
Color - Green
Element - Wood
Note - F/Tone - "A"
PB - Heart, Blood, Vegus
Nerve, Ciruiatory System,
Thymus Gland, Skin, Arms,
Hands
EMSB
Centre of compassion,
altruism, forgiveness,
gentleness, acceptance
of reality as it is,
Anger, Resentment,
Shouting

THROAT
Color - Sky Blue
Elements - Metal/Air
Note - G/Tone - "I"
PB - Thyroid, Throat, Mouth,
Bronchial & Vocal System, Lungs
EMSB
Grief, Guilt, Regret
Crying, Deep Sighing
concrete perceptions
Centre of communication,
speech, wisdom, kindness

SOLAR PLEXUS
Color - Yellow/Gold
Element - Sun
Note - C/Tone- "AAH"
PB- Stomach, Liver, Pancreas,
gall bladder, Muscles, Nervous
System,
EMSB
Centre of self-respect, willpower
confidence,
physical energy,
self-control.

ROOT
Color - Red/Black
Element - Earth
Note - C/Tone- HU
PB- legs, feet, large intestine
spinal column, bones
EMSB-
Centre of survival instinct,
Courage, stability, Empathy,
physical health,
sense of belonging,
family, community,
material world

THE WORKINGS OF THE 7 ELEMENTS THEORY

In Lemurian Medicine humanities cosmic and earthly energetic and physical associations were taught. It was common knowledge that the functions, and attributes of the internal organs and chakras and their functions, characteristics and attributes were directly impacted by the seven elements of nature and of the universe. The following chart reveals how each life force element corresponds to a respective chakra and a set of partnering organs energetically and the ways in which the corresponding elements help to regulate and balance the body.

OUR EARTHLY NATURE

According to my observations of nature, the elements their functions, sentience, and connections within humanity and the ways in which our human bodies and behaviors correlate, I came to experience certain insights, awareness' and innerstandings as to just how they operate in, as and through us; not just physically but psychologically. I came to innerstand the following about nature and its presence and role within us on the following psychological levels. There are many variations of how this happens.

What keeps our bodies alive is the oxygen/carbon exchange that allows us to live off of the air we breathe, the heat of the sun, the water we drink, the mineral and/or nutritional content within the food from the plant life grown within the Earths soil, and the cosmic and energetic vibrational frequencies. These 7 components of nature feed and sustain our energetic or subtle bodies which create and maintain the complete composition of our physical body's molecular and energetic structure allowing our spirit to express itself externally through the body and soul. The following list demonstrates some of these psychological associations.

7 Elements of Nature

8. **Air** – thought, consciousness/ awareness
9. **Water** – flow, movement, progressive action of movement
10. **Fire** – passion or desire, anger and frustration
11. **Mineral** –mental clarity and concrete perceptions of visions and dreams,
12. **Earth** – daily nourishment, sustenance, grounded-ness, fixed sense of self
13. **Wood/Vegetation** – energy that fuels and supports our visions and passions
14. **Sound** – vibrational intensity or power behind our words spoken that help to manifest them in form.

OUR COSMIC NATURE

The elements of the universe provide the energetic circuitry of the soul. Though subtle, they are what allow us to consciously and unconsciously interact with all that exists within our physical environment. The law of attraction, the communication network of our nervous system that sparks, directs, and controls the inner electrical network of the mind/body allows us to operate the physical as well as the psychological mechanics of our being. Light is the life force of our spirit or ka body and is maintained by the energetic frequencies that work and move through us. The ethers both within and without, allow us to tap into that which Creates or is responsible for the creative process whether from the Cosmic Universe of our internal Universe of the mind/body. The etheric space provides the incubational environment necessary for life to formulate and materialize. It's where the intangible transforms into the tangible giving material form and substance to all things and from where all material things are birthed. Like gaseous matter our thoughts and visualizations, though not seen, are real and are the stuff from which ALL physical matter has derived from. The vibrational impact that our Spoken word coupled with our though intentions has in the process of what we manifest into physical form is similar to the way in which liquid when frozen takes on the shape of its container.

7 Element of the Universe

1. **Intelligence** – consciousness, order, applied wisdom, knowledge & ability to create
2. **Ether** – the meditative incubation or contemplations of thought that creates via vision
3. **Magnetism** – our ability to connect to and attract thoughts, vibrations, people, intentions etc.
4. **Electricity** – our energetic frequency levels
5. **Light** – the radiance of the spirit and/or Divine life force within us
6. **Vibration/Sound** – the ability to verbalize or vocally express that which gives conscious visual or mental form to our thoughts, and emotions and eventually physical form.
7. **Matter** – embodiment or material manifestation of one's thoughts, intentions or one's contemplations/meditations

SENSORY MECHANICS

Again, our sensory mechanic are the physical gateways of our entire body that allow us to interpret, interact with, and store the information concerning our relationship to our surroundings, each other and the Elements of Divine Life Force. We combine and utilize all of them in order to have this human experience on earth. They teach us who and what we are, as well as the design, the knowledge and the purpose of the divine laws of creation. Whether physical, cosmic, spiritual, social, or material there are divine laws that exist to maintain order for life to take place. The following is a brief list of our Extra and Ultra Sensory Mechanism that we have been equipped with however some of which have atrophied due to religious and societal mandates that forbid the recognition of and/or the natural practice of by making the practice of these ultra-sensory aspects of our true nature punishable by death.

1. **The eyes** (visual Intake)
2. **The Nose** (Intake of smell)
3. **The Ears** (Intake by Hearing)
4. **The Tongue** (Intake through taste) and
5. **The Hands & Feet** (Intake through touch).
6. **Vestibular** (balance)
7. **Proprioception** (propulsion)
8. **Interception** (internal warning signals)
9. **Clairvoyance**
10. **Clairsentience**
11. **Clairaudience**

12. **Claircognizance**
13. **Mental telepathy**
    a.   **Latent Telepathy**
    b.   **Retro-cognitive Telepathy**
    c.   **Precognitive Telepathy**
    d.   **Intuitive Telepathy**
    e.   **Emotive Telepathy**
    f.   **Super-conscious Telepathy**
    g.   **Ancestral Sentience or Telepathy**
    h.   **Cellular Sentience**
(Please refer to pages 13 through 15 for their detailed explanations.)

Another quite important dynamic that directly influences the function-ability of the chakras is the type of inner and outer environment that one is exposed to throughout one's life, most importantly from childhood. One's family and community dynamics, its traditions, beliefs and value systems, rituals, practices, societal influences and natural setting -whether urban, suburban, rural, tropical or otherwise, along with the predominant collective consciousness that one is exposed to. This all influences the quality of life force by which our chakras ingest, conceptualize, interpret, and act upon on all levels but especially within our personal development and their level of healthy functioning. There are key components that exist within a close-knit community that allow one to thrive and maintain a sense of belonging, productivity, acceptance and support that one is able to recreate no matter where they go. When one does not feel a sense of connectedness and support from one's community it triggers subconscious fear that causes one to react from a heightened fear-based awareness, survival tactics and coping skills versus discernment and healthy interaction and responsiveness. This is all due to our inherent knowing that harmony and balance are a part of the spirit/soul's natural blueprint despite how much we as a species have strayed from it.

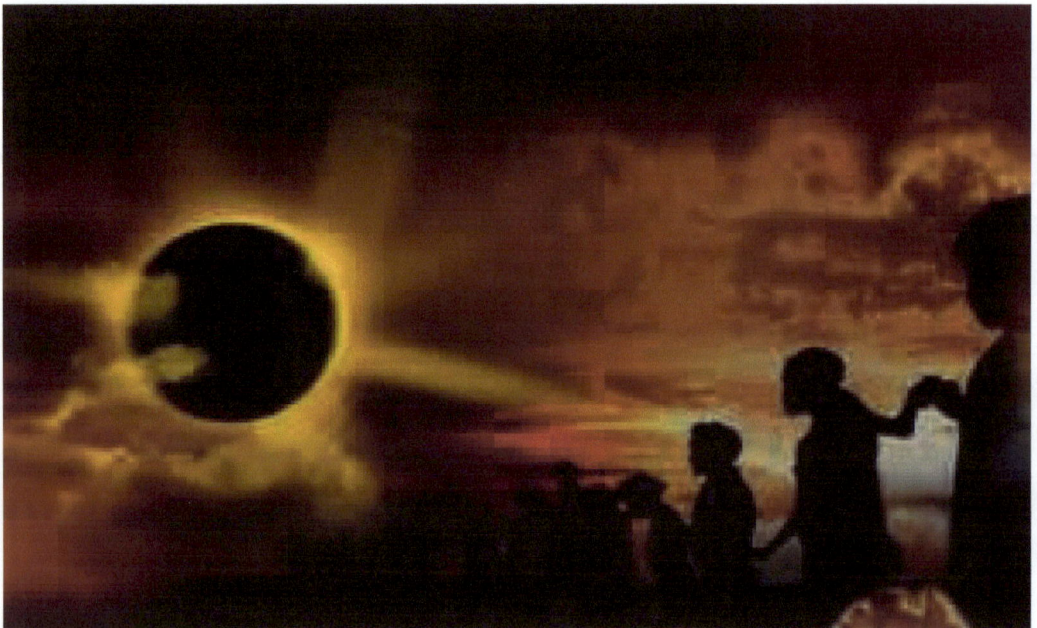

THE UNIVERSAL CYCLES OF SEVEN

There are underlying universal patterns of behavior, rhythms or ciphers of life that are consistent throughout the universe and throughout time yet are unique to each occurrence in its effects. These cycles apply to all aspects of life whether cosmic, earthly, or on a human level, these cyclical components are an integral thread to all of existence. So far, I've come to see these cycles reflected on seven levels which are listed below along with their components. The following material explains the 7 various aspects of life force and how they relate to our bodily functions, processes, e-motional expression and their effects upon and within our physical and subtle bodies throughout life.

7 ELEMENTS OF THE UNIVERSE

1. **Magnetism** – the universal energy force of gravity or the law of attraction within all things, which draws people or things near or them away each other
2. **Electricity** – our neurological and energetic functionality & design of our nervous systems
3. **Light** – the radiance of our true Self, our Spirit and its Divine life force design
4. **Ether** – our minds where the incubation or contemplations of thought is created in vision
5. **Sound** – our vibrational resonance, our vocalized expressions that helps to transition the conscious visual or mental form of our thoughts, and emotions into physical form.
6. **Intelligence** – discernment & innerstanding of how to act upon information or applied wisdom & knowledge
7. **Matter** – embodiment or material manifestation of one's thoughts, intentions or one's contemplations/meditations

7 ATMOSPHERIC LAYERS OF EARTH

1. **Troposphere** – The lowest portion of Earth's atmosphere which contains 75% of the atmospheres mass and 99% of its vaporous water content.
2. **Stratosphere** – the second layer of Earth's atmosphere which contains the ozone layer and is where the absorption of ultraviolet radiation occurs.
3. **Mesosphere** – the third highest layer of Earth's atmosphere and is the coldest place and is also where most meteors burn up upon entrance into Earth's atmosphere
4. **Thermosphere** – Second highest layer of Earth's atmosphere which is completely devoid of water vapor due to its extreme low pressure. It is also where the absorption of energetic ultraviolet and X-Ray radiation from the sun occurs.
5. **Ionosphere** – the Earth's magnetic field of atmospheric electricity and solar winds. It reflects and absorbs radio waves.
6. **Exosphere & Magnetosphere** – the outermost layer of Earth's atmosphere which contains extremely low densities of hydrogen, helium, nitrogen, oxygen, carbon dioxide and several other molecules that escape into the Ionosphere and outer space. This region of the atmosphere surrounds the earth and is where charged particles spiral along the magnetic field lines.

7. **Outer Space** – The Dark Void (also referred to as the "Wombniverse" or "Dark Matter") that exists between celestial bodies. A plasma where hydrogen, helium, electromagnetic radiation, magnetic fields, neutrinos, dust and cosmic rays reside. Plasma being a state of matter in which an ionized gaseous substance becomes highly electrically conductive to the point that long-range electric and magnetic fields dominate the behavior of the matter. (Wikipedia)

7 ELEMENTS OF NATURE
1. **Air** – thought, consciousness/awareness
2. **Fire** – passion, desire, intense feeling of emotion or excitement
3. **water** – flow, direction, progressive action of movement
4. **Mineral** –mental clarity and concrete perceptions of visions and dreams,
5. **Earth** – daily nourishment, cultivation, and sustenance of one's visions or dreams
6. **Wood/Vegetation** – energy that fuels and supports our visions and passions
7. **Sound** – vibrational intensity or resonance of one's words spoken that help solidify one's vision into form.

7 CHARACTERISTICS OF MOTHER NATURE
1. **Fertilization/Conception** – The fusing of two like yet separate entities or beings into one new entity or being that contains a combination of the DNA of both entities fused
2. **Incubation/Germination** – the formation or development of an entity from the time that its conception until it has reached its full formation
3. **Birth** – The process by which the host of an entity in incubation is expelled so that it can become an individualized organism
4. **Growth** – the developmental process of maturation
5. **Reproduction** -The continuation of a life form through sexually mating with a genetically compatible entity
6. **Death** – the cessation of all biological functions that sustain a living organism or the exhaustion of life within a living organism. The transition from one's physical form into a state of energetic form of existence.
7. **Decomposition/Transmutation** – the breaking down of the physical form as an organic substance into its basic cellular components that then become absorbed into other organisms.

7 CHARACTERISTICS OF HUMAN & ANIMAL NATURE
1. **Sentient** – the ability to feel, perceive, or experience subjective feelings or sensations from others and within one's environment.
2. **Instinctual** – innate behavior or inherent inclination of a living organism towards survival or Self preservation
3. **Anatomy** – the physical structure of a living animate entity whose body and systems thrive off the life force elements of its natural environment or habitat.
4. **Psychological** – The personality, which made up of the id which represents the impulsive subconscious drives and hidden memories, our superego or moral conscience imprinted upon us by our parents and societal codes of conduct learned in our early years. and the ego is our sense of reason that mediates

between the id and the superego. It's our ability to empathize, express and respond to various emotional characteristics such as compassion, empathy, altruism, aggression, and fear to name a few.
5. **Co-habitational -** Naturally living in intimate groups or collectives made of those within their own descendants and species
6. **Reproductive** – All offspring are reproduced from within the womb or the portal of life through the Female who is responsible for the continuation of the species.
7. **Survival-** striving for food and inhabitable environment in order to sustain one's individual and collective existence.

7 ELEMENTS OF COMMUNITY
1. **Ecological -** the natural environment, animals within that environment and the earth's natural resources available in the area or region.
2. **Cultural** – the customs, arts, social institutions, and achievements of a particular people, social group, or nation
3. **Structural** – the architectural set up, and use of natural resources
4. **Societal** – an aggregate of people living together in an ordered community
5. **Spiritual** – the sacred and ethical belief systems and practice that are held within a collective community, culture, or society
6. **Medical** – the theories and practices of treating physical, mental, emotional ailments and trauma's,
7. **Economical** – the economic structure of a society (trade/sale, import/export cultivation of natural resources, industrial complex, and labor structure.)

7 COMMON CORE CHAKRAS
1. **Crown** – our spiritual center that allows us to receive spiritual insights and the sense of connectedness with the God-Self or Spiritual Intelligence
2. **1st Eye** – our center of visualization by which we create material reflections of the intangible imagery within our minds where spiritual sight takes place.
3. **Throat** – the energy center that is responsible for our ability to express ourselves outwardly both vocally or physically.
4. **Heart** – the center that is responsible for the embodiment and expression of the divine attributes of love and connectedness holistically
5. **Solar Plexus** – the energy center by which we connect with the divine within and ourselves and each other as well as the center of our personal identity and power
6. **Navel** – the emotional center where our ancestral and life experiential memories reside
7. **Root** – our connection to our roots, the earth, that of family and community and our sense of belonging within these dynamics

7 SUBTLE BODY LAYERS OF APPLICATION

1. **The Physical Body** – material form or embodiment of oneself
2. **The Etheric Body (or energetic duplicate of the physical body)** – Ka body that provides the vitality, health, life and organization to the physical body
3. **The Emotional or Astral Body** – where desires, emotions, imagination, psychic abilities reside.
4. **The Mental Body** – Where thought, cognition, intelligence, and spiritual innerstanding resides from access to (The One Mind) resides
5. **The Causal Body** – Higher Soul where Akashic Records of all of one's lifetimes and incarnations reside.
6. **The Buddhic Body** – where one is beyond individuality, selfless, where one is dedicated to the evolution of the soul group consciousness beyond the sense of any personal desires.
7. **The Atmic Body** – Undifferentiated awareness that enlivens as well as observes and acts through every living being. Where perfect self-mastery is attained

These cycles are integrally weaved within one's self and one's environment and through every aspect of hu-man life on earth. Kun Qi assists in the re-awakening, re-alignment, and reconstruction of the original blueprint of these structures in their unadulterated form within one's own inner vision and innerstanding of their divine purpose and original intentions along with the desire and the means to recreate them in modern times. You will find yourself working with all aspects of the Universal Cycles of 7 in various ways within the8 directional cipher meditations that are to follow. These sequences of Kun Qi Kung will allow you to shift your experience of the outer and inner dynamics of life and self-mastery to that of your divine nature more easily.

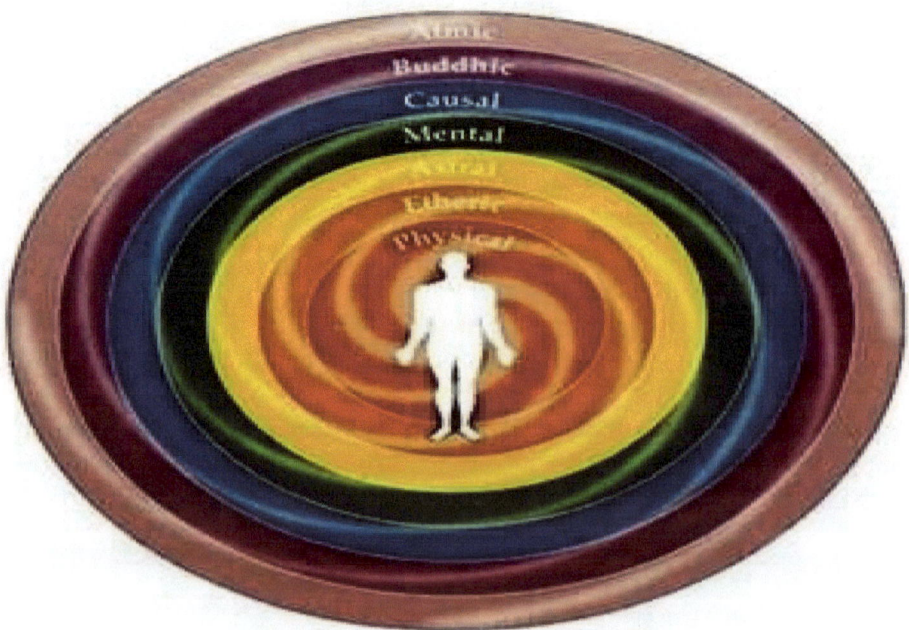

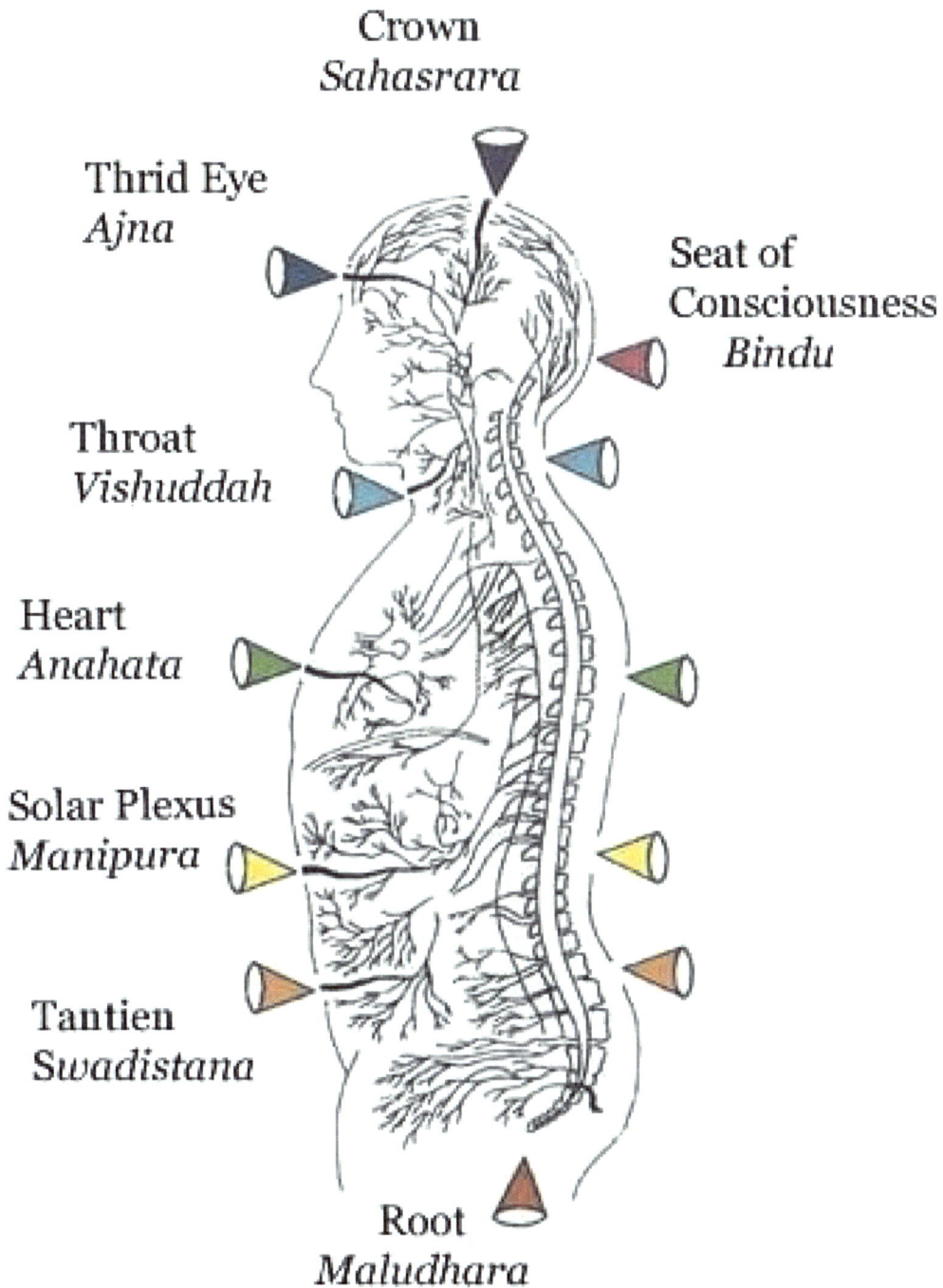

Chakras

Crown
Sahasrara

Thrid Eye
Ajna

Seat of
Consciousness
Bindu

Throat
Vishuddah

Heart
Anahata

Solar Plexus
Manipura

Tantien
Swadistana

Root
Maludhara

61

THE WORKINGS OF THE CHAKRAS

A WORD OF CAUTION HERE: THE CHAKRA CENTERS ARE EXTREMELY POWERFUL. Understanding how the chakras work, how to identify imbalance within them, and natural ways in which one can balance them oneself will help you to work more effectively with the chakras in an interactive and integrated manner. The following information is designed to give you some general and specific understanding of the chakra system such as, what chakras are, where they reside within the body, what their functions are and how one's conscious awareness in regards to their functions and operations can assist in accelerating one's personal healing process.

WHAT ARE CHAKRAS?

The word 'chakra' derives from the Old Indo-Iranian language of Vedic Sanskrit. They are energy points or more accurately defined as "Spiraling Vortex" within the subtle body. If you could visually see your chakras you would perceive various sized spinning or pulsing vortexes of energy that spin inward drawing combined life force energies into you from the front -- similar to a black hole-- of the body towards the spinal column and its electrical network then outward through the back from that same Information Relay Network. These energies download & upload information from the life forces around us through the chakras into the kundalini system, which is the psychic network within the spinal column. Looking from the side they would look like funnels whose mouths face outward. The relay network of the chakras relays conscious and subconscious sentient information through intelligence, clairvoyance or intuitive communication that contains knowledge concerning the reality being experienced by all.

These wheels of energetic intelligence have the ability to make us aware of all realities within our life, past, present, or future, on earth and beyond. Chakra's allow us to identify and discern between our own truth and the opinions we're fed about who you are and how you're meant to act by others. It also connects us physically, mentally, emotionally, psychically, and spiritually because they are levels of consciousness affected by our mental states.

Each chakra has a particular state of consciousness, which it holds and effects. The planetary magnetics within The Universe energetically directly impact our inherent personalities through our chakras. As the planets, stars, and celestial bodies within the Milky Way - especially our solar system - shift, their magnetic frequencies shift which cause varying degrees of energetic sedation and/or stimulation. These shifts affect the ways in which we perceive innerstand, and act upon things. This is why our chakras are extremely important and integral to sustaining our life force. The more knowledgeable one becomes about the physical, mental, emotional, spiritual and cosmic functions the more aware of one's personality blueprint and divine design one becomes. These centers of energy may be fast or slow, pulsating or radiant, expanded or contracted at any given time. Chakras are not energy centers working independently, rather they are responsible for differing aspects of the whole systems operations reflecting who we are and what we think and feel.

So, how do we work with them? Since chakras are energy centers, and energy follows conscious and unconscious thought, it stands that first we must tune into the thoughts, feelings and levels of consciousness within the chakras in order to discern their current state to know what needs to be released, embraced, altered, and transcended to align them. If we don't do this all-important step, all other work on these centers will be fruitless, for the condition of the chakras will only revert back to the way they were before the work was done. While working on the thoughts and emotional adjustments needed there are many other things that can and do help to balance these centers as these major energy vortexes allow us to perceive and relate to the world around and within us.

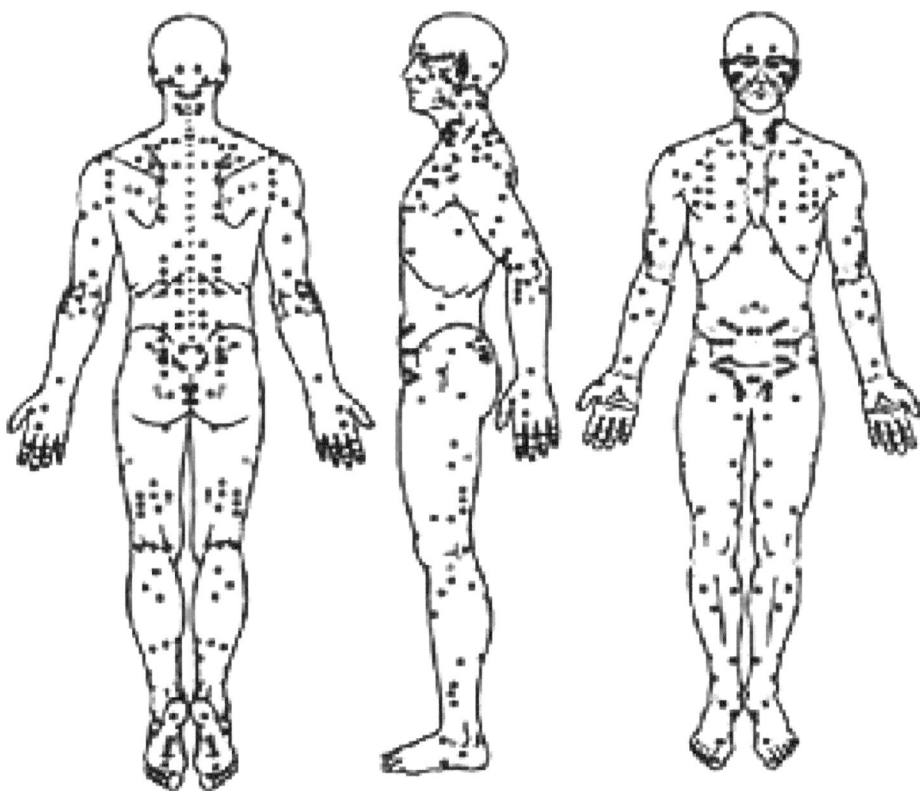

Our bodies have hundreds of chakra portals some being major portals that relate to major organs or subtle body functions while others that are minor operate more as energy release portals. The major chakras reside along the spine and within the joints while the minor chakras, also known as acupuncture points, are scattered throughout the body as pictured above. All chakras are designed to release and recalibrate the flow of chi within the related organs and areas of the physical and subtle body that connect and associate with each other in order to maintain harmony and proper function of the body. Within the meditative movement series, we will be working mainly with the 8 major chakras along the spinal column and the 13 sub-major chakras within the joints of the body. The 13 secondary chakras respond to actions and physicality while the eight primary chakras deal with mental, emotional and spiritual processing. The primary chakras influence your health greatly because they are our filtering system that regulates the ways we discern, decipher, interpret, and respond to input from our outer and inner environments. There is a direct correspondence between the quality of life force and information that is coming into these centers and the effect on the health and function-ability of the body. Each chakra relates strongly to specific parts of the body especially the nervous and reproductive systems, as well as the filtering and processing of specific emotional, mental, and spiritual insights and intelligence. Over stimulation or repression in the emotional, mental or spiritual bodies create imbalances within the electrical circuitry of the chakra system causing imbalances in the chakras themselves and often time manifests into physical ailment depending on what areas of the body the chakra that is imbalanced rules.

Since chakras are energy vortexes, they are affected by what is encountered by our senses whether it be the impressions through sight, sound, taste, feel, or thought perceptions etc. In looking at pictures of chakras, they often look like colored dots or various multi petal flowers sitting on the body, but in truth, they are spiraling vortices of energy that are multi-dimensional. With practice it is entirely possible to regulate the flow of energy through the chakras   and the entire physical and subtle body fields. Though extremely rare, there are those who have come to master the bodily functions through the mind in ways that allow them to survive in environments that would otherwise be impossible for the human body to survive. Various Spiritual masters whose lives were dedicated to spiritual self-mastery within the Asian, Egyptian, African and Eastern Indian esoteric practices throughout time have been able to extend and/or compress their auric and energetic field in various ways or on various levels using various spiritual teachings and practices in order to alter the effects of extreme conditions. One of the recorded tests was performed in Tibet with some of the spiritual initiates there. During a certain Initiation, a monk was taken out into the snow where they were witnessed being able to generate enough internal/external qi to melt a large area of snow measuring approximately 50 feet. In places like India and Egypt yogi's and initiates have been recorded demonstrating the ability to consciously manipulate and control the internal organ functions in order to survive within an environment that normally would end in certain death such as conditions of extreme walking on fire or extremely hot stones, open exposure to extreme weather conditions, oxygen deprivation, contorting their body to fit into a small box space, etc. They not only survived but come out unscathed.

EXPECTATIONS

One of the most common misperceptions by persons seeking to experience or receive chakra work that are not familiar with the dynamics and functions of the chakras is the expectation that a practitioner can permanently "Balance" or "Align" one's chakras with one treatment. This expectation derives from the fact that in Western society very little has been taught about the dynamics of the chakras or how they in truth operate within us as a regulatory system. The balancing and regulating of the chakras are a lifelong process which has to do with our experiences past, present and otherwise and their impact on our cellular memory accumulated over lifetimes. The energetic imprint from our thoughts, words, actions and experiences that one's been exposed to and/or has interacted with, can have long term affect that require time to access, innerstand, transform, transcend and transmute into their divine purpose. This process is different for everyone and depends on their degree of conscious awareness of what is happening around them and the purpose for its presence in their life at the time.

People are always coming into greater and greater awareness of Self physically, psychically, and spiritually. When presented visually through 1 or 2 dimensional charts, chakras look distinct in their separation of area and color however, the chakra colors are intertwined and mutational and in a constant fluid movement that surround the entire body. The physical and etheric body are one body and therefore one living chakra with varying sub levels of multiple chakras branching throughout the body as a whole. One's goal is to increase, purify and radiate higher frequencies of life force energies through them so that indeed, you become a pure channel of Divine Life Force/Consciousness that can transmute and transport as Divine Light.

One more thing that is important; chakras can become distorted. The major reason is lack of flow or movement of fluids and life force through the spinal column. This refers to movement on all levels, the blocking of energy, whether it be physical, mental, emotional, or spiritual. Lack of movement can distort or clog the chakras creating a sort of stagnant condition. Being blocked or stagnated, at any level is going to affect the chakras. Also, physical traumas such as injury, surgeries, or chronic dis-ease affect the chakras and their functionality. Kun Qi regardless of what level of physical fitness and or condition one is in can be used as a tool that stimulates the circulation of healthy life force and improves ones total body strength and function-ability from the inside out as well as increase ones levels of mental, emotional, and spiritual clarity.

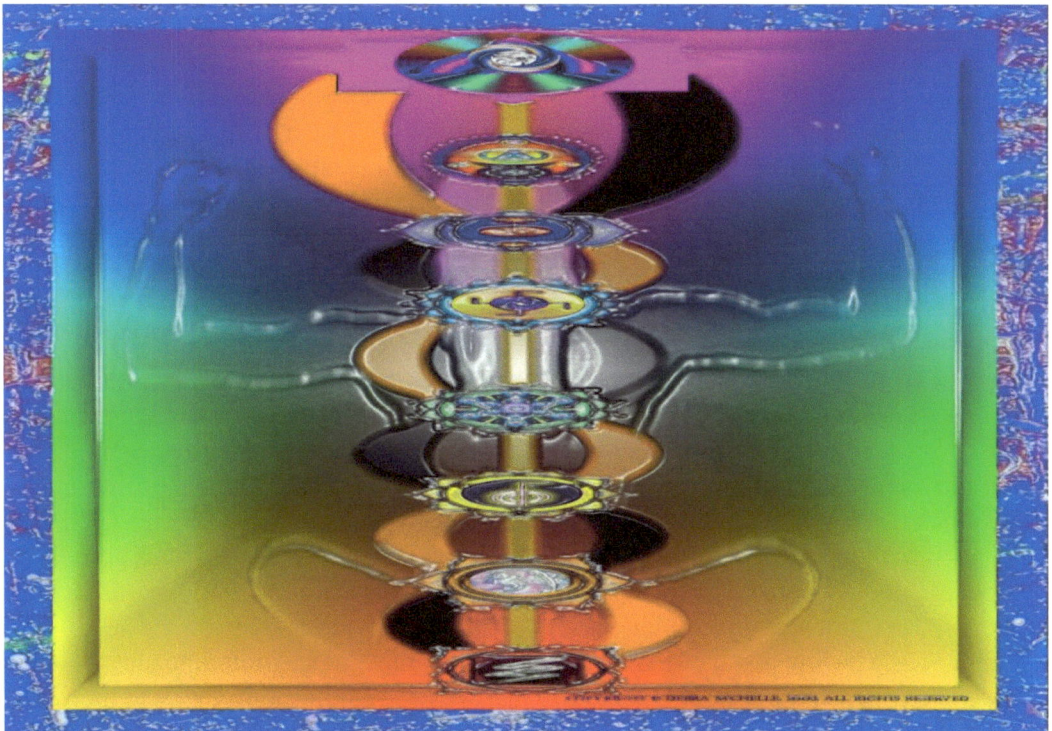

65

CHAKRA LOCATIONS

Our chakras reside in the subtle or etheric body. The 8 major chakras align subtly along the spine starting at the base of the spine within the pelvic floor and at specific central locations along the spine going up through the head. The channel that life force energy flows through is commonly known in eastern & Kemetic philosophy as kundalini. Kundalini is an energy that is coiled in alignment with the base of the spine that has been there since birth and tends to lie dormant in most unless awakened. **Kundalini is the ultimate life force. Creative power, divine feminine energy. Put simply, it is our "inner fire" that once activated flows up through the major chakras, giving each of them a "boost".** The kundalini energy resembles a staff and has been depicted in many spiritual and medical codex as the symbol of the caduceus. Many spiritualists believe that the Twenty-third Psalm of The Bible is speaking of the kundalini. Almost all religions believe in the spiritual energy power within the human body but not all referred to them as chakras. The previous diagram is a visual depiction of the chakra codex and the flow of kundalini energy takes along the spine.

CHAKRA VIBRATIONS

Each chakra has a different vibrational resonance that generates a sacred geometrical patterns, hues, and size specific to each chakra's resonant frequency. When a chakra is balanced, clear, and energized it emits a strong vibration, radiates clear hues of color, and spins optimally for that chakra's functionality. There are many ways to align and harmonize the vibrational resonance of the chakras such as vocal toning, singing, drumming, music, chants, mantras, being in nature, the vibrational energy of colors, and gemstones, movement and most of all, our thoughts. At the root of all colors, sounds, and movement is vibrations. By immersing oneself with the sounds and colors of the chakra your chakras become rejuvenated and balanced. The colors of the chakras are that of the rainbow as shown in the picture on the previous page.

Each chakra needs to function at its correct frequency independently. Each needs to be clear, balanced, energized, and properly spinning for us to operate as our higher Self. At the times when all the chakras reach a level of unison the entire physical, emotional, mental, intellectual, and spiritual vibration of the human body is raised; to maintain this state of alignment takes years of focused cultivation and practice and learning non-attachment to the e-motional body. Like a musical scale, each chakra matches the corresponding tone for each whole note on the scale. Once each individual chakra is resonating at its proper corresponding tonal note your entire physical, emotional, mental, and spiritual body raises into its own new vibrational level to match that of the chakras. It is important to remember we are in essential truth, a spiritual being that has chosen to take on human form in order to experience the human experience. We also chose to embody in human form in order to fulfill those aspects of one's evolutionary intentions that inspire the innerstanding of Oneness from an experiential perspective. As we embody into human form we first chose the blueprint that will serve our purpose for embodiment, the appropriate vessels and alignments that will best empower us to fulfill that purpose (our parents, our planetary birth alignment, our tendencies and set of skills), We then slow down our vibration by adding the molecular components that each possess to produce the components of life that we need for our journey. The more work we do that helps to keep our bodies and minds clear and functioning properly the higher levels of spiritual and/or cosmic awareness or enlightenment our mind/body will access and resonate at while still occupying our physical human form.

BALANCED CHAKRAS = HAPPINESS & HEALTH

Universal Love, Energy, and Knowledge is meant to flow freely through the chakras. It is important that you try to maintain the correct energy flow through each chakra since you could also negatively be affected by a chakra being too open. Remember that balance in each, and balance in all in comparison to one another is what you seek. When the chakras are aligned and balanced, the energy flows freely from the spiritual center to the primal base allowing us to apply the insights from our communication with our higher spiritual influences. An example of the way this is reflected in real life terms would be relationship patterns that we find ourselves repeating despite our having vowed never to repeat it. If one continues in a dysfunctional relationship it will continue to drain one's energy and cause the body to breakdown creating illness and various stress related physical conditions. This is due to not identifying and resolving the unhealthy behaviors and their indicators from previous relationships and learning tools of cultivating healthy long-lasting communication and relating like setting personal practices and boundaries.

UNBALANCED AND BLOCKED CHAKRAS = ILLNESS

When the mind, body, soul aspects that our chakras relate to are causing them to vibrate or spin improperly one becomes unable to move their physical, emotional, or mental body onto a higher spiritual level. When we are born, we can have a perfect balance or have an imbalance from past lives that we bring into this lifetime. Although the human body is a vessel and acts more like a biogenetic machine it seldom breaks down due to manufacturer's flaws and/or natural biological causes. *"The subtle nature of the etheric (and other), energies influence the physical cellular network through the meridians which are carriers of etherically-based biological information. When the flow of chi or life force to a particular organ is deficient or unbalanced, patterns of cellular disruption occur." Richard Gerber, Vibrational Medicine*

On an ascended level of conscious awareness, illnesses more often then realized, have been chosen by us as a catalyst for us, or those around us, to learn higher lessons and transcend outdated beliefs, practices, and ways of operating or viewing life and the world within and around us. We are given intuitive messages and hints all the time about what we could be doing in order to live more harmoniously with the flow of our lives, but we often ignore these signals, and signs. We are too often caught up in the drama of physicality, being driven by the exterior voices like the impression of the media and material world versus listening to our inner selves. Because of this, the chakras eventually shift out of balance and become misaligned and too opened or closed to operate optimally as designed. When one is distracted by these impressions, distortions within the chakras begin to manifest in one's physical body and or into one's personal expressions as pain, emotional turmoil, confusion or dissatisfaction.

Each chakra regulates different parts of the body and the root cause of almost all illness stems from poor chakra health. When your chakras are blocked the circulation of life-force within the body slows down, you can become more emotionally sensitive, mentally and/or emotionally overloaded and your spiritual connection becomes weakened. You may feel depressed, out of touch, like you lost something, tired, overwhelmed and unable to think clearly. You may get angry for no reason, be afraid, be unsure of yourself, lack self-confidence, be unhappy without a direct innerstood reason, and have a general negative outlook on life. All of these are indications that the chakras are not aligned and there is a lack of cohesive flow between them. This can either inspire a negative outlook on life or spur one to seek out ways to heal.

HEAL YOURSELF THROUGH CHAKRA BALANCING

The majority of illnesses and ailments derive from imbalances within our emotional body which directly corresponds to the chakras. Think about times when you feel uncomfortable in a situation or scared, and how your stomach starts to feel queasy, or you get that butterfly nervous sensation in your gut. This is your emotions, your chakra emotions, manifesting into physical form as an inner vibrational sensation. When you feel safe and no longer scared or anxious your stomach eases and the butterfly feeling in your gut goes away. Or when you're mentally stressed by worry or having pressing matters like deadlines on your mind, you may feel agitated, confused and frustrated, your neck and shoulders get tense and you may even unconsciously grit your teeth. This is a natural physical response that occurs during mental stress. Your whole body can be affected over time depending on whether you are aware of these natural holding patterns.

Childhood and past life issues are another source of inner tension that you may not be consciously aware of, that have been found to be root causes of illness and dis-ease. I am not saying that every single thing wrong physically is a chakra issue. We as humans are physical beings that are affected by nature and our physical environment and flukes happen. But on a spiritual level we choose the body we are in for this lifetime, or Spirit chooses this body for us, for a reason and for lessons to be learned through them. Chakra work is not always easy or painless unless one has achieved a higher level of spiritual development enabling them to transcend emotional pain patterns. We often think we have resolved an issue mentally when there may still be residual emotional trauma that still resides on a deeper level within the chakra since we as humans have a tendency to bury our emotions and those emotions are transferred to a cellular level in our bodies. If those issues are not addressed, they then follow and resurface in future lives. This is how psychological as well as physical traits are transferred genetically and from between incarnations.

Any of us who have done major chakra work will tell you that "I got it all fixed" is not something that happens. When one raises to a new physical vibrational level the feelings of being in two places at once must be transcended before one can settle into their new physical vibrational level. Then when one thinks they have it all together they will find other chakra issues to deal with.

Like an onion, there are layers to issues and its necessary to peel away the layers in order to get to the core issue so that it can be recalibrated and healed. You will know when an issue is totally cleared when you experience the release on all four levels.
- Physically - moving from tension to relaxation and feeling healthy and energized physically

- Emotionally - moving from heavy intense emotions to peaceful positive emotions
- Mentally - understanding the situations, yourself, and others as being the vehicle that was needed to teach you certain lessons about self. (i.e. how to view and respond to life in more productive ad constructive ways.)
- Spiritually - feeling your emotions and mindset transmuted into that of compassion, understanding and unconditional love for onesself 1st, and then others.
- Financially – obtaining the knowledge and financial wisdom to take full responsibility for one's life by making the right decision that will allow you to manifest and live one's dreams and aspirations

But fair warning... chakra imbalances can come back if fall back into unconstructive habits or subject yourself to toxic people, places, or practices. Deep emotional or spiritually rooted trauma that tend to have repeated over and over in your life may require multiple treatments to completely transcend. When one comes to innerstand the power and value of

- ❖ self-knowledge,
- ❖ self-respect,
- ❖ active self-healing,
- ❖ financial investment stability
- ❖ personal development practices

for the purpose of self-mastery and is willing to take the time and expend the energy necessary to integrate what one has come to learn, than one is able to transform one's sense of self enough to not only avoid repeating the past outdated pattern but to consciously transform and create the type of healthy relationship patterns that are physically, mentally, emotionally, financially, socially, and spiritually healthy, and fulfilling. Without taking time to recognize and reflect on our emotional triggers and the traumatic experiences we've buried and neglected to address, one will not be able to see their part in repeatedly attracting the same unhealthy relationships behaviors by subconscious subjection.

As one progresses to deeper levels of healing, they may need assistance with working through the deeper more traumatic issues that rise to the surface. Psychologists, psychiatrists and life coaches can help with insights to overcome destructive behavioral patterns, or unproductive thought patterns or beliefs which will also help balance the chakras. Spiritual leaders, practitioners, as well as reading and studying spiritually motivating and enlightening material can assist on the spiritual level. Holistic medical physicians and healing arts practitioners are available to address and provide tools to care for our physical being. Each in turn can provide forms of treatment that will be effective in your healing journey. When you have incorporated the things that assist with healing and becoming empowered to heal yourself then you are making true advancements within each chakra and your whole being and your spiritual purpose.

The following diagram provides a detailed list of the 7 major chakras, with the associations, operations and physical and psychological functions that each is responsible for.

CHAKRA DETAILS	PHYSICAL BODY DETAILS	EMOTIONAL, MENTAL & SPIRITUAL BODY DETAILS
ROOT CHAKRA: • Color - Red/Black, • Element – Earth/Fire • Resonance – 91 hz - 104 hz • Tonal Note - C • Intonation – HU	**Location:** L5 – Coccyx – Gastrocnemius, Soleus, Peroneus, ankles, feet, descending colon, spinal column, bones, hip bones, buttocks, Rectum, Anus, blood, immune system. **Affects:** Rectal and colon problems, immune system disorders, base of spine/lower back problems, varicose veins, feet and leg problems, cramping in legs, tightness in Glutes, quads, IT Bands, Tensor Fascia Late and hamstring musculature.	Survival, tribal associations, instinct, past life memories, family, marriage, parenting, correct behavior, society, ability to provide basic needs for living. Following the establishment of or what family rules. Doing what your family/spouse wants. Trying to fit in. Compromises to these issues, depression, problems with decision making.
NAVEL CHAKRA: • Color - Orange • Element – Water/Earth • Resonance – 107 hz - 116 hz • Tonal Note - D • Intonation – "O"	**Location:** T10 – L4 Reproductive organs, Kidneys, urinary bladder, small intestines, lymph circulation, inguinal rings, appendix, rectus, oblique & transverse abdominals, Quadratus Lumborum, quads, hamstrings, glutes, sacral spinalis, Peroneus, Anterior/posterior Tibial's, Illiacus/Psoas, hips and knees, prostate gland, lower back muscles, sciatic nerve. **Affects:** menstrual cycle problems, cancers in this area, impotency. Pelvic and lower back pains, urinary and bladder problems, chronic tiredness, gas pains, sterility, difficult breathing, varicose veins, constipation, colitis, diarrhea, hernias, Sciatica, lumbago, hip problems.	Power, creativity, sexual matters, blame, control, passion, ethics, money, greed, honor in relationship matters, fidelity, feelings of repression or wrongness in sexual matters. Reproduction issues. Birthing new ideas.
SOLAR PLEXUS CHAKRA: • Color – Yellow/Gold • Element – Sun/Air • Resonance – 118 hz - 124 hz • Tonal Note - E • Intonation – "AAH"	**Location:** T4 – T9 – gallbladder, liver, solar plexus, circulation, stomach, pancreas, duodenum, spleen, adrenal and suprarenal glands, Latissimus Dorsi, Erector Spinae, upper Quadratus Lumborum, Rib Cage. **Affects:** gallstones, jaundice, shingles, arthritis, circulation problems, ulcers, heartburn, indigestion, gastric reflux, duodenal ulcers, gastritis, lowered resistance to infection, anemia, allergies, hives, skin conditions, eczema, Indigestion, stomach, intestinal, and colon problems. Eating disorders. Diabetes, adrenal, pancreas, liver dysfunctions, gall bladder, kidneys, and ulcers. Spleen and middle of back problems.	Responsibility issues, caring for others, trust, fear, guilt, career, intimidation, personal honor, victimization feelings, and courage. Self-concern issues; self-respect, sensitivity to criticism, self-esteem, self-worth and own confidence, independence, reliability, decision making.

HEART CHAKRA: • Color - Green • Element – Wood/Earth • Resonance – 129 hz–139 hz • Tonal Note - F Intonation – "Hu" or "A"	**Location:** C7 – T3 – Thyroid/parathyroid glands, shoulders, trapezius, rhomboids, rotator cuff, Pectoralis Major/minor, Upper Latissimus Dorsi region, subscapularis, elbows, muscles of the arms, hands, wrists, and fingers, esophagus, trachea, heart, valves, coronary arteries, lungs, chest, and breasts. **Affects:** Bursitis, colds, thyroid conditions, asthma, pneumonia, bronchitis, upper back/shoulder/arm weakness and structural misalignments, difficulty breathing, pain in lower arms and hands, heart conditions, chest conditions, circulatory system conditions, Bronchitis, pleurisy, pneumonia, congestion, influenza,	Love, happiness, desire for happiness, sadness, anger, hatred, prejudice, loneliness, forgiveness, compassion, hopes, desires, wants, grief, resentments, inability or resistance to reach out to others, commitment, trust in your close interpersonal relationships. Choices in love.
THROAT CHAKRA: • Color – Turquoise/Sky Blue • Element – Metal/Air • Resonance – 142 hz - 149hz • Tonal Note - G • Intonation – "I" (eye)	**Location:** C4 - C6 – Nose, Nasal Cavity, lips, jaw, mouth, Tongue, Eustachian tube, Vocal cords, neck glands, Neck Muscles, shoulders, tonsils, Larynx. **Affects:** Hay fever, runny nose, hearing loss, tooth aches, deterioration of the teeth and gums, canker sores, herpes of the mouth, laryngitis, hoarseness, sore throat, thyroid and gland problems, hiatal hernias, choking, gagging, chronic neck problems, subluxation in cervical vertebrae, stiff neck, pain in upper arms, carpal tunnel, chronic cough, winged scapula, upper back pain, atrophying of the PMC low oxygenation to the brain and head.	Communication, expressing yourself, telling truth, following your dreams and being true to yourself. Addictions, habits, judgment, faith, making decisions, knowing and being yourself, criticism, will power, doing what you said you would do. All forms of expression & communication.
THIRD EYE CHAKRA: • Color - Indigo • Element - Ether • Resonance – 159 hz–175 hz • Tonal Note - A A⁻ • Intonation – "EEE"	**Location:** C2 - C3 – eyes, optic nerves, auditory nerves, sinuses, jaw bones, cheeks, outer ear, face, teeth, facial nerves. **Affects:** sinus problems, allergies, pain around the eyes, fainting spells, crossed eyes, deafness, eye weakness, earaches, Tinnitus, ringing in the ears, pressure on brain stem, nervous system, full spinal problems, learning problems, Bell's Palsy, acne or pimples, eczema.	Truth, knowledge, intellect, intuitive powers, learning from experience, feeling inadequate, inner wisdom, knowing yourself and self-evaluation, open-mindedness, accepting yourself and others. Listening and seeing openly.

CROWN CHAKRA: • Color – Violet/White • Element – Light/Vibration • Resonance - 180 hz–244 hz • Tonation - B/B~ • Intonation – "EEE"	**Location:** C1 – Head, Pituitary Gland, bones of the face, inner/middle ear, brain. **Affects:** Headaches, migraines, nervousness, insomnia, head colds, high blood pressure, dizziness, memory loss, energy/exhaustion problems, increased dysfunction of mental/emotional faculties, skin and muscles systems.	Spirituality, devotion to spiritual and personal matters. Unconditional love to self, the earth, and to others. Empathy, humanitarianism, selflessness, values, and ethics. Connection with ULEK™, ability to go with the flow of life and to see the larger picture, inspiration without wants. The Higher Self. Mystical depression, searching feelings, sensitivity to the environmental elements, (sun, light, sound)
BINDU CHAKRA: • Color - Magenta • Element – Magnetism/Electricity • Resonance - 254 hz + • Tonal Note - ↑C – • Intonation – "AUM"	Brain, nervous system Pineal Gland.	Knowledge of past lives, akashic records of past lives, Divine design and higher purpose Seat of the soul, center where we communicate with our ancestors who have left physicality. Higher Self

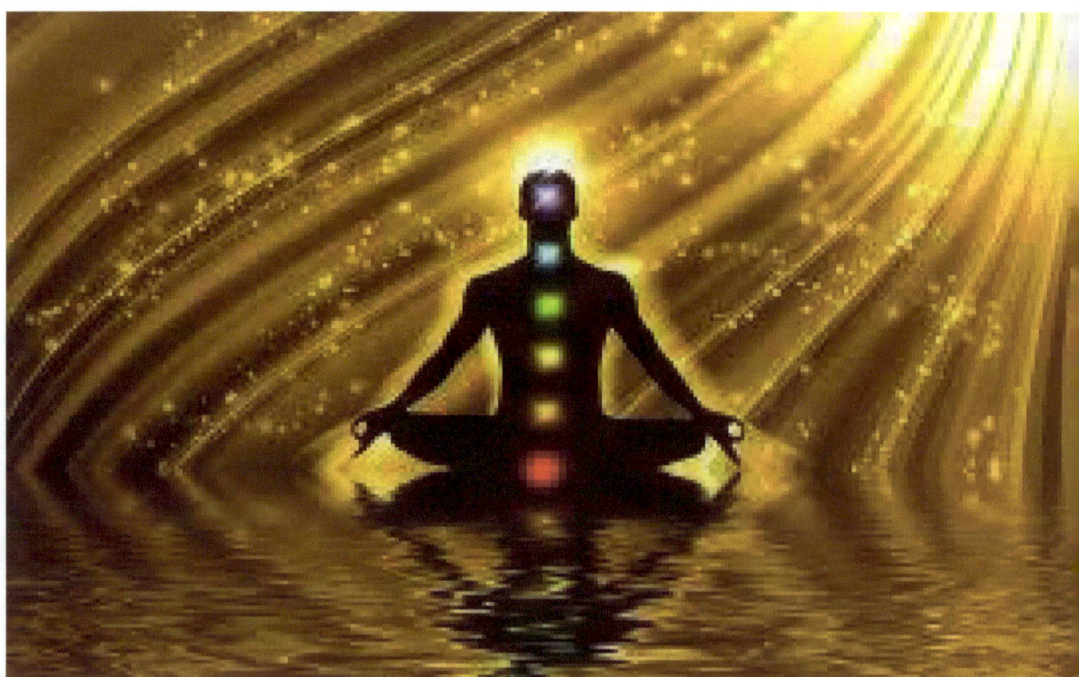

72

CHAKRA ASSOCIATION TO THE 7 ELEMENTS

In Lemurian Medicine the chakra system and its functions, characteristics and attributes were a reflection of the seven elements of nature and the way in which these elements interact with and balance our chakra and organ systems. In Atlantean Medicine the body, soul, and spirit were a reflection of the seven elements of the universe. KUN CHI meditative movement sequences work to attune you to these same elements of nature and the universe by the way in which these associated forces operate throughout the function of our tangible and intangible systems.

"Wind", represents things that slow and accelerate, rise and fall, expand and contract, and enjoy freedom of movement. Wind along with air, smoke, and the like, best represent the human mind where changing currents of thoughts, clouds of confusion, the stillness of silent meditation and focused intention take place. As one grows physically, they also grow in conscious awareness and innerstanding of life around them by learning which causes one to expand mentally in terms of our knowledge, our experiences, and our personalities. *Wind* also represents breathing, and the internal processes associated with respiration. Mentally, emotionally, and spiritually it represents an "open-minded" attitude, trust in the unknown and the carefree feeling of faith. It can be associated with will, elusiveness, evasiveness, benevolence, compassion, wisdom, and intensity.

"Fire", represents the energetic intensity behind passion, the forcefulness of power behind assertion or aggression, and the momentum of movement created by the constant change of our situations and conditions. This can be seen in animals, particularly predators or patriarchal governments intrinsically driven by a desire to dominate. Both are full of impulsive aggressive actions of forcefulness that consume at the expense of another. They are primary examples of fire or *ka* objects. Bodily, fire or *ka* represents our metabolism and body heat, and in the mental and emotional realms, it represents drive and passion. Fire can be associated with motivation, desire, intention, cleverness and an out-going spirit.

"Water", represents the fluid, flowing, formless shifting things in the world that are in constant flux. Outside of the obvious example of rivers and the like, plants are also categorized under *water*, as they adapt to their environment, growing and changing according to the direction of the sun and the changing seasons. Blood and other bodily fluids are represented by *sui*, as are our mental or emotional tendencies towards adaptation and change whether driven by a survival or recreational purpose. *Water* is associated with emotion; those of defensiveness, adaptability, flexibility, suppleness, magnetism, responsiveness and sensitivity.

"Earth", represents the hard, solid, stationary or fixed objects of the world. The most basic example of Earth is stone. Stone is highly resistant to movement or change, as is anything heavily influenced by earth. Within the physical body the bones, muscles and tissues are represented by earth. On an emotional level, earth is predominantly associated with stubbornness, stability, physicality, and gravity. It is a desire to have things remain as they are; a resistance to change while on the mental level it is seen as self-confidence. When under the influence of this earth mode or "mood", we are fixed in

73

our attitudes, desires, and rituals; we are aware of our own physicality, beliefs, and sureness of action as physical matter.

"Void", represents "The Ethers", "The Womb", "Deep Waters", or "The Heavens" and represents the dark incubative spaces where all things are formed from nothing. It's the triple darkness of tangible and intangible form within the inner and outer universe where unconscious and conscious thoughts and desires form into matter and movement, particularly those things composed of pure energy. Atoms, their component particles, and atomic forces fall under this category, as do people in a transcendental state of consciousness.

Mentally, void represents the incubational space where spirit, thought, and creative energy resides. It represents our ability to think, to communicate, and to create. It also associates with our sense of power, intelligence, creativity, spontaneity, and inventiveness.

Physically, void is represented by the womb; the incubational chamber where life is formed, developed and birthed from. Void is of particular importance as it is the highest of the elements. In martial arts, particularly in fictional tales where the fighting discipline is blended with magic or the occult. Practitioners often invoke the power of the Void to connect to the quintessential creative energy of the world. A warrior properly attuned to the Void can sense his surrounding and respond appropriately to situations around them without thinking, and without using his physical senses. This aspect of "Void" is represented within the universe as ether and can also include all the various types of vibration/sound waves as its byproduct. Both are a consistent presence within the universe that are obvious and evident as an integral part of the function-ability of the universe and all that is within it.

THE ENERGETIC ROOT OF TENSION/STRESS/ILLNESS
When the organs or musculature are deficient in life force, it causes changes in the function-ability of that organ and its partnering organ either increasing or decreasing the rate in which that organ performs it function. Conditions such as sickness, inactivity of the body parts that relate to an organ, and/or mental/emotional trauma can over stimulate or overly sedate the organ. High levels of mental, emotional, or environmental stress and lack of exposure to natural healthy life force energy either from nature or the universe, can over stimulates or diminish the organs activities in order to compensate. This may force the organ and musculoskeletal systems to work harder for longer periods of time creating undue stress on these systems. When this happens their ability to function properly start to breakdown, physical energy and mental processes start to become challenged and the body mind starts to deteriorate when energy starts to stagnate wherever there is tension, dis-ease and misuse of the body's natural organic rhythms, fuel, and harmonious environments.

What we pick up through our physical senses, of sight, hearing, tasting, smelling and touch can have the same energetic influence on the body that causes it to respond and react physically; thus the emotions of fear, of anger, of lust, and of love can create reactions and responses inside the whole body that can generate an overwhelming need to release the feeling or emotion by some sort of physical act. These integrations stimulate the brain-cells, the ductless glands, and other parts of the endocrine system to energize secretions. (of which epinephrine, thyroid and hypophyseal secretions are a part of). These secretions are thrown into the bloodstream along with the most available fuel, glycogen, which is also mobilized in the blood. This body-wide preparation for action may be a designated kinetic reaction.

Anger, fear, and grief are also strong excitants and stimuli to involuntary and voluntary motor reaction/response. The fact that emotional reactions is more injurious to the body than muscular action is well known, the difference being the fact that when one reacts by physical activity to the increases in adrenaline due to heightened emotional stimulation the energetic impact is consumed. Without using physical activity as a release valve, the increases in adrenaline due to heightened emotional stimulation are not consumed therefore they build up in the body as toxic waste products. Anger, fear, and grief are also strong excitants and stimuli to involuntary and voluntary motor reaction/response. It is obvious that whatever the excitant the physio-chemical action of the brain and the ductless glands cannot be reversed--the effect of the stimulus cannot be recalled, therefore either a purposeful muscular act or a neutralizing act must be performed or else the liberated energy will smolder in the various organs and associated parts of the body.

As shown in the following 7 Phase Elemental Meridian Chart, each element corresponds to a respective chakra and a set of partnering organs that reflect the energy of each corresponding element and the ways in which they help to regulate and balance within the body. The following chart depicts the elements, seasons, and gamma ray colors as they relate to the internal functions of the organs, the chakras, and the mental, emotional and spiritual bodies.

7 PHASE ELEMENTAL MERIDIAN CHART

YIN (SOLID) ORGANS

(- HT) HEART
(- PC) PERICARDIUM
(- SP) SPLEEN
(- LU) LUNGS
(- KI) KIDNEY
(- LV) LIVER
(GV) GOVERNING VESSEL

YANG (HOLLOW) ORGANS

SMALL INTESTINE(+ SI)
TRIPPLE WARMER (+ TW)
STOMACH (+ ST)
LARGE INTESTINE (+ LI)
URINARY BLADDER (+ UB)
GALL BLADDER (+ GB)
CONCEPTION VESSEL (CV)

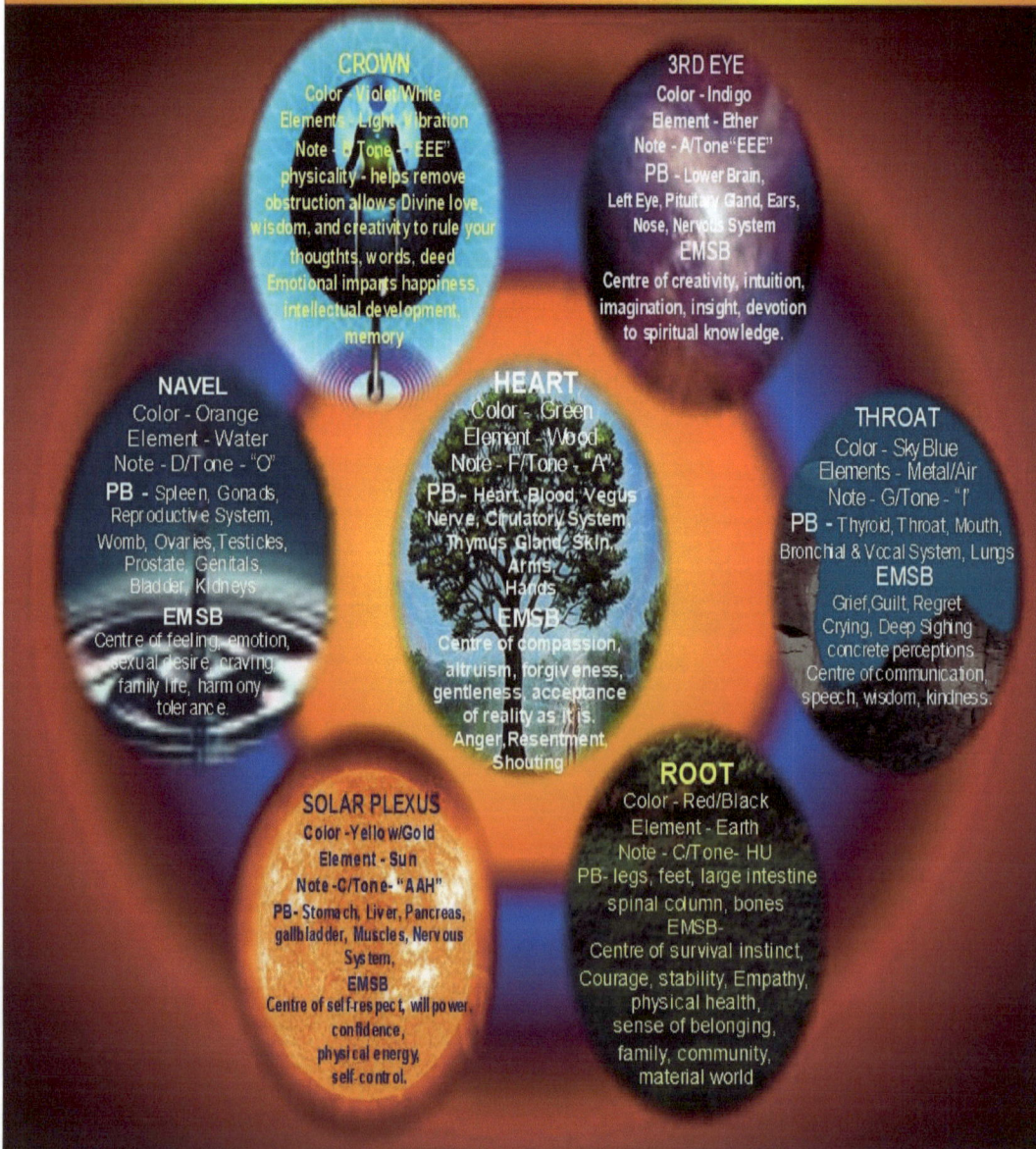

CROWN
Color - Violet/White
Elements - Light, Vibration
Note - B Tone - "EEE"
physicality - helps remove
obstruction allows Divine love,
wisdom, and creativity to rule your
thoughts, words, deed
Emotional imparts happiness,
intellectual development,
memory

3RD EYE
Color - Indigo
Element - Ether
Note - A/Tone "EEE"
PB - Lower Brain,
Left Eye, Pituitary Gland, Ears,
Nose, Nervous System
EMSB
Centre of creativity, intuition,
imagination, insight, devotion
to spiritual knowledge.

NAVEL
Color - Orange
Element - Water
Note - D/Tone - "O"
PB - Spleen, Gonads,
Reproductive System,
Womb, Ovaries, Testicles,
Prostate, Genitals,
Bladder, Kidneys
EMSB
Centre of feeling, emotion,
sexual desire, craving,
family life, harmony,
tolerance.

HEART
Color - Green
Element - Wood
Note - F/Tone - "A"
PB - Heart, Blood, Vegus
Nerve, Cirulatory System,
Thymus Gland, Skin,
Arms,
Hands
EMSB
Centre of compassion,
altruism, forgiveness,
gentleness, acceptance
of reality as it is.
Anger, Resentment,
Shouting

THROAT
Color - Sky Blue
Elements - Metal/Air
Note - G/Tone - "I"
PB - Thyroid, Throat, Mouth,
Bronchial & Vocal System, Lungs
EMSB
Grief, Guilt, Regret
Crying, Deep Sighing
concrete perceptions
Centre of communication,
speech, wisdom, kindness.

SOLAR PLEXUS
Color - Yellow/Gold
Element - Sun
Note - C/Tone- "AAH"
PB- Stomach, Liver, Pancreas,
gallbladder, Muscles, Nervous
System,
EMSB
Centre of self-respect, will power,
confidence,
physical energy,
self-control.

ROOT
Color - Red/Black
Element - Earth
Note - C/Tone- HU
PB- legs, feet, large intestine
spinal column, bones
EMSB-
Centre of survival instinct,
Courage, stability, Empathy,
physical health,
sense of belonging,
family, community,
material world

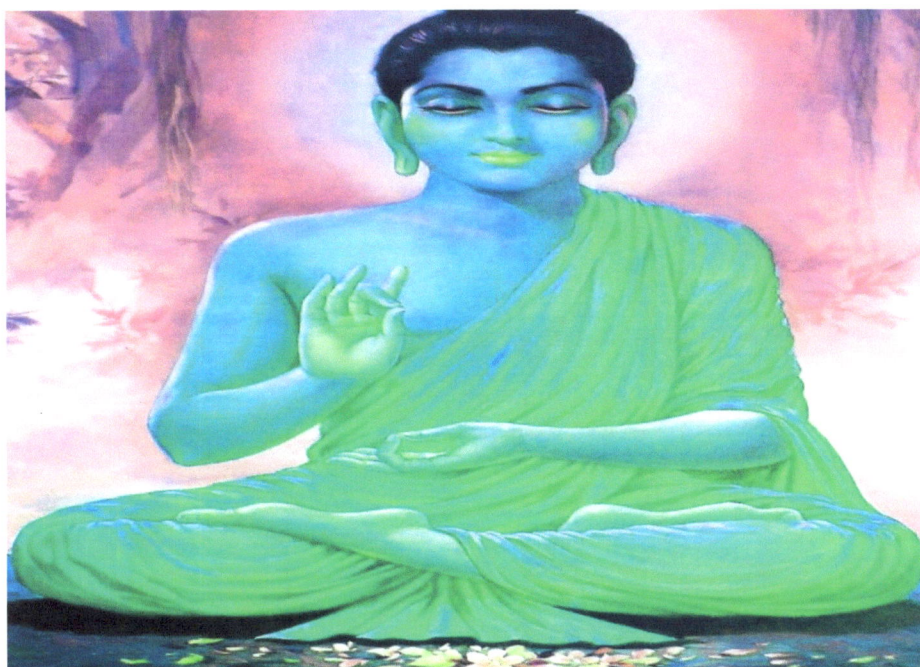

THE USE OF MUDRAS

The fingertips of every living being have many concentrated nerve endings which are free energy discharge points. Science also confirms that around every tip there is a concentration of free electrons. By touching the tips of the fingers together or touching the fingertips to other parts of the palms this free energy (Prana) is redirected back into the body along specified channels that flow back up to the brain. The redirected energy traveling through the nerves stimulates the various chakras. Keeping the hands on the knees stimulates the hidden channel (Gupta Nadi) from the knees to the Perineum, and makes the energy start from the Root (Mooladhara) Chakra.

Thus, the tension applied to the nerves and/or the neural or psycho-neural circuits formed by the mudras help in balancing the seven basic elemental building blocks. This posture whether sitting or standing balances and redirects the tension of the internal energy which increases the circulation of life force into the veins, tendons, glands, and sensory organs, to bring the body back to a healthy state.

The use of Mudras add a very powerful and unique benefit when integrated with meditation and breathe work. Mudras allow one to awaken the command points to the organs and various anatomical regions and function-ability of the brain and body and their connection to the elements of nature and the universe. When pressure is applied to these command points one's healing intentions can be accessed more directly within the internal and subtle bodies stimulating the flow of life force energy along each associated meridian thus having a deeper more deliberate healing effect. The chart below shows where the reflexology regions for some of the major organ and glands reside within the hands that can be used as a guide for stimulating qi and releasing blockages within the associated areas.

साइनस Sinus

आँख Eye
मस्तिष्क Brain

कान Ear

फेफड़ा Lung

कन्धा
Shoulder

पिट्यूटरी ग्रन्थि
Pituitary Gland

यकृत
Liver

पित्ताशय
Gall Bladder

अग्नाशय
Pancreas

आमाशय Stomach

बड़ी आँत
Colon

छोटी आँत
Intestines

वृक्क Kidney

मूत्राशय
Urinary Bladder

थाइरॉइड व पैराथाइरॉइड ग्रन्थियाँ
Thyroid & Parathyroids

डिम्ब ग्रन्थि
Ovary

गर्भाशय Uterus

पुरःस्थ ग्रन्थि Prostate

अण्डकोश
Testis

शिश्न Penis

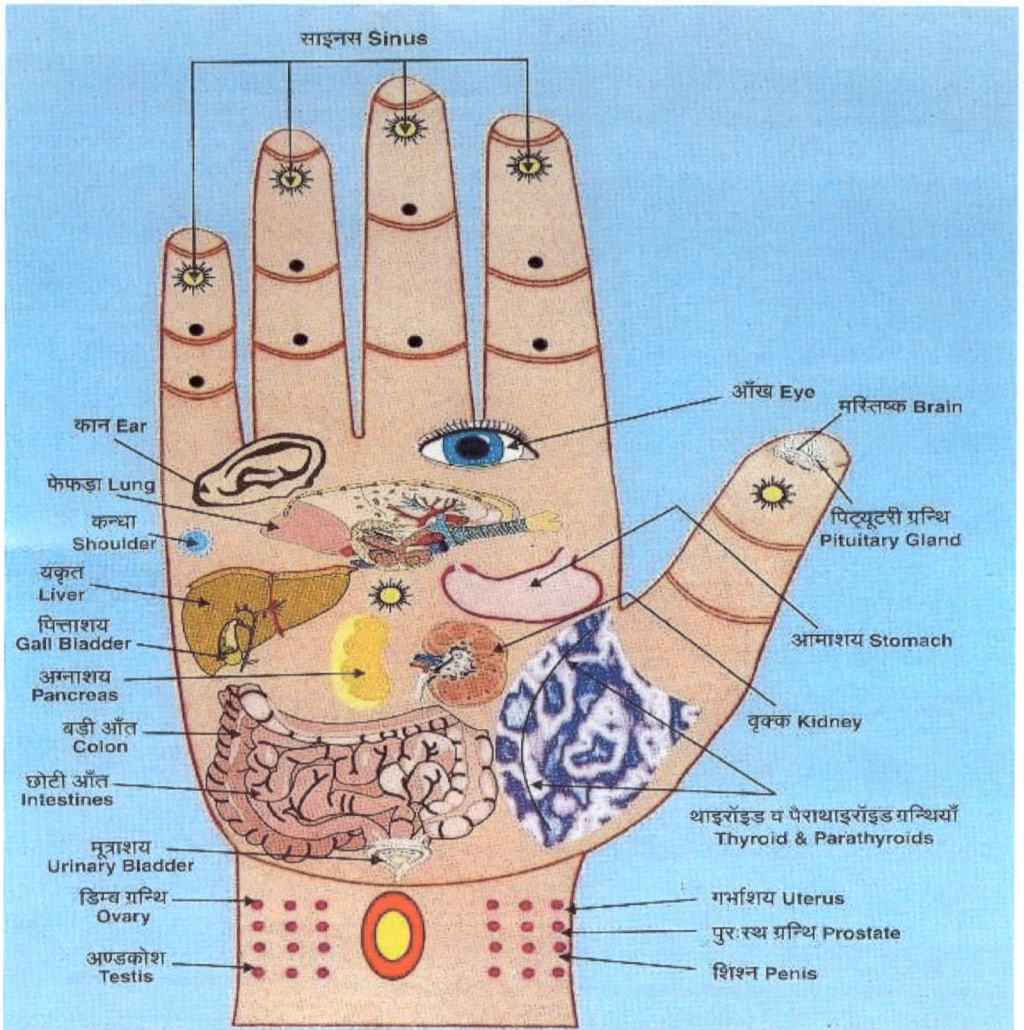

THE HISTORY OF MUDRAS

Mudra in Sanskrit means "a postural seal" or "closed electrical circuits" of the physical and subtle body channels. In short Mudras are systematic modes of communication and self-expression consisting of hand gestures and finger postures that retain the efficacy and interconnectedness of the internal body systems. Mudras have also been used as a means of nonverbal communication or external expression of inner resolve, suggesting that such non-verbal communications are more powerful than the spoken word and are as natural as the subconscious movements and functions that our bodies perform on a daily basis.

No one knows for sure where and how mudras originated. They have been in use for millenniums and have been found to be practiced on all continents, by people of all religions as well as those professing none. The following are a few specific mudras that have historically been linked to specific belief systems.

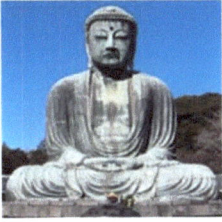

In the Orient mudras were and are still observed in the rituals and rites of the cultural traditions of Hinduism and Buddhism in India, Tibet, China, Japan Indonesia etc. The paintings in the caves of Ajanta and sculptures in the Ellora caves, dating back to 2nd. and 1st. centuries BC show innumerable mudras. Hinduism shows the earliest recorded knowledge and analysis of Mudras. The earliest documentations are found in Mantra Shastra (the book of incantations), Upasana Shastra (the book of worship and prayers) and the Nritya Shastra (the book of classical dances). The following verse from Srimad Bhagwad Gita mentions that Lord Krishna was in the posture of Gyan Mudra when he bestowed the knowledge of Gita to Arjuna.

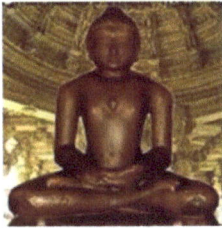

In Jainism, the spiritual path of Amhimsa -nonviolence towards all living beings - Swami Mahavir Jain and in Sikkhism, Guru Nanak Devji are always shown in Gyan or Dhyan Mudra. The Dhyāna mudrā is the gesture of meditation, of the concentration of the Good Law. The hands and fingers form the shape of a triangle, which is symbolic of the spiritual fire or the triune spirit. Sometimes the Dhyāna mudrā is used in certain representations of the Medicine Buddha, with a medicine bowl placed on the hands. It originated in India and in China during the Wei period. This mudra was used long before the Buddha as yogis have used it during their concentration, healing, and meditation exercises. It is heavily used in Southeast Asia in Theravāda Buddhism; however, the thumbs are placed against the palms.

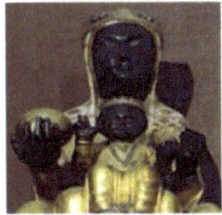

In Christian art Yeshua (Jesus) is often show displaying the hand mudra of benediction or blessing, Mother Mary is shown holding an ancient Catholic mudra known as The "hand of the blessing" was a Roman sign of "The Hand of the All Goddess". It was later adopted by Christian clergymen. In Islam it is called the "Hand of Fatima". This is one and the same as Hamsa. The palm-shaped amulet depicting a open right hand as a defense against the evil eye.Among the Shiites, the fingers of the hand of Fatima also represent the 'five holy persons' of the Prophet's family: Muhammed, Fatima, Ali, Hassan, Hussein. Ali's name or those of The Twelve Imams are sometimes engraves on metal Hands of Fatima. Hamsas can also include a heart, a hexagram, or the word Allah inscribed in the palm of the hand. Egypt used it to evoke the protection of the parental spirits. The index finger is the Mother-Goddess, the middle finger is the Father-Godhead, and the thumb with an acorn seed on it is the Child, Horus, the newborn sun of each day.

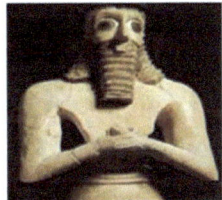

The anciet Babylonian time the Sun God Damuzi was shown depicting this Mudra while descending into the underworld. Damuzi, in Sumerian mythology, was the god of vegetation and was the partner of the Mesopotamian Goddess, Inanna or Ishtar . The mudra used in this ancient carving was similar to if not the same as that depicted as Dhyan commonly used in East Indian culture.

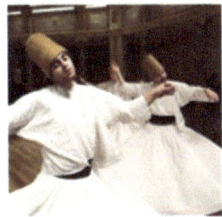

In Islam, the mystical Whirling Dervishes used Hand signs or Mudras for Sufi whirling (or Sufi spinning) is a form of Sama or physically active meditation which originated among Sufis, and which is still practiced by the Sufi Dervishes of the Mevlevi order. It is a customary dance performed within the worship ceremony, through which dervishes (also called semazens) aim to reach the source of all perfection. This is sought through abandoning one's nafs, egos or personal desires, by listening to the music, focusing on God, and spinning one's body in repetitive circles, which has been seen as a symbolic imitation of planets in the Solar System orbiting the sun.[1] As explained by Sufis:,. At the beginning of the Sema, by holding one's arms crosswise, the semazen appears to represent the number one, thus testifying to God's unity. While whirling, his arms are open: his right arm is directed to the sky, ready to receive God's beneficence; his left hand, upon which his eyes are fastened, is turned toward the earth.

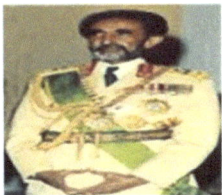

In Rastafarianism – The DivineEmporer of Ethiopia Haile Selassie, referred to as "The Lion of Judah" often held a particular Mudra when photographed This mudra, is noted to symbolize rulership, and is often seen (as previously noted) by spiritual figure heads in various cultures and religions.(Hinduism, Bhudhism, Jainism, etc.)

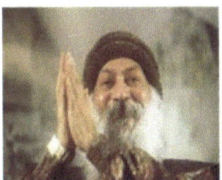

In Modern Mysticism/Spiritualism - Acharya Rahneesh known as the social/spiritual mystic "Osho" philosopher, mystic, international guru is depicting the 'Praying Hands' Mudra There is a common prayer gesture among Christian and western religion which is called praying hands or the hands clasped or folded together before the heart. Such a prayer gesture is a symbol of obedience, submission, sincerity and repentance. There are others who raise their prayer hands as a symbol of gratitude and reverence to The Divine Creator within and around us.

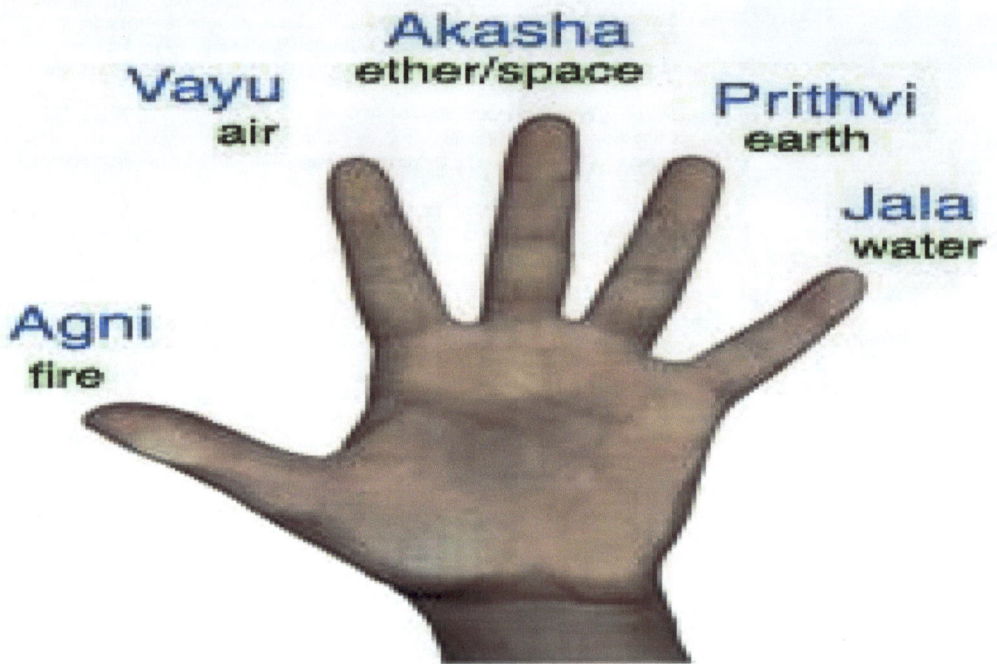

Akasha ether/space

Vayu air

Prithvi earth

Jala water

Agni fire

A SCIENTIFIC LOOK

Within East Indian Culture there are various supreme Sacred Sciences that furthers the investigations on and into the human mind and body. These sacred sciences have been studied, researched, practiced and continue to be within these cultures. Some of which have been not only introduced to Western society but are becoming a regular part of American culture.

- ➢ Tatva Vigyan   The science of elements
- ➢ Mudra Vigyan The science of finger postures
- ➢ Kayakalpa Vigyan   The science of rejuvenation
- ➢ Brahma Vidya   Theosophy – Divine Knowledge
- ➢ Pranvinimaya Vdiya   The science of curing sickness and the defective
- ➢ Surya Vigyan   The science of solar energy
- ➢ Punarjanma Vigyan   The science of reincarnation
- ➢ Deerghavu Vidya   The science of longevity
- ➢ Swar Vigyan   The science of sounds
- ➢ Rasayan Vigyan   The science of Alchemy
- ➢ Mantra Vigyan   The science of spiritual incantation
- ➢ Samyad Preshan Vidya The science of Telepathy etc.

According to Chinese palmistry, various life force elements correspond to the fingers and thumbs. Though there are only 5 recognized elements of the body that are distinguished by Ayurveda or Chinese medicine, there are 7 actual elements represented within the hand itself.

1. **THE THUMB** – symbolizes the Earth and controls the meridian channels to the lungs
2. **THE FOREFINGER** – symbolizes Wood and Plants and controls the meridian channels to the large intestine
3. **THE MIDDLE FINGER** – Symbolizes Fire and controls the meridian openings to the pericardium and reproductive systems.
4. **THE RING FINGER** – symbolizes Metal and controls the meridian openings to the respiratory, digestive and eliminatory systems.
5. **THE PINKY FINGER** – symbolizes Water and controls the meridian opening to the heart and small intestines.
6. **THE PALM** – symbolizes the Ethers and controls and activates creativity
7. **THE NERVOUS SYSTEM** – symbolic of the air & fire and all its Life force activities.

The palm of the hand, which is the root of the fingers, and the nerves that ignite their movement also possess associated elements, which need to be considered. As mentioned before, the fingertips of every living being have many concentrated nerve root endings which are energy discharge points. Science also confirms that around every tip there is a concentration of free electrons. By touching the tips of the fingers to other fingertips and parts of the palms this free energy (Prana) is redirected back into the body along specified channels that flow back up to the brain. The redirected energy traveling through the nerves stimulates the various chakras. Thus, the tension applied to the nerve/s and/or the psycho-neural circuits formed by the mudras help in balancing the five basic elemental building blocks. This balancing of the tension, and redirection of the internal energy increases the flow of life force in veins, tendons, glands, and sensory organs, to bring the body back to a healthy state.

Keeping specified nerves stretched for specified periods tones up the nervous system. Folding the fingers of each hand in certain specific postures provides the required tension on the nerves. The fingers of each individual are different in their shape, size, and patterning. These are determined and provided by nature as a tool to bring the cosmic and earthly elements into prime condition when affected adversely via the nerves. Thus, it produces a different 'end tension' on the nerves when different individuals fold their fingers or the same individual folds the fingers by different methods in different Mudras. This is exactly the tension required by that individual for each particular application. Nature has already bestowed us with the tools to be used to keep us healthy.

A WORD OF WARNING: Mudras should be learned from a practiced Master; someone who has dedicated years in practice and study of their science and its nuances, in the same way that one would study with yoga, tai chi, or qi kung. Mudras are nature's way of healing, as intended by nature and therefore, the mandates of nature are to be followed. These are no instant pills, which provide temporary relief with a variety of potential contraindications and negative side effects that cause greater harm in the long run. While some Mudras do give instant relief, for permanent and long term gains they should be done with sincerity and belief consistently over time. Remember, the gains from all Intentional Movement modalities can be long lasting and achieved without interfering with the natural working of the body mind or spirit through consistent application. Once you innerstand the basic principles of each mudra and its principles and nuances, you will generally be able to do most of the Mudra's yourself.

Compare this with Acupressure where the nerves are influenced by the application of pressure on certain points or Acupuncture, where slight electrical impulses are conveyed through needles inserted in the body. The advantage in Mudras is that the pressure to be applied on the nerves is automatic and controlled by the shape and size of the fingers and not by external agencies. Because Mudras are the mechanics for reaching the neurological network of all the systems inside and around the body; they are considered to be the link between our humanness and our Godhood.

NEURAL SCIENCE
Mudra Vigyan is also a science based on the principles of the Ayurvedic (East Indian) Medical Science which lays down three factors primarily responsible for the body's ills, wind (Vata), bile (Pitta) and Phlegm (Kapha).

YOGA TATVA mudra vigyan (Yoga related to the elements)
- The use of Mudra is built upon the knowledge of the five fingers of the human hand.
- Detailed descriptions are on the art of many ancient sculptures.
- Mudra is a very exact and scientific yogic function by which one can develop or even change, one's internal and external dispositions viz. mental (anger, emotional disturbance, intelligence etc.), spiritual (concentration, meditation) or physical (in various diseases, illnesses).
- Mudras can bring miraculous mental, spiritual and physical changes and improvements in our body. They help in quickly balancing the elements of the body.
- Mudras effect changes in veins, tendons, glands and sense organs.
- Mudras need no prior preparation. They can be done (mostly but with exceptions) at anytime, anywhere and under virtually any circumstances.
- They are like literal remote-control switches bringing quick and effective changes.
- They help bring about permanent changes.
- A constant practice of Mudras can stop or slow down the destructive changes in the human body. It can help develop a virtuous, socially amiable, non-violent, pious and courteous disposition.
- Some of the Mudras can balance the elements of the body within 45 minutes; some react within a few seconds on the human body.
- The ancients believed there were 24 diagnostic elements. The 24 words of the Gayatri Mantra have a special relationship with 24 mudras known as GAYATRI MUDRAS. They have different names and formations. The importance of Mudras is also clear from the grim qualifier to these:
- Mudras awaken the cosmic energy and help unite the atman (soul) with the Paramatama (the cosmic soul).

CHAKRA MUDRAS FOR MEDITATIVE MOVEMENT

The following mudras are used in conjunction with Kun Qi Kung in order to enhance and amplify the healing effects of the movement. Each chosen mudra has direct associative purposes to the chakras allowing the spiritual body to reside within the physical body. These mudras are used specifically with the 8 Directional Series as a means of linking the energy channels of both the internal and the subtle body systems and to increase the flow of life force through them.

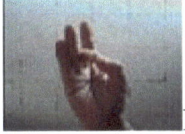 **BINDU**

AAKASH (ETHER): aligns with the Bindu (8th) Chakra. The use of this mudra helps to remove weakness of the bones and deficiencies in hearing. **Caution:** This Mudra should not be done while walking. This mudra helps to stabilize the chakra of the universe within you.

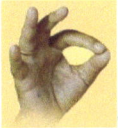 **CROWN**

GYAN (DIVINE LIFE FORCE KNOWLEDGE) is associated to the Crown Chakra (7th) and is the mudra of spiritual knowledge. This mudra heightens communication with and receptivity to Divine Inspiration. The tip of the thumb contains the command point that leads to the pituitary and pineal glands. When we press these centers by index finger the two glands work actively. The benefits of this mudra are many. It increases concentration, mental peace, sharpens memory, enriches spirituality, and has been used for treating insomnia, mental disorders, stress, depression, anger issues and drowsiness. It helps in the development of telepathic, clairvoyant, and extra-sensory abilities.

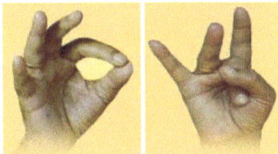 **1ST EYE**

GYAN & SUNYA (ETHERS OF THE MIND) correlates to the 1st Eye Chakra (6th) and represents the deep dark quiet stillness of the night. It represents the inner chamber of the mind where thoughts and ideas are formed, incubate, and are birthed from within our imagination. In the body, Sunya mudra represents the brains inner chambers and the brain stem that deciphers information to and from the nervous system. Shunya has and can be used to reduce numbness in the body, help those with impaired hearing and as a means of relieving earaches. It is useful for the deaf and mentally challenged, but not for those with inborn conditions. If there is no physical defect, the mudra, if practiced regularly, has been known to assist in the restoration of one hearing power. It has also been used for relieving the sensations of nausea and vomiting while driving on winding hilly curves, taking off or landing in aircrafts and with problems of vertigo. The mudra should not be continued after the problem has been removed.

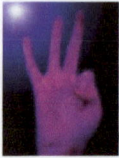

THROAT

VAYU (AIR/WIND/BREATH) corresponds to the Throat Chakra (5th) and represents things that are intangible yet build up, expand, and enjoy freedom of movement. *Vayu* represents breathing, and the internal processes associated with respiration. As we grow physically, we learn and expand mentally as well, in terms of our knowledge, our experiences, and our personalities. Mentally and emotionally, it represents an "open-minded" attitude and carefree feeling. It can be associated with will, elusiveness, evasiveness, benevolence, compassion, wisdom, and electricity.

On a physical level Vayu has been known to help in the prevention of all diseases that occur due to the imbalances within the quality of air and its inner circulation. It has been used as a treatment for Rheumatism, Sciatica, Arthritis, Gout, Parkinson's disease and paralysis without any medicine. It is useful for Cervical Spondylitis, paralysis of the face and catching of nerve in neck and in correcting disorders associated with gas in the stomach. Depending on one's physiology, it may take anywhere from 1 minute to 15 minutes or so to effectively expel all accumulated wind in the stomach without the use of an anti-flatulent. The Mudra should be stopped when the trouble abates.

Considering that almost 80% of the body's aches and pains are due to wind, the practice of this Mudra is an essential recourse that should be added to other treatments and has been known to be very effective with Parkinson's disease (an ailment of the nerves where the patient's body, head and limbs shake uncontrollably).

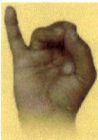

HEART

MRIT SANJIVINI APAAN VAYU MUDRA corresponds to the Heart Chakra (4th). In the case of severe heart issues, this life-giving divine Mudra can help to provide relief within a few seconds. They are a helping hand for Cardiac disease and first aid for heart problems. They strengthen the heart. It also improves self-confidence, normalizes blood pressure, and has been used to help treat menstruation related problems. Mrit Sanjivani Apaan Vayu can be used as tools for purification of the entire body. This finger position works like an injection in cases of a heart attack. Regular practice is insurance in preventing heart attacks, Tachycardia, palpitations, depressions, sinking feeling of the heart. It is also known as the Mrit Sanjivani Mudra for arresting heart attack.

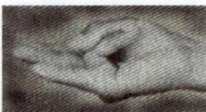

SOLAR PLEXUS

SURYA/PRANA (SUN or FIRE/METAL LIFE FORCE) relates to the Solar Plexus Chakra (3rd) and represents the energetic, forceful, moving things in the world. Animals, particularly predators, are primary examples of *fire* objects capable of movement and full of powerful energy. Bodily, *fire* represents our metabolism and body heat, and in the mental and emotional realms, it represents drive and passion. *Fire* can be associated with motivation, desire, intention, and an outgoing spirit. This Mudra sharpens the center in the thyroid gland. It reduces cholesterol and the accumulated fat in the body helping to reduce weight. It can also reduce anxiety and help to correct indigestion problems.

PRANA (METAL/LIFE FORCE), is known as the mudra of life as it integrates the power of life-force at a cellular level. It helps weak people to become strong and reduces the clamps in blood vessels. If one practices it regularly, it can help to restore one's energy bank improving vitality of the body physically, and psychologically. Prana Mudra also helps to improve the immune system, inner vision and the power of the eyes as well as reduces eye related diseases. This mudra has been use to help treat dizziness, improve circulation and brings clarity in thought improving concentration. Prana also helps to lower blood pressure, regulate breathing, control eating habits, and open blocked veins. It has been said to help in the removal of vitamin deficiency and fatigue. This finger position is a useful Mudra and can be done for any length of time at any time and in any place, which adds to its benefits. This is the mudra which, along with the Apaan Mudra, precedes any efforts at higher meditation by the Yogis and saints. This mudra helps to increase the Shakti "Life force" increasing the bodies vitality and sustenance when deprived of food and water. Other functions of Prana mudra are increasing self-confidence and improving weak eyesight and quiescence (motionlessness) of the eyes.

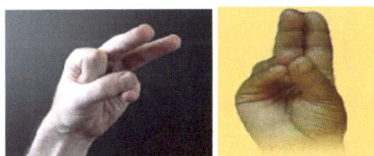NAVEL

VARUNA/PRANA (WATER/LIFE FORCE) is associated to the Navel Chakra (2nd) and represents the fluid, flowing, formless things in the world. Outside of the obvious example of rivers and the like, plants are also categorized under *water*, as they adapt to their environment, growing and changing according to the direction of the sun and the changing seasons. Blood and other bodily fluids are represented by *Varuna* as are mental or emotional tendencies towards adaptation and change. Varuna helps to retain purity in the blood by balancing the water content in the body. It helps prevent the pains of Gastroenteritis and Muscle Shrinkage. *Varuna* can be associated with defensiveness, adaptability, flexibility, suppleness, and magnetism. It is used to enhance beauty, remove impurities from the blood, restore moisture to skin, relieves painful cramps, treat diarrhea and dehydration.

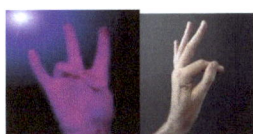ROOT

PRITHVI – (EARTH EMBODIMENT) correlates to the Root Chakra (1st) representing the hard, solid objects of the world. In people, the bones, muscles and tissues are represented by *earth*. Mentally it is confidence. *Earth* is predominantly associated with stubbornness, stability, physicality, and gravity. Emotionally it is a desire to have things remain as they are; a resistance to change. When under the influence of this mode or "mood", we are aware of our own physicality and sureness of action. **This mudra has been used to help reduce physical weaknesses.** It can help improves the complexion of skin and makes the skin to glow. It energizes the body increasing activity and helps to keep it healthy. It also helps to improve one's sense of Inner stability, Self-Assurance, calms the stomach, Strengthens the body and mind and Increases one's energy. This mudra increases solidity in the body. Removes weakness and lack of body solidity and helps gain for those underweight, chronic fatigue and weakness.

APAAN (VEGETATION/EMBODIMENT) plays an important role in our health as it regulates the excretory system. It has been used by some to regulate diabetes. It has been used in the treatment of constipation and piles and to help regulate normal regular waste excretion. Apaan can help provide relief in urinary problems, as it facilitates discharge of waste material from the body.

Apaan can be used to assist in the cleansing & purifying of the liver and gall bladder improving their function ability, by helping to encourage the removal of toxic waste products from the body, regulate bladder problems, and balances the mind increasing one self-confidence, patience, sense of serenity and inner harmony. Helps in purification of the body, urinary problems, easy secretion of excreta, regulating menstruation and painless discharge, easy child delivery, Piles, Diabetes and kidney disorders.

Caution: This Mudra should not be done by pregnant women before completing 8 months. After that, a 10 minutes practice 3 to 4 times a day will help to encourage a normal delivery.

The use of Mudras works best as a preventative measure for improving and sustaining good health. If one has been diagnosed with a physically debilitating condition, first give the body a chance to heal itself before giving it invasive medicines and drugs, which will have some side effects. If one has been prescribed medications as treatment, then mudras can be used in conjunction with the prescribed treatment as ones condition improves.

MUDRA MEANINGS AND PROPERTIES ARE IN APPENDIX C

THE 8 DIRECTIONAL CIPHER OF KUN QI
(CHAKRA REJUVENATION, EMPOWERMENT & HEALING)

The human organism, like the earth itself is a being of interactive multidimensional energy. The following levels of the Kun Qi Kung meditation are very powerfully healing and regenerative sequences of movements as they connect the divine healing energy of Tanran Reiki with the power of the seven elements of Earth. The planetary vibrations within our own solar system and the star formations of the cosmos within this galaxy such as Sirius, Orion's Belt, and the Pleiades known as Cosmic Qi, or Da Qi (The Cosmic Breath). If you are open and aware of your cosmic/galactic origin you can generate a direct line of energetic frequencies through mudras and the power of visualization. Drawing on these energies allows you to become a channel of Divine Guidance and otherworldly wisdom, love, compassion, and power, which embeds these energies into the physical body healing and rejuvenating your chakra centers, internal organs, physical ka body and subtle bodies with life force and empowering you to ground them on earth. This chakra sequence combines the sentient energy within the elements, the use of specific chakra mudras, circular breathing, directional movements, and visualization. The combination of these healing modalities is quite intentional in their purpose. The ways in which they serve to compliment and support the purpose and function of each other makes for a more complete, holistic system of movement.

THE PURPOSES OF THE DIRECTIONAL CIPHERS OF MOVEMENT

Before I explain the sequence itself, I'd like to go deeper into how all the components of meditative movement work together. How the body functions internally is directly related to the emotional state that we are in, and those things outside ourselves that trigger these emotional responses. On a cellular level, every thought or emotionally charged memory remains lodged within our cells (also referred to as cellular memory). Unless the emotional charges within the cellular memory have had an opportunity to release physically, it becomes lodged in the subconscious and continues to cycle into our perceptions of love, life, and relationships unconsciously. Examples of this would be our inner mental dialog about life, self, and situations at hand. Kun Qi introduces the 7 elements of life force, and their connection to the processing and expression of our emotions and their healing impact upon and within our physical and subtle bodies. They can be utilized as a means by which one can tap into their Higher Soul, which is at One with Universal Intelligence, and reveal the deeper intentions and soul lessons that one's life experiences were designed to teach. It is also able to reveal the inherent power all possess to change circumstances and the world around them by changing their perceptions about things to that of a higher perspective where one is able to envision universally beneficial conditions and the means by which these conditions can be made manifest through implementation.

This meditative movement sequences works with the 7 elements of nature and the universe and I believe derives from the ancient Tehuti wisdom system that was practiced in ancient Kamet (Egypt). Vibrational attunement with the elements is achieved over time through focused awareness and direct unadulterated exposure to the elements coupled with deep circular breathing and inner visualization. The more exposure to the elements of nature that you are able to come into contact with the more you can feel their vibrational frequencies as a very present sentient energy in a deeper more consistent way. As one regains this awareness and becomes more open to receive the personal wisdoms that nature speaks concerning the natural synchronicity of all of life and our kinship with it, the more one is able to see beyond the constructs of society to gain the insights to one's True origins and higher purpose for existing. Remember, all of creation is connected on an energetic and a molecular level thus the conditions of the many are directly impacted by the actions of the one.

Periodic Table by Article Value

December 2008

Quality legend:

	High	Mid	Low
Views High	Showcase		Blemish
Views Mid			
Views Low	Treasure		Under the Rug

1 H (Hydrogen)																	2 He (Helium)
3 Li (Lithium)	4 Be (Beryllium)											5 B (Boron)	6 C (Carbon)	7 N (Nitrogen)	8 O (Oxygen)	9 F (Fluorine)	10 Ne (Neon)
11 Na (Sodium)	12 Mg (Magnesium)											13 Al (Aluminum)	14 Si (Silicon)	15 P (Phosphorous)	16 S (Sulfur)	17 Cl (Chlorine)	18 Ar (Argon)
19 K (Potassium)	20 Ca (Calcium)	21 Sc (Scandium)	22 Ti (Titanium)	23 V (Vanadium)	24 Cr (Chromium)	25 Mn (Manganese)	26 Fe (Iron)	27 Co (Cobalt)	28 Ni (Nickel)	29 Cu (Copper)	30 Zn (Zinc)	31 Ga (Gallium)	32 Ge (Germanium)	33 As (Arsenic)	34 Se (Selenium)	35 Br (Bromine)	36 Kr (Krypton)
37 Rb (Rubidium)	38 Sr (Strontium)	39 Y (Yttrium)	40 Zr (Zirconium)	41 Nb (Niobium)	42 Mo (Molybdenum)	43 Tc (Technetium)	44 Ru (Ruthenium)	45 Rh (Rhodium)	46 Pd (Palladium)	47 Ag (Silver)	48 Cd (Cadmium)	49 In (Indium)	50 Sn (Tin)	51 Sb (Antimony)	52 Te (Tellurium)	53 I (Iodine)	54 Xe (Xenon)
55 Cs (Caesium)	56 Ba (Barium)	57 * La (Lanthanum)	72 Hf (Hafnium)	73 Ta (Tantalum)	74 W (Tungsten)	75 Re (Rhenium)	76 Os (Osmium)	77 Ir (Iridium)	78 Pt (Platinum)	79 Au (Gold)	80 Hg (Mercury)	81 Tl (Thallium)	82 Pb (Lead)	83 Bi (Bismuth)	84 Po (Polonium)	85 At (Astatine)	86 Rn (Radon)
87 Fr (Francium)	88 Ra (Radium)	89 ** Ac (Actinium)	104 Rf (Rutherfordium)	105 Db (Dubnium)	106 Sg (Seaborgium)	107 Bh (Bohrium)	108 Hs (Hassium)	109 Mt (Meitnerium)	110 Ds (Darmstadtium)	111 Rg (Roentgenium)	112 Uub (Ununbium)	113 Uut (Ununtrium)	114 Uuq (Ununquadium)	115 Uup (Ununpentium)	116 Uuh (Ununhexium)	117 Uus (Ununseptium)	118 Uuo (Ununoctium)

* Lanthanides:

58 Ce (Cerium)	59 Pr (Praseodymium)	60 Nd (Neodymium)	61 Pm (Promethium)	62 Sm (Samarium)	63 Eu (Europium)	64 Gd (Gadolinium)	65 Tb (Terbium)	66 Dy (Dysprosium)	67 Ho (Holmium)	68 Er (Erbium)	69 Tm (Thulium)	70 Yb (Ytterbium)	71 Lu (Lutetium)

** Actinides:

90 Th (Thorium)	91 Pa (Protactinium)	92 U (Uranium)	93 Np (Neptunium)	94 Pu (Plutonium)	95 Am (Americium)	96 Cm (Curium)	97 Bk (Berkelium)	98 Cf (Californium)	99 Es (Einsteinium)	100 Fm (Fermium)	101 Md (Mendelevium)	102 No (Nobelium)	103 Lr (Lawrencium)

Everything that exists in form is made up of atoms, electrons, neutrons, protons, quarks, zedes etc. which are reflected in the components of the Universe. Chemically the only difference is the combination of component within its cellular structure. Every living organism on earth including human beings is made up of the same components just in differing quantities and combinations of elements. The sun, the moon, the stars, the galaxies… the multi-universe itself contains the same Life Force Elements that we do in some semblance and operates in the same way as the cell within the human body. This is what is known as the macrocosmic/microcosmic relationship.

Kun Qi helps to re-establish that connection to become at one again in one's bond with Mother Earth and the elementals that govern nature's rhythms and our purposes for being here as a part of Her evolution. These components of the meditative movements are performed in respect to the following 8 directional ciphers with the symbols of Tanran Reiki that correspond with the 8 major Chakras. As they incorporate and align with the life force energy from the 7 elements of Nature and the 7 elements of the Universe, they provide a very powerful healing vibration both within oneself and outside oneself. It creates a sentient energetic force field that both penetrates and alters dis-eased mental, emotional, and physical structures on both a tangible and intangible level that can be seen and felt within one's self and seen within one's life as they purify all atomic and subtle body structures on a molecular level traveling in all directions endlessly. This opens portals to Divine vision and intuition that allow you to access guidance from higher dimensions.

The following chart demonstrates the 8 directional patterns used in each of the following Kun Qi Kung Sequences with south being the direction in which one begins and ends. This sequence of movements is the foundation of movement for each of the following series of Kun Qi Kung which was introduced to me by Fabien Manmann.

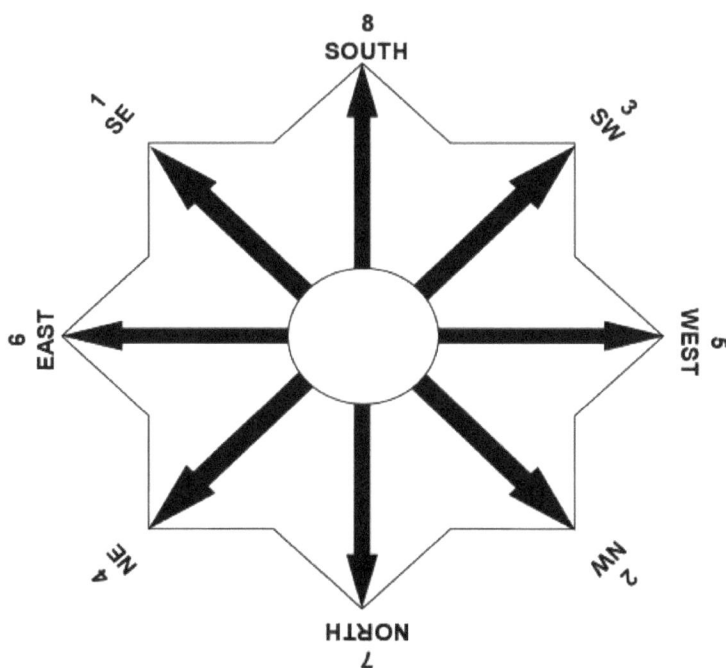

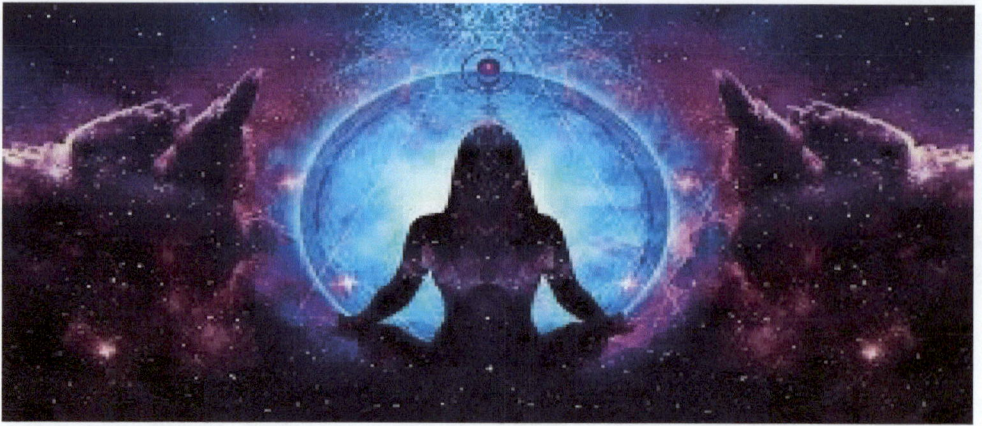

THE 8 EXTRAORDINARY MERIDIANS AND PLANETARY EMISSARIES OF THE 8 DIRECTIONAL CIPHER

The 8 extraordinary Meridians represent the body's deepest level of energetic structuring. These meridians are the first to form in utero and are the carriers of Yuan Qi – the ancestral energy which corresponds to our genetic inheritance. They function as deeper reservoirs from which the 12 main meridians can be replenished, and into which the latter can drain their excesses.

SOUTHEAST:
- **Emissary - "Orumila", "Tehuti", "Maat",**
  - Life giving power behind the spoken word
  - Healing through the power of mantras
  -
- **Yin Quiao Mai** – "Yin Movement Channel"
  - Runs between the head and the ankles
  - Connects with all the Yin meridians and dominates the interior of the body
- **Rigel** – "The Traveler" or "The Legs of the Giant" influences the seas on our planet.
  - Is linked with the adrenals

NORTHWEST:
- **Emissary – Yemonja, Auset**
- **Yang Quiao Mai** – "Yang Movement Channel"
  - Runs between the head and the ankles
  - Connects with all the Yang meridians and dominates the exterior of the body
- **Antares** – "The Way of Action" or "The Warriors Way"
  - Brings the physical, astral, and mental bodies into balance when attuned and initiated to this star.
  - Linked with the pituitary gland

SOUTHWEST:
- **Emissary – Oshun, Het-Heru**
- **Yin Wei Mai** – "Yin Regulating Channel" or "Guardian Vessel"
- **Regulus** – "The Heart of the Lion" or "The House of the Sun"
  - Influences the gonads in the physical body
  - Those attuned to this star are initiated into "The Royal Way"

NORTHEAST:
- **Emissary – Elegba, Eshu, Sebek,**
- **Yang Wei Mai** – "Yang Regulating Channel"
- **Altair** – "The Flying Eagle"
  - First star of the Aquarian Age and is related to the Innate Qi.
  - Associated with the Crown Chakra and the Barathary Gland

WEST:
- **Emissary – Heru, Qebhsennuf,**
- **Dai Mai** – "The Belt Channel" or "The Girding Vessel"
  - Circles the waist, and is the only horizontally flowing meridian
  - Acts like a kind of belt that contains the other vertically flowing meridians
  - Used in Tai Yin Fa Series III exercises to spiral the Dai Meridian up to connect with the energy of the planets, stars, and galaxies, and then down to connect with the core of the earth.
- **Arcturus** – "The Druid Star" or "The Guardian of Old Knowledge and the Grail"
  - Has a physical resonance to the pancreas

EAST:
- **Emissary – Babalu Aye', Auset, Seker, Tuamutef,**
- **Chong Mai** – "The Penetration Vessel" or "Thrusting Vessel"
  - Flows vertically deep within the body, along the front of the spine and is most closely associated with Yuan Qi (Our Ancestral energy)
  - The Chong has a close resonance with our energetic core.
- **Aldebaran** - "Star of the East" "One Who Sees" or "The Eye of God"
  - Taoism, The Wisdom Systems of Tehuti have their divine roots in the initiations of this star.
  - Linked to the Hypothalamus

NORTH:
- **Emissary – Ogun, Herukhuti, Hapi,**
- **Du Mai** – "The Governing Vessel"
  - Flows from the perineum up along the midline of the back to the head and stops on the inside of the upper lip
  - Responsible for governing the qi for all the yang meridian inside the body
  - Has close relationship with the brain, spinal cord and kidney
- **Vega** – "Star of the Sound Initiations"
  - Connected to the Pineal Gland, music, speaking, and the Kabbalah

SOUTH:
- **Emissary – Amset,**
- **Ren Mai** – "The Conception Vessel"
  - Runs from the perineum up along the front midline of the torso, and ends in the lower mouth.
  - Partners with Du Mai in the microcosmic orbit as a continuous circuit which is how energy circulates when we are inside our mother's womb.
  - Meets all the yin meridians
  - Responsible for receiving and bearing the qi of the yin meridians
- **Sirius** – "The Keeper of the Egyptian Knowledge" and "Show-er of the Spiritual Way"
  - Syrius is connected to the thymus

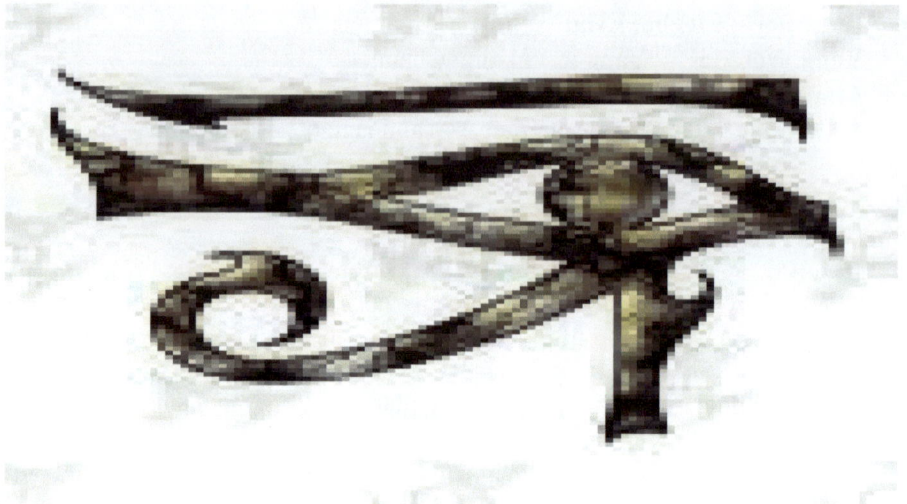

SACRED SPACE INVOCATION

CREATING SACRED SPACE
Please note that this is not a religious ritual and performing this sacred space sequence is optional

Creating Sacred Space both within oneself and within one's environment is one of the most important aspects of personal healing on one's spiritual journey towards ascension into one's Higher Self that one can do. Our ability to call in life force from the ascended realms as well as the Cosmic and Earthly Life forces and those that have chosen to be of service in the healing and ascension of humankind and all that resides here on planet earth is our divine right. Creating Sacred Space is a very important part of performing healing work. It helps to clear and protect oneself within the area one chooses to work in and increases the vibration to match that of your healing intentions by welcoming in the sentient aspects of nature and the spiritual beings, ancestors, and totems that have chosen to be of assistance to you that you hold in a place of divine reverence and honor. Following are two short and simple sacred space invocations that are quite effective that can be used if you do not have one that you feel more comfortable with; "The Violet Flame Invocation" of sacred space and the "Tanran Reiki Invocation".

THE VIOLET FLAME SACRED SPACE INVOCATION:

First take a moment to quiet and center yourself by focusing on the rhythm of your breathing. Breathe deep and to a slow count of 4 or five counts both in and out stilling your mind. If you have ways of creating protection around yourself and a space invoke them at this time. If not, envision a violet beam or flame of light surrounding you. Within this flame envision a bubble of light blue light around your body. To affirms your healing intentions welcoming higher levels of consciousness to bring greater Self-awareness and personal insights during your healing sessions by inviting your spiritual guides, ascended healing masters, ancestors, animal totems, and light beings to be present, to surround you with their Divine protection so that divine healing may take place and to guide you in your journey towards divine health.

INVOCATION OF THE 7 WINDS

Totems have been used since the recorded history of humankind, in many cultures from all over the world as messengers of our oneness with nature and the animal kingdom. A **totem** is a being, object, or symbol representing an animal, plant, or entity that serves as an emblem of a group of people, such as a family, clan, group, lineage, or tribe, reminding them of their kinship, descent, ancestry (or mythic past). By inviting the spiritual guides and totems of the 8 directions and their sentient wisdom, (the life-sustaining light rays of the sun, the cosmic energies from the planets and stars, and the sentient wisdom from the animal, plant, and mineral kingdoms and Mother Earth who nourishes us with the sustenance we need to feed our body and the beauty needed to feed our souls) we come to recognize their presence within us and our Oneness with them. I often use this invocation of sacred space when doing movement as I find that it feels more attuning and in sync with my personal style of sacred communion and honoring my Creator, my ancestors, and all our relations.

Totems have been used since the recorded history of humankind, in many cultures from all over the world as messengers of our oneness with nature and the animal kingdom. A **totem** is a being, object, or symbol representing an animal, plant, or entity that serves as an emblem of a group of people, such as a family, clan, group, lineage, or tribe, reminding them of their kinship, descent, ancestry (or mythic past). By inviting the spiritual guides and totems of the 8 directions and their sentient wisdom, (the life-sustaining light rays of the sun, the cosmic energies from the planets and stars, and the sentient wisdom from the animal, plant, and mineral kingdoms and Mother Earth who nourishes us with the sustenance we need to feed our body and the beauty needed to feed our souls) we come to recognize their presence within us and our Oneness with them.

This method of creating sacred space is one that is performed as a means of honoring the indigenous life forms to earth and to the Spirit that gives life to all things based on the beliefs and practices of the Original ancestors of the America's. The wisdom within the cyclical and energetic patterns of nature and various animal totems and the universe itself were honored and esteemed for their influence and guidance as to the natural flow of life and how-to live-in sync with it peacefully. The patterns of nature, when recognized and acknowledged, are still very powerful sources of life force energy and wisdom as to our oneness with them and how we were originally designed to operate in alignment with them as a part of the whole of nature itself.

The following invocation is used to help one re-attune with the sentience of nature and to deepen our innerstanding of its Divine purpose and the deep relationship we share with it within ourselves.

Invoking the Winds is a Native American ritual that acknowledges the spirit totems of the Seven cardinal directions. (South, West, North, East, Above, Below, and Within). It is meant to invite the spiritual guardians to assist, protect and provide us with the wisdom and divine sentience within the nature of each totem and how they are reflected within our own essential being. There is a fluid movement sequence that can be performed along with the salutation that tends to express outwardly the sacred tone of welcoming in those who are of a higher dimensional frequency and are here to assisting us in our intentions of going deeper into our journey of self-awareness, self-healing and self-mastery. There is a sense of tranquil peace and protection that one experiences from time to time while performing this sequence that is sweet, blissful and beyond words. You can feel the ancestors, animal spirits, and cosmic counsel right there with you, empowering you to be a channel of even greater healing light and vibration.

 I have found that by performing the movements while repeating the salutation of the 7 directions I have felt a deep opening of my heart and spirit that revealed the characteristics of Divine Source, the transcended and ascended Beings and the spirit of the animal totems that are honored by it and how these characteristics are being called upon and addressed in my life at the time. In other words, *how they speak to the same nature within me and how they are guiding me through the phases of my life as I pay attention to their subtle messages that are revealed by their presence around me.

OPENING THE DOOR TO EACH DIRECTION

To begin this opening meditation, fix your gaze in front of you (or close your eyes) and move your hands into a prayer pose in front of your heart. While holding this prayer pose, in sacred meditation, draw in your breath deeply and slowly, focusing your inner awareness to that of your spiritual heart allowing a sense of calm and peace to embody your consciousness. Maintain this sense of centered energy as you slowly exhale, moving hands upwards with great intentionality reaching up past your forehead so that your palms are together above your head at your eighth charka, "The seat of the soul". Envision the suns radiance, as you inhale, enveloping your entire body as you drop your hands away from each other, open your arms until they are shoulder height, and parallel to ground. With palms upward, start to bend your elbows drawing your hands in toward the body as if balancing two birds on your palms. Bring them in towards your head as if to hear them whisper in your ears. While hands are in this position, rotate them in front dropping them down to the level of your heart and extend your arms fully forward in front of you offering your love and acknowledgement as gifts from your heart towards the direction of the wind you are speaking the salutation to.

With arms stretched out in front of you fan your arms out to your sides again, in welcoming the presence of the elementals into the space. Once your arms are out to your sides again turn the palms over so that they are facing down towards the earth. Bring your arms down towards the earth as if drawing a half circle from the outer edges to the middle gathering energy between them from Mother Earth until your hands are back together in front of you, then as you bring your palms together, flip them upright and bring them back up in front of your heart. This sequence is performed in each direction in accompaniment with each invocation of the 7 winds.

The following salutation can be used to invoke the energies of each direction either verbally or from within yourself while you perform the accompanying movements or upon completing the movement for each direction whichever feels most comfortable for you. Start facing south and turning ¼ turn to the right (west) and so on until you are facing south again. The last three salutations can be done facing south or in any direction that you feel led to begin them.

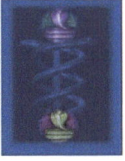

To the Winds of the South - Great Kundalini Serpent & Caterpillar

"Spirit of Knowledge, sexuality and the healing powers of nature; awaken your kundalini light within me. Fill me with your wisdom and innerstanding of the flow of Divine life and how to remain one with it. Help me shed what no longer serves my highest good, in the same way that you shed your skin, releasing the old paradigms of this world while embracing the new visions of living as one with divine life, innerstanding and embodying what it is to live as my divine Self. Thank you for teaching me to move silently on this earth plane, with the eyes to recognize the purpose and beauty of all things with appreciation for the lessons learned, the truth revealed, and the freedom to choose anew. Aho!"

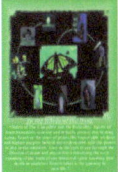

To the Winds of the West - The Butterfly

"Spirit of Transformation create in me the peaceful acceptance and ability to embrace without fear, the endless cycles of death, metamorphosis, renewal and rebirth. Protect me during the times of transformation. Provide for me the safe space and self-time for the healing, metamorphosis and renewal of my spirit, soul, body, and mind that I need in order to embody fully Your Divine Nature within me that I am designed to reflect. Thank you for teaching me the ways of peace and the impeccable wisdom and higher purpose behind my experiences with the power to live fully present in the moment with no attachments to what was, is, and shall be. I thank you for giving me the eyes to see through the illusion of death and physicality embodying the over-standing of the truth of my immortal spirit knowing that death, in whatever form it takes, is a gateway to a new higher life. Aho!"

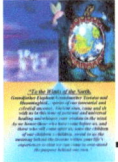

To the Winds of the North - The Elephant and The Tortoise

"Spirits of my extraterrestrial, celestial, and terrestrial ancestors, Ancient ones, come… commune with me in this time of personal and universal transformation and ascension and whisper your wisdom in the winds of my mind. So much honor and gratitude to all of you who have come before me, and all who will come after… unto the children of my children's children. Reveal to me the meaning behind the lessons within your life's experiences, the wisdom gained and the akashic knowledge of creation so that I can come to inner-stand and fulfill the purpose behind my own with your guidance to creating the future that your wisdom contains for the healing of our people and harmonizing of all life forms on this earth plane and throughout the universe, eternity and beyond. Aho!"

95

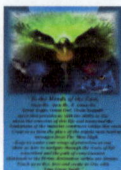

To the Winds of the East - "Amun Re, Atum Re, Atun Re"
The Eagle, The Owl, and The Seagull

May your spirits provide me with the ability to rise above the concerns of this life and transcend the limitations of the psychological and material constructs within the manmade world. Come to me from The Most High… from the place of the Triple suns… Keep me under your wings of protection and the light of your wisdom as you show me how to navigate through the rivers of life unscathed and the path of consciousness that leads to the Divine destination within my dreams. Thank you for teaching me how to live, love, heal and create as One, free in Your Great Spirit."

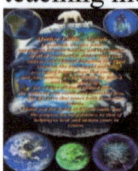

To Mother Earth, Earth Elementals and All My Relations… Gaiah

"In gratitude I offer forth my prayers for your healing and the healing and harmonizing of all of creation that abides within your embrace, the Mineral Kingdom, the Plant kingdom, the four-legged and the two-legged beings, those that creep and crawl among us, the finned, the furred, and the winged ones, for we have all been birthed from the waters of your womb and are nourished from the life force that issues forth from your breasts. Thank you, Mother Earth, for giving us life here. May the purpose for my embodiment be that of helping to heal and sustain yours in return as well as all of my relations for you have revealed to me the wisdom within nature and taught me to respect its beauty and simplicity as my own. "

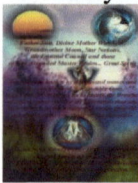

To Father Sun, Divine Mother Wombyin, Grandmother Moon, Star Nations, The Orisha, Elohim, Reiki Guides and Those of the Ascended Master Realm…

"You who are known by a thousand names and You who are the Un-nameable Ones, thank you for allowing me to breathe the Breath of Life for another day, for all of the loving creations that You have made, and the beauty that comes from the creative insights You share within my soul. Surround me with your presence… Speak to me through Your Divinity within me and guide me along the path of Right-Us-Ness through Divine knowledge, order, and healthy creative expression."

96

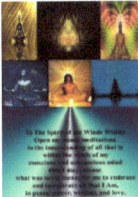

To The Spirit of the Winds Within

"Open my minds meditations to the innerstanding of all that is within the winds of my conscious and unconscious mind. Thank you for allowing me to release what was never meant for me to embrace and to embrace all that I Am in You in spirit, soul, body, and mind with peace, power, wisdom, and love abundantly. Inspire me to take action on the insights that you awaken in me and reveal from On High so that I may live in complete alignment with my Divine Purpose as my Divine Self."

In gratitude I speak this prayer to the Spirits in the directions of the north, south, east, west, above, below… and within…
Ashe', Ashe', Ashe'

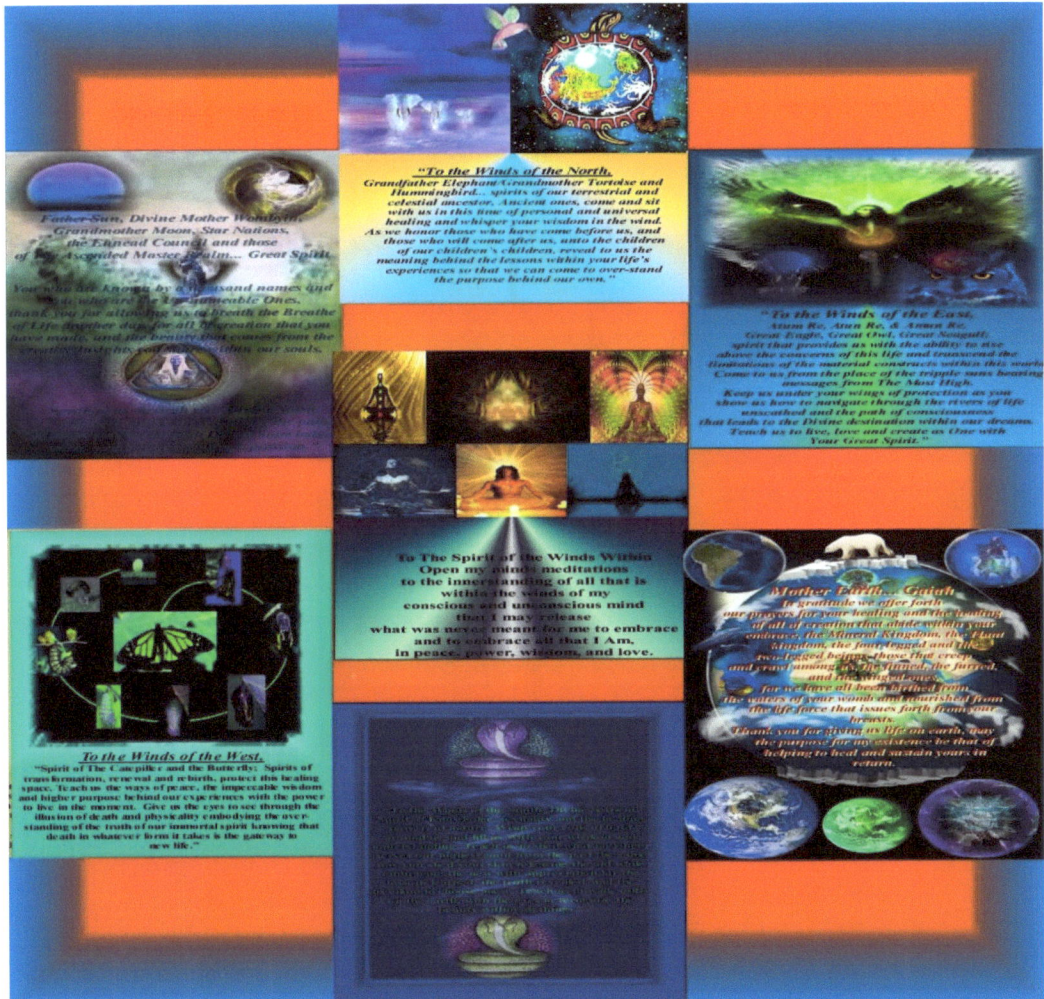

(Detailed information on each animal totem can be found in appendix E)

97

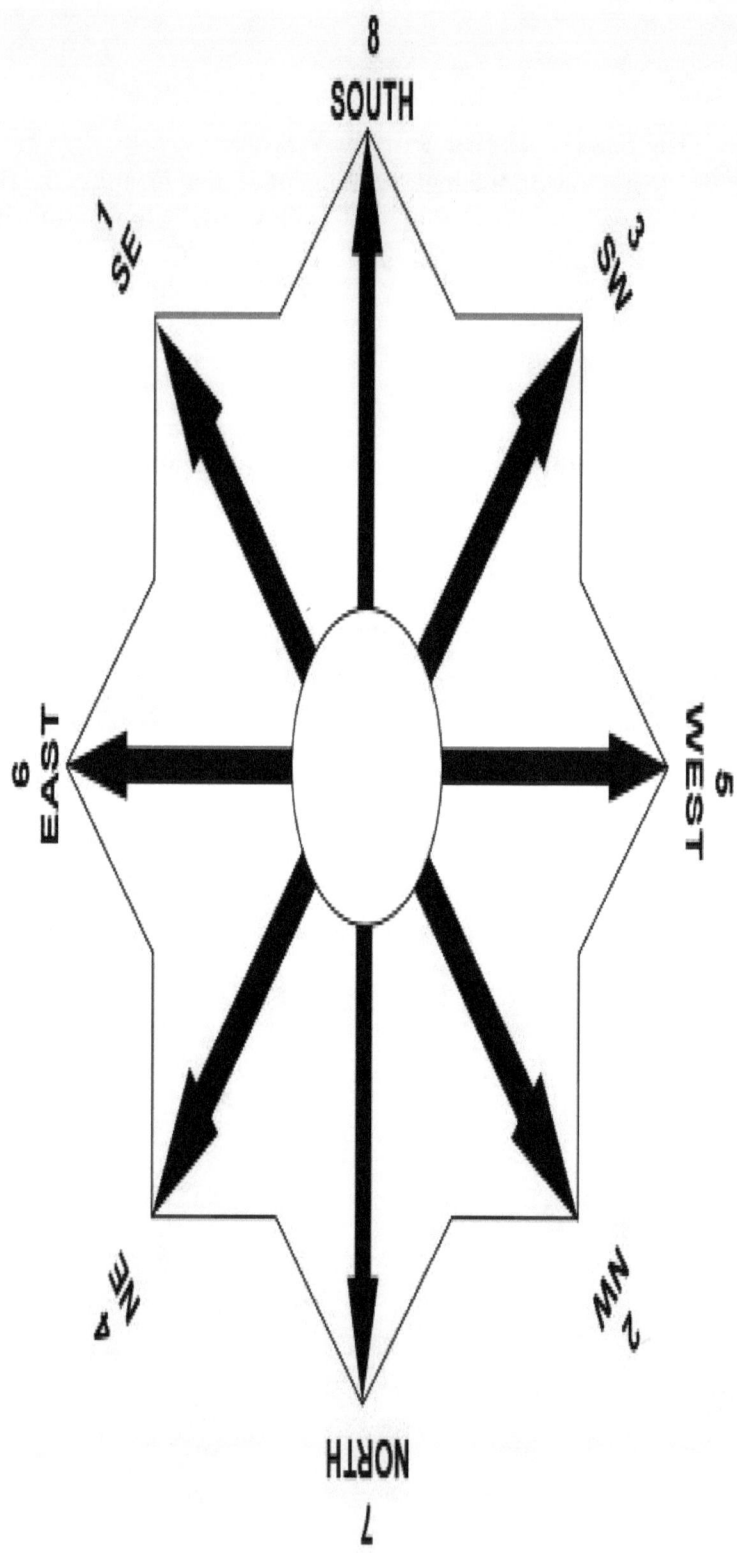

SOUTH
8

SE
1

SW
3

EAST
9

WEST
5

NE
4

NW
2

NORTH
7

8 DIRECTIONAL CIPHER SEQUENCE I - SITUATIONAL CLEARING

The steps for the situational clearing sequence do not require much movement or space thus, circular breathing works best. It also will assist you in achieving a meditative state as you will focus more on visualization versus movement. Exhaling as you lunge into each direction allows you to send the creative power of your visualizations out with greater power and lifeforce for manifestation. It also sends more carbon dioxide out to feed the environment. Inhalation as you rock back and as you make the turns allows you to draw in the life force from the elements into your subtle and physical body fields aligning their life giving energies with your chakras which we will go into more detail later.

Start by standing facing in the direction of the south. Place the palms of your hands inward over the dantien and begin circular breathing. Using the inverted heart mudra works well also in creating a greater loving energy vibration to work with.

Bring to mind a situation or circumstance that you would like to gain clarity on, change, or improve. Spend a moment visualizing the situation as it is then when you feel ready shift your focus to what you would like to have happen or how you would like to see things become while rotating the hands around each other in front of you. This will start to generate and build qi energy between the palms. At this point, inhale deep into your belly and step out in the direction of southeast leading with the left foot. Step forward in that direction pivoting the front of your body in that direction so that your left knee is leaning directly over its big toe. Upon inhalation, rock back shifting your weight to the right leg. While the right leg is holding your weight, turn the left foot in towards your body about 120 degrees then turn your right leg 90 degrees, this should have you facing in the direction of the northwest and repeat the previous pivoting motion. Once you are facing northwest, exhale while lunging forward in that direction. This time as you pivot back on the left foot inhaling, you will then rock forward again onto the right so that the left foot is free to move. At this point lift the left foot and shift your body so that you are facing in the 3rd direction of southwest. Repeat the same sequence of movements moving from southwest to north east then moving into the direction of the east to west and lastly from north to south.

During the rhythmic movements of each directional ciphers envision the highest most positive outcome that you would like to experience with the situation that you are considering. With your intentions send loving vibrations to the situation from your heart out through your breath into the environment in each direction allowing yourself to feel the convictions of your desires and prayers. Let yourself feel the way you would want to feel were everything resolved and everyone or everything involved were aligned with the most positive and productive outcome for all. Continue this circular movement pattern throughout the entire meditation until you feel that your situation has become cleared within yourself and you are able to see and feel it resolved with the most positive outcome imaginable. Perform one last complete rotation to seal the healing intention and to send it peace, faith, and acceptance, then end the sequence facing where you started, in the direction of the south. Repeat this sequence as many times as you feel the need to in order to feel release and resolution with the situation you have chosen to clear and give Thanks to all your spirit guides, ancestors, and Orisha for the manifestation of your intentions.

ADVANCED MOVEMENT FOR 8 DIRECTIONAL CIPHER SEQUENCE

This advance section can be integrated into the 8 directional movement cipher to tone the musculature and increase one's fitness levels. While rotating the hand in front of you, inhale deep into your belly then upon exhalation step out in the direction of southeast leading with the left foot. Lunge forward in that direction pivoting the front of your body in that direction so that your left knee is lunging directly over its big toe. While in this forward lunged position go deeper into the lunge by doing 3 pulsing lunges with that left leg. During inhalation, rock back shifting your weight to the right leg. In this position do 3 pulsations during exhalation sinking into and pressing forward with your right quad. Sink back as far as your quad will hold you then, press forward slightly using the heel and the quad of your right leg as if doing a reverse lunge. Now, while the right leg is holding your weight, turn the left foot in towards your body 90 degrees then turn your right leg 90 degrees, this should have the front of your body facing in the direction of the southwest. In this position, shift your weight to your right leg sinking down into it like a squat while allowing your left leg to straighten. This is called a half-sided squat. Exhale slowly while you do 3 squatting pulsations to the right then shift your weight to the left and do the same squatting pulsation while slowly and deeply inhaling. With your left leg holding your weight, shift your right foot another 90 degrees away from your body and allow your entire body to follow until you are facing Northwest corner directly. Exhale while lunging forward in that direction. This time as you rock back on the left foot doing the 3 pulsations and inhaling you will then rock forward fully onto the right so that you are standing on your right leg and your left leg is free to move. At this time lift the left foot and step your left foot in towards your body then move into a lunging position with the left foot into the 3rd direction of southwest. Repeat the same sequence of movements moving from southwest to north east then moving into the direction of the east to west and then again for the north to south, continuing this circular movement pattern throughout the entire meditation until you've moved through the 8 directions. End the sequence facing where you started, in the direction of the south. while standing in this direction become aware of your breath taking some time to center in your breathing and allow your mind to open up to any insights and higher awareness' that come. Take note of them when done by journaling them down once you've completed the entire series, or when you feel guided. I've received many profound insight and messages when I've allowed myself this time to sit at the end of each rotation especially when doing the 8 directional cipher for the chakras.

Once you have attuned and awakened your connection to the Life Force energy within the surrounding elements of nature and the universe, take a few moments to direct their combined flow of life force energy through your meridian channels by riding your breath using the power of visualization. This will help you to become aware of your ability to direct the flow of life force through the energetic circuitry of the internal organ systems better known as the meridian channels.

Meditation on the chakra and their mental, emotional, and physical components is one of the first steps in identifying the areas of disharmony within. The more one is aware of the characteristics of the chakras and one's own current physical, mental, emotional, spiritual states of mind, the more insights as to how to address imbalances and re-align them with the optimal state of health and well-being based on one's own personal condition. There are many holistic "tools" that we can use rebalance the chakra centers. Exercise, massage, energy work, yoga, internal cleansing, organic food, herbs, and focused meditation can be used as natural alternative methods of bringing about homeostasis within the body/mind especially if you focus your intentions on the result you have in mind. Know that energy follows thought. By implementing high frequency substances like stone essences, pure essential oils, botanical essences, holistic healing herbs and other plants you're better able to purify your internal systems from built up cellular matter keeping your mind/body system functioning at higher levels. The use of therapeutic quality pure essential oils may be used in massage and aromatherapy to affect the areas, as well as with sound therapy and/or energy work. Please do not confuse food grade oils or "fragrance" oils for this purpose. Only pure grade essential oils such as YOUNG LIVING and BE YOUNG made from non-chemically treated organic produce that contain the full spectrum of holistic properties to fully achieve the goals here. Of course, the higher the rate of vibration or frequency of the treatments used, the better the result will be.

Being conscious of the function of what each chakra regulates helps you to be more effective in your healing practice. The integration of Tanran Reiki with the 8 directional cipher enhances the effects of clearing and healing the physical and energetic bodies in their entirety. It brings about a deeper overall healing while helping to open the inner channels of consciousness to be able to see how the elements of the Universe and the Earth work in conjunction with our physical psychological systems to heal and align our personal mind/body energy to reconnect with these elements with conscious awareness. Knowledge is power, and the more one is aware of the ways in which the Divine Sources of life force works within and around us and allow ourselves to trust it enough to tap into the Source within ourselves the more able we are to create that which we desire to experience instead by choice and the healthier our lives become on all levels of existence.

The combination of our intentions, inner state of mind, and intentional breath work coupled with movement provides the direction for the electrical current to flow by sending our mentally generated life force, (chi) to specific areas within and without. As you focus your intentions and inner visualization to match the rhythm of the breath you are able to literally send the heartfelt vibrations where they need to go within the physical body and out into the world while consciously drawing in the life force frequencies of the etheric and elemental vibrations.

Rhythmic breathing and movement create a calming flow that moves one into an alpha state where mental chatter ceases, and the body begins to move on its own. The use of specific hand mudras ignites and activate the command points to the various internal organs stimulating the flow of life force through their respective meridians helping to rebalance the emotional aspects of the organs which has a healing effect. Vocalizing healing mantra's integrates the use of sound, (the one shared component between the elements of Earth and the universe). This creates an inner vibration that stimulates movement within the inner workings of the body that can be felt. When the tonal note of each chakra is intentionally used in combination with the corresponding mudras, visualization, circular breathing and movement, it amplifies and magnifies the power and intensity of the new life force that is being ingested and generated. Visualizing one's healing intention comes from one's Higher Self or Higher Mind and directly integrating and activating It's sentient healing purpose allowing your minds meditations and intentions to become a living healing frequency that radiates from within. This healing energy not only generates healing within oneself, it can also be sent out into the environment you are in and on throughout the universe through intention, visualization and exhalation of breath. Remember… sound has the ability to travel through whatever it comes into contact with. Thought intention coupled with these aforementioned frequencies will connect to and intensify all other frequencies that resonate at the same vibration. And because healing energy and intentions are of a higher and lighter vibration, they also have the ability to move through heavier negative energies transforming them or lightening them as they move through. Thus, meditative movement, used as a tool for intentional healing, has the power to change our inner and outer experiences to provide the sense of inner peace, clarity, and overall wellbeing that we envision.

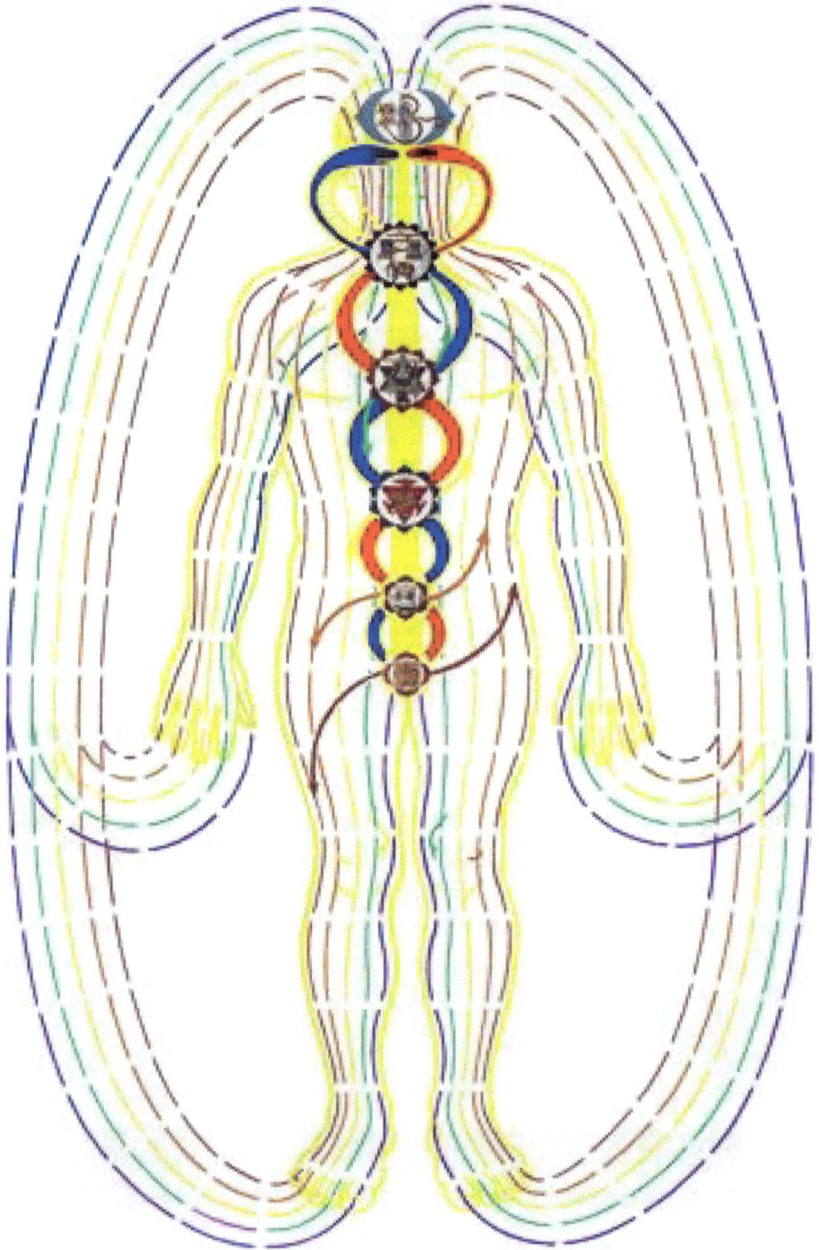

8 DIRECTIONAL CIPHER SEQUENCE II
CHAKRA CLEARING

This sequence combines visualization of the color spectrum of the gamma rays from the sun along with the chakras using the 8 directional movement sequence, and circular breathing as a means of clearing and aligning one's chakras. By refocusing the movements, visualization, and breath work, from the organs and their meridian system to the chakra system we combine the physical with the subtle bodies starting with the bindu and going down to the root. It's important to create sacred space around you and to align with the elementals as it is this which will recharge and rejuvenate your chakras and the electrical circuitry of the nervous system that connects to the physical anatomy that they regulate.

Once you've created sacred space, begin by facing the direction of the south. Focus for a few moments on circular breathing and relax the body/mind even deeper allowing it to align you more deeply with the element of air and wind. Once you've become relaxed, focus inwardly bringing your inner attention to your Bindu or 8th Chakra above and slightly behind your head. Visualize its color, (Magenta) streaming down from the sun into this chakra to fill and activate it. Once you feel ready, begin your 1st cipher of the 8 directional movement by moving the left foot into the direction of Southeast. Continue the 8 directional cipher in each direction inhaling as you lunge outward in each direction and exhaling as you rock back and pivot into the next direction. If you are performing the advance movements then you will adjust the breath work to align with the extra middle movement. Once you've completed the sequence for the Bindu or 8th Chakra move your focus down to the Crown chakra envision the color of Violet flowing down into your Crown chakra and repeat the 8 directional cipher. Perform the same for the following chakras using the following colors and ending/beginning each cipher facing the direction of the south allowing yourself time to open up to any new insights and awareness' that you may receive.

- Bindu – Magenta
- Crown – Violet or Purple
- 1st Eye – Indigo
- Throat – Aqua Blue
- Heart – light Green
- Solar Plexus – Yellow or gold
- Navel – Orange
- Root – Red or Black

VOCAL TONING FOR CHAKRA AND MERIDIAN CLEARING

The use of the voice to tone during meditation creates inner vibrational frequencies that break up, release, and heal various blockages within the body. By vocalizing in the tonal note that corresponds to a specific area of the body with intention and focus, we're able to send that vibrational resonance directly to that area of the body to assist it in rebalancing. For example, while performing the first round within the 8 directional sequence while focusing on circulating life force into and through the root chakra, vocalize the word "HU" in the tonal note of C. You'll notice that you can fell the vibration vibrating in various areas of the body. These areas, more often than not, correspond to the Root Chakra. Vocal toning works especially well when combined with the 8 directional sequence covered later.

CHAKRA TONAL NOTES & VOCALIZATIONS

- **BINDU –**
  - Note – B/B#
  - Vocalization – AUM/OM
  - Anatomy – Brain, Nervous System, Pineal Gland
- **CROWN –**
  - Note – B
  - Vocalization – EEE
  - Anatomy – Pituitary Gland, Head, Bones of face, Inner/Middle Ear, Brain
- **1ST EYE –**
  - Note – A/A#
  - Vocalization – EEE
  - Anatomy – Eyes, Optic Nerves, Auditory Nerves, Sinuses, Jaw Bones, Cheeks, Outer Ear, Face, Teeth, Facial Nerves
- **THROAT –**
  - Note – G/G#
  - Vocalization – I (EYE)
  - Anatomy - Nose, Nasal Cavity, Lips, Jaw, Mouth, Tongue, Neck Glands, Vocal Cords, Neck Musculature, Larynx, Shoulders
- **HEART –**
  - Note – F/F#
  - Vocalization – AAY
  - Anatomy – Thyroid, Parathyroid Glands, Muscles of the Shoulders, Chest, Upper Back, Elbows, Arms, Hands, Wrists, and Fingers, Esophagus, Trachea, Heart, Valves, Coronary Arteries, Lungs, Breasts
- **SOLAR PLEXUS –**
  - Note – E
  - Vocalization – AAAH

- Anatomy – Gallbladder, Liver, Solar Plexus, Circulatory System, Stomach, Pancreas, Duodenum, Spleen, Adrenal & Suprarenal Glands, Erector Spinae, Upper Quadratus Lumborum, Rib Cage
- **NAVEL –**
  - Note – D/D#
  - Vocalization – OH
  - Anatomy – Reproductive Organs, Kidneys, Urinary Bladder, Small Intestines, Lymph Circulation Inguinal Rings, Appendix, Rectus, Abdominals, Quadratus Lumborum, Musculature of the Pelvic Girdle & Upper Legs, Knees, Sciatic Nerve
- **ROOT –**
  - Note – C/C#
  - Vocalization – H<u>U</u> or OOOH
  - Anatomy – Coccyx, Musculature of the Lower Legs, Ankles, Feet, Hip Bones, Glutes, Rectum, Anus, Blood, Immune System

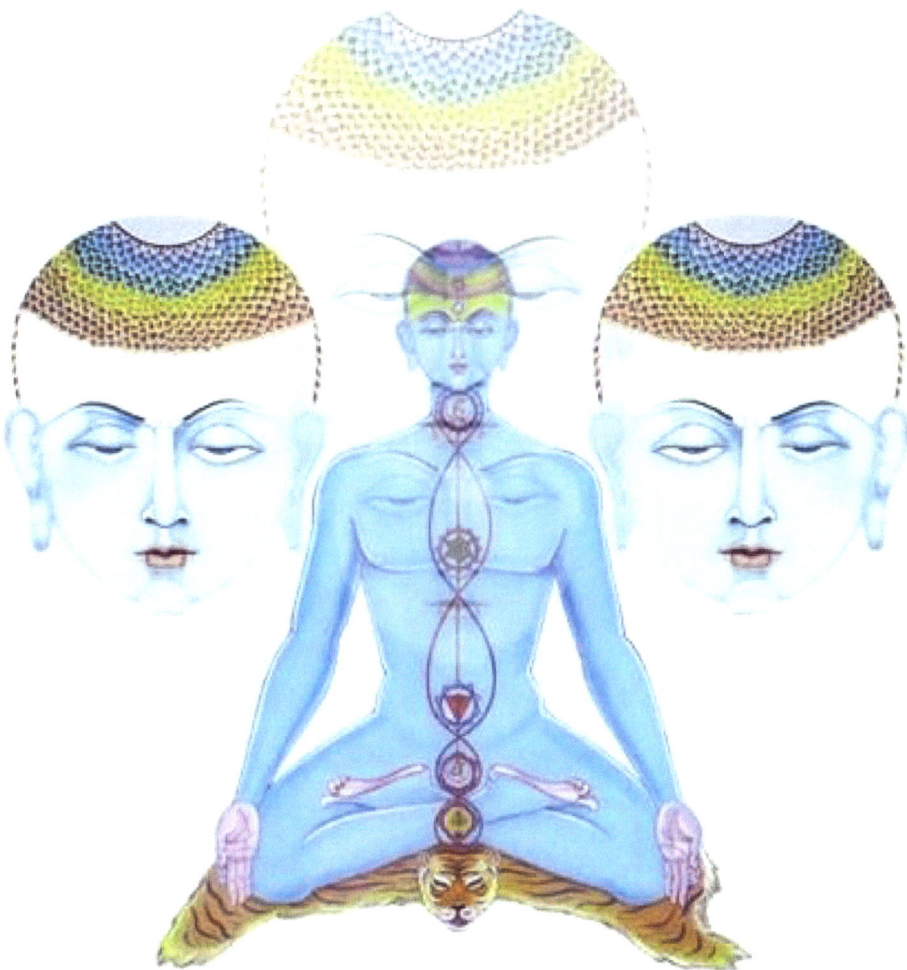

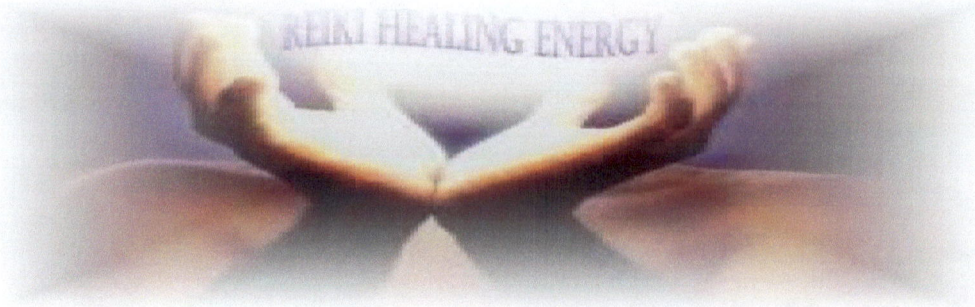

THE HISTORY OF TANRAN REIKI

Reiki is a Powerful healing technique for stress reduction, internal healing, and life transformation that promotes health & wellbeing within ones internal and external environment. The word Reiki is made of two Japanese words - Rei which means "God's Wisdom or the Higher Power" and Ki which is "life force energy". Therefore, Reiki is " Divinely Intelligent life force energy." Therefore, though Reiki is spiritual in its configuration, it is not a religion. Reiki has no dogma, and there is nothing you must believe in order to learn and use Reiki. In fact, just like gravity, Reiki is not dependent on belief at all and will work whether you believe in it or not. Because Reiki comes from God, The Creator or the Universal Source of all that exists, many people find that using Reiki puts them more in touch with the experience of their religious and spiritual beliefs rather than having only an intellectual concept of it. It is still important to live and act in ways that promotes harmony with others. Reiki has been known for its transformative work with hospice patients in providing personal soul transformations within their death process which has allowed many to make that transformation in peace and embrace their dying as a transition into the next phase of life for them. Reiki not only provides a sense of peace, and completion for the one passing onto the next realm but to their love ones left behind.

Reiki is an ancient form of energy healing that was re-introduced to society by Mikao Usui of Japan around 1922. Dr. Usui had received the symbols from an ancient Buddhist text. Through meditation on the symbols and text during a 21 day fast, Usui had not only learned their purpose but found that he became embodied by their healing power. The healing system of Reiki pre-dates back to the Atlantean and Lemurian time period. Prior to their destruction, some of the records of this system were taken to the Andes, Himalayas, Egypt, and other spiritual sanctuaries for safekeeping by various Athlantian/Lemurian Priests and spiritualists. Many of the records of their existence were either stolen or destroyed during various wars, overthrows and land disputes between ruling countries like in the destruction of the Great Library of Alexandria which was created by Ptolemy I Soter, who was a Macedonian general and the successor of Alexander the Great. As a symbol of the wealth and power of Egypt, it employed many scribes to steal books from around the known world from various temple orders. Once acquired the materials were copied, kept, and used to gain spiritual supremacy. Thus, the Alexandria Library was the only place where much of the ancient knowledge that was transcribed, mostly on papyrus scrolls, were kept.

This Historically vast ancient library was set afire by Julius Caesar in 48 BC, and attack by Aurelian around the 270 AD resulting in the loss of many of the ancient scrolls and books, written concerning these teachings and symbols along with the destruction of the cultural knowledge of the African and cosmic origins of humanity that existed and were known in ancient times. Also, according to Socrates of Constantinople, Coptic Pope Theophilus destroyed the Serapeum in 391 AD. The Serapeum of Alexandria was a temple built by Ptolemy III (who reigned from 246–222 BCE) which was the largest and most magnificent of all temples in the Greek quarter of Alexandria. which housed an offshoot collection of the great Library of Alexandria. Nothing of this library now remains above ground.

Reiki in and of itself is based on the principles of life force energy that flows from The Source of Creation throughout ALL life forms and is a gentle healing system that allows spiritual energy to flow through its initiates who have committed themselves to be conduits of its healing energy and intentions. In and of itself the energy is intelligent, loving, and creates the maximum amount of healing a person is able to receive at any given time. All the receiver has to do is be receptive giving permission for whatever changes which want to happen to be experienced. The energy is nonviolent and therefore only works to the degree that one allows it.

No divine knowledge or experience surfaces to our conscious awareness unless we are ready and willing to objectively look at the experience in order to learn its purpose for our evolution and move beyond it. Also, each session builds on the previous session so there tends to be a progressive evolution to one's healing process. People will usually feel calm, peaceful, and relaxed with warmth being felt within their bodies. Although Tanran Reiki is the only form of system of Reiki that I'm aware of that aligns directly with the human chakra system, it is not necessary to know much about the chakras, meridians, or the physical or subtle bodies. All that is required is one's permission to be an open channel for the energy to flow. The basic premise is that Reiki energy itself is intelligent. We do not have to guide the energy with our mental knowledge but can instead allow ourselves to be guided by the energy to use knowledge of the practitioner and the practitioner themselves to support what it wants to do to heal the receiver."
"Reiki applies to and addresses the person as a whole unit; body, emotions, mind and spirit creating many beneficial effects that include improved health, relaxation, greater self-awareness and feelings of peace, security and alignment with one's Divine design. It begins the reawakening of one's divine blueprint of being a vehicle of Divinely guided life force through its attunement process. It's a simple, natural and safe method of physical healing and spiritual ascension for everyone regardless of one's spiritual path. It has been effective in helping virtually every known illness and malady and always creates a beneficial effect with many who have reported miraculous results.

Tanran Reiki also works in conjunction with all other medical or therapeutic techniques to relieve side effects and promote recovery. In order for the Reiki healing energies to have lasting results, one must come to a place of accepting responsibility for her or his healing and take an active part in it. Therefore, the Tanran system of Reiki is more than the use of the Reiki energy. It also includes an active commitment to improve oneself in order for it to be a complete system. The ideals are both guidelines for living a gracious life and virtues worthy of practice for their inherent value."

TANRAN VS OTHER FORMS OF REIKI AND ENERGY SYSTEMS

"Tanran Reiki is an offshoot of Traditional Usui Reiki with additional symbols that correspondence with the chakra systems energy vortices within the subtle body. Usui's form of Reiki was not able to do this, due to there being too few symbols to make such a correspondence. Because of this development the attunements power levels that anchor them into the chakras, is stronger and the specific Universal Life Force Energy that each symbol represents can flood through each channel thus expanding the healing effects on all levels simultaneously. The symbols are activations of specific healing processes designed to transmute unwholesome energy into healthy energy by its Divine Source. For instance, Sei He Ki is designed to heal inner child wounds, mainly by providing on an energetic level, certain things that were not fully provided as needed in childhood, like validation, loving attention, nurturing, approval, connection, bonding, and permission to be oneself. Most of us have experienced some deficiency in this area and can benefit from this kind of focused session which opens the doors into one's life for one to come into contact with these types of affirming experiences."

"Tanran Reiki differs from some energy healing traditions that teach people to generate and send healing energy. Although the results gained from people who generate and send energy may be good, this kind of energy is not always guided and regulated by the wisdom of the Divine Universal Loving Energy and can be limited in its results or be more overwhelming to experience. With Reiki The wisdom of the Universal Loving Energy regulates the process so that what arises is never too much healing to handle. I say, "differs from some energy healing traditions," for a reason, because I do believe that there are other similar healing traditions that are like Tanran Reiki that also channel the Universal Loving Energy through them. If the intention is to channel the Divinely Intelligent loving power greater than oneself, then it will have the same flavor."

"The Tanran Reiki system also differs in a more extensive use of chanting and breathing. Chanting the names of the symbols is used during the attunements, along with visualizations of the symbols, and/or drawing the symbols through invocational miming. The breathing taught is a mild form of Rebirthing breathwork which often happens naturally when the energy flows through someone. In general, energy follows our breath and our breath follows the energy. Chanting or intoning sounds help energy blocks to dissolve more quickly as well as deepen the feeling of being surrounded by warm loving vibrations."

Tanran Reiki combined with Kun Qi Kung meditative movements enables one to circulate Divine Universal healing life force of each symbol consciously enabling healing to take place on all levels internally and externally, simultaneously. Once you attune to The Divine healing characteristics of each symbol you become empowered to activate, embody, and channel their life force energies directly to the associated chakras and throughout all the physical and subtle body levels aligning them in a way that creates their healing manifestations. The following chapter gives you more detailed information concerning the Reiki symbols, how they relate to the body and the chakras, and the accompanying details as to how to work with them within the series of meditative movements. This works in seated and group meditations just as effectively which makes this form of healing adaptable to any environment and any physical condition.

TANRAN REIKI SACRED SPACE INVOCATION

By invoking the Reiki Guides and the Symbol Doh Yah Noh around one's auric field it creates a seal around you that protects one's energy fields from any negative or unhealthy outside energy other than that of the surrounding life force around oneself and from within. This is designed to be done in sync with circular breathing when setting sacred space before one starts meditative movement. This keeps one consciously connected to receive guidance from the energy during the entire sequence. You can also use the Reiki symbols of Cho Ku Rei, Zee Gah Nah, and Dai Ko Myo to seal and protect the healing space that you're working in. I find these two methods of protecting oneself and one's healing space creates an inner sense of peaceful welcoming and safety for everyone who enters into the space. Many have commented on the fact that they feel safe and surrounded with a loving peaceful vibration.

CREATING SACRED SPACE WITH TANRAN REIKI

When using Tanran Reiki to create sacred space call upon the Reiki guides, healing masters, and/or Divine Elders and invite them to prepare your energy field to receive their light energy and to bless and activate the sentient life force of each symbol so that their healing energy can work within you as a universal healing force. **First, envision or draw the symbol Zee Gah Nah, once in front of you and once behind you or on either side of you**. Zee Gah Nah is a spinning triple vortex that works similar to a black hole vacuuming out low frequency energies such as sorrow, anger, and confusion transmuting them into higher, lighter frequencies of wisdom, inner-standing, and gratitude for the purpose for all things. When spun counter clockwise, Zee Gah Nah suctions out and removes non-productive or toxic energy that is being release during your active meditation. When spun clockwise it works in reverse sending out energy that has been transmuted into healthy love encompassing life force which allows for the healing chi of the elements to penetrate unhindered into your chakras and/or auric field. **Next, envision Cho Ku Rei in the 8 corners surrounding you** (like a cube) at the top and bottom of you auric space or the space that you inhabit, (southwest, southeast, northwest, and northeast). This helps define the space and creates a protective field around you. **Next envision Dai Ko Myo within the middle of the sacred space you are preparing.** The power and intention of this master symbol draws in the sacred energy of the infinite realms and raises the vibration as it encompasses all of the 7 elements within the universe and within nature and represents the Divine workings of all things above and below. Once done, seal the space by envisioning Doh Yah Noh around the entire area to reinforce the protection of your auric field. The following charts are a visual representation of what this may look like.

On the following page is a diagram of the Tanran symbols used to create sacred space. Those that have been attuned to the symbols can utilize this very effective tool for creating protective sacred space prior to working on a client or oneself. It can also be used on a regular daily basis to protect ones energy field when going out among the general public. It can help to keep you auric field protected from feeling overwhelmed in crowded places and/or to assist you in remaining detached thus allowing you to remain in a peaceful state amongst the chaos.

If you have not been attuned to Tanran Reiki, the use of the Violet Flame or the Invocation of the Winds invocations will meet your requirements. For those wanting to become attuned to activate Tanran Reiki the training process for level 1 & 2 of the Tanran system is a 2 day workshop that will cover the Origins and a more thorough history of Tanran Reiki, its systems, the similarities and differences of Tanran Reiki as opposed to other systems of Reiki, a review of the Tanran symbols, their applications and functions, how they connect with the chakra system, and attune you to the energy.

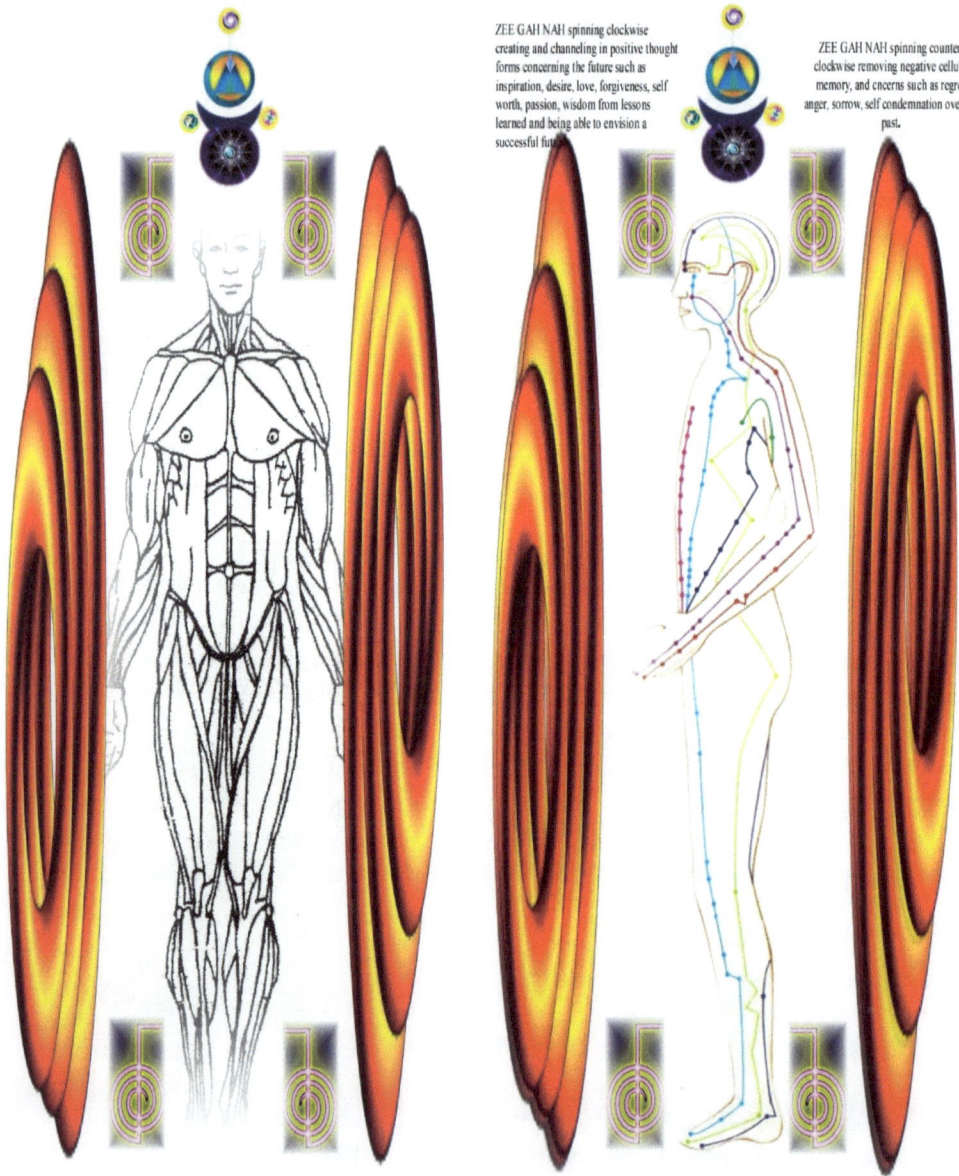

ZEE GAH NAH spinning clockwise creating and channeling in positive thought forms concerning the future such as inspiration, desire, love, forgiveness, self worth, passion, wisdom from lessons learned and being able to envision a successful future.

ZEE GAH NAH spinning counter-clockwise removing negative cellular memory, and cncerns such as regret, anger, sorrow, self condemnation over the past.

TANRAN SACRED SPACE INVOCATION DIAGRAM

TANRAN REIKI ATUN-MENT PRAYER AND HEALING SALUTATION
BE THE UTTERANCE THAT CARRIES THE MIRACLE OF ETERNAL HEALING INTO THE UNIVERSE.

"Here and now I invoke the presence of the Reiki Guides, the healing and Ascended Masters, and the healing vibrations of the earthly and the universal elements to bless this space as they work in, as, and through me healing all impropriety and dis-ease within my spirit, mind, and body and that of all life forms within the universe."

"I allow and envision the healing powers of love, life and the sentient life force of Our Creators within the Reiki symbols to enter through the "Seat of the Soul" above my head, to re-activate each symbol within each respective chakra, radiating throughout my body to awaken, cleanse, and heal my life force and to release Their healing energy into the world touching the hearts of those to whom it's being sent, as well as Mother Earth, The Elements, and all within the infinite expanse of the Universe."

"I take in the Prana of life as my life force, visualizing, intoning, and merging the aspects of each symbol, each element, each attribute, each mudra. As I breathe in, embody, and release this healing life force to radiate throughout My entire body and the entire universe with divine unconditionally loving healing intentions, I invoke these affirmations and embrace their healing intentions within my entire being both conscious and unconscious becoming one with them." "As I move and become Kun Chi I allow it to transform my life to reflect the personification of divine health, wealth, knowledge of Self and that of creation throughout The Universe and all of Creation."

Perform this salutation with the meditative movement sequence of the 8 directions after creating sacred space. I've found that the combination of breath work, visualization and movement in this sequence are synchronized and even more powerful in their healing and transformative effects. This sequence also integrates the visioning power of the mind with the various internal/external systems of the body through the breath and the healing life force energy of Tanran Reiki deepening the healing effect multi-dimensionally.

You will again be using the 8directional movement pattern in this and the following Kun sequences however we will be slowing the movement down while intensifying the movements in order to better synchronize and internalize the sentient power of the symbols.

Stand facing south and begin circular breathing Atun-ing yourself to the Reiki Guides, your inner vision and your breath. Ask the Guides to bless and activate sacred space around you as you visualize the symbol set for sacred space from page the previous page. Once you've activated sacred space bring your attention to the crown.

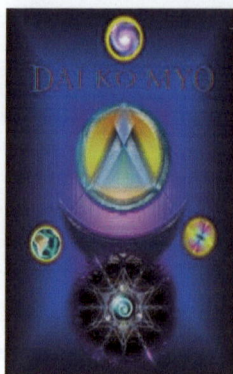

SEQUENCE V ~ SITUATIONAL CLEARING WITH DAI KO MYO

When DAI KO MYO is used during situational clearing it can open the channels for pure wisdom, unconditional love, and absolute truth from Divine Source to create phenomenal and immediate changes based on ones level of faith in the miraculous and the collective intelligence that flows throughout all that exists within the Universe. We are meant to non-dogmatically access absolute truth based on our inherent connection to Divine Source and our spiritual beliefs and practices as it remains nonverbal and beyond all opinions. It is pure knowingness. When connected to Dai Ko Myo, through intention and meditation we are able to access absolute truth and reach greater levels of peace, understanding of various spiritual knowledge, and application of the insights and spiritual principles revealed. Absolute Truth can never be the property of a concept capturing mind; this would be like trying to put the Ocean in a cup for a concept does not include the whole. But we can be plugged into absolute truth as living and pure wisdom energy. As we radiant light we unite with the truth that beyond all conflicts and illusions is where eternal peace resides. Making this domain part of our conscious experience is part of the healing of this world.

ATTRIBUTES OF THE SYMBOL

Each element of the symbol has meaning. This applies to each of the Tanran symbols as a symbol is only a visual representation of a deeper conceptualization. The Tripod figure at the top of the symbol represents the Universal Oneness of all Creation also known as The Divine Source from which all of creation derives. The center triangle reflects the Divine Trinity of love, wisdom, and power, surrounded by a protective hermitic field. It contains not only Divine Love, Intelligence, and Action, but Divine Truth and Divine Protection and or intervention. The top sphere represents the principles that govern the universe which is the source from which the akashic records reside. The bottom left, represents Pure or Divine Wisdom, the life force we derive from the planet and access all knowledge of medicinal remedies to ailments, and the bottom right, Divine Creativity. The cup portion that contains the tripod figure represents the receptive holding principle that houses or holds the Divine power of the tripod or triune aspects of the Divine Absolute contained within Dai Ko Myo. This represents also the holding space where we receive Divine inspiration from the Source, where we are able to access the akashic records, and all Higher Knowledge, Divine Inspiration and Guidance. The spiral within the symbol of Dai Ko Myo represents the divine unfolding, the internal processing, and the transcendence and transmutation of thought. It consists of three spiral turns, one for cosmic intelligence, one for cellular intelligence, and one for earth intelligence. It simultaneously represents the spiritual or mental body, the emotional body, and the physical body and symbolizes the way in which Divine Source descends into our being. Dai Ko Myo in its entirety symbolizes the Great Light and infinite Creative Potential and contains all the other Reiki symbols within it. Because you are a part of this infinite light you are able to manifest your desires that are in alignment with its principles, through it.

The difference between using Daikomyo with situational clearing and doing situational clearing without Daikomyo is that the focus of the situation is released to Divine Will thus you allow yourself to become open to innerstand and accept the higher purpose for the situation to unfold versus a specific desired outcome. Sometimes a situation that seems negative comes to us because there is a pattern of behavior or emotional trigger that we have been unconsciously operating by that is creating the situation. By opening ourselves to see through the eyes and mind of Divine Source, our part in creating it we can then innerstand the purpose of the situation and what it is meant to teach or inspire us to do differently in order to evolve and restore balance to one's self and to the situation. Doing this when in movement, and while being attuned to cosmic and earthly life force, the toxicity gets circulated out of the areas of the body that hold the cellular memory triggers by transmuting the toxicity with healthy life force energy.

After you've centered yourself within your breathing and intention activate the symbol by invoking the Reiki guides and giving them permission to bless and activate Daikomyo within your crown chakra. Once you feel centered in this connection allow your mind to shift into the focus of the situation of concern that you are wanting to resolve and perform the 8 directional movement sequence until you feel clear.

KUN QI SEQUENCE VI -
TANRAN PERSONAL & UNIVERSAL HEALING

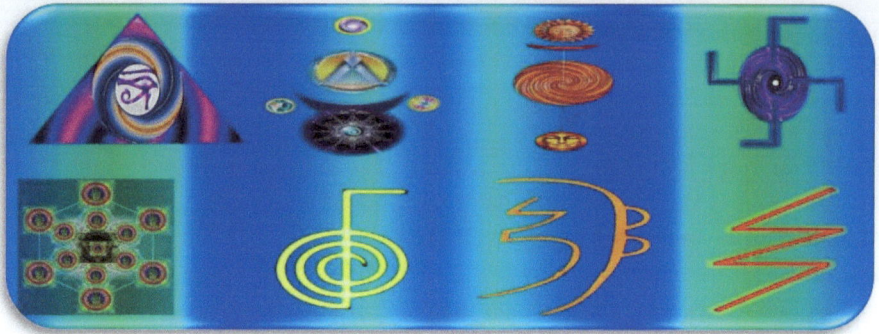

Tanran Reiki combined with Kun Qi Kung meditative movements enables one to circulate Divine Universal healing life force consciously enabling healing to take place on all levels simultaneously. One you attune to The Divine healing characteristics of each symbol you become empowered to activate, embody, and channel their life force energies directly to the associated chakras and throughout all the physical and subtle body levels aligning them in a way that creates their healing manifestations.

The meditational movement sequence for the next four series of Kun Qi Reiki Qi Kung will be perform in the same manner as the 8 directional cipher used for the chakra clearing sequence only during these sequences of Kun Qi the visualization and meditation will be on the symbol associated to each chakra and its attributes versus the color within the spectrum of the gamma rays.

There are two ways in which you can perform the following sequences. The first way is to work with the corresponding symbol to each chakra. This will work to re-attune that symbol within its related chakra strengthening its attributes within the function ability of that chakra and the expression of it attributes throughout your day. The other way to use the symbols while performing the 8 directional chakra sequences is to focus on attuning each symbol, within all of the chakras, one at a time. For example, you would attune to the Bindu Chakra with the Dohyahnoh symbol and then perform 1 cipher of the 8 direction movement starting and ending by facing the south. Next you would move your attention down to the 1st eye chakra while still attuned to the symbol of Dohyahnoh and again perform the next cipher of the 8 directional sequence for that chakra and so on. You will continue to attune each chakra by performing the 8 directional cipher while focused on Dohyahnoh until each chakra has been attuned to that symbol. Then you will start all over again with the next symbol and repeat the same sequence for that chakra. Remember, it is very important to allow time after each 8 directional cipher to take note of any imagery, insights and/or awakenings that rise into your consciousness concerning the chakra/symbol connection and activation within you paying attention to the messages revealed. The following chapter gives you more detailed information concerning the Reiki symbols, how they relate to the body and the chakras, and the accompanying details as to how to work with them within the series of meditative movements. This works in seated and group meditations just as effectively which makes this form of healing adaptable to any environment and any physical condition.

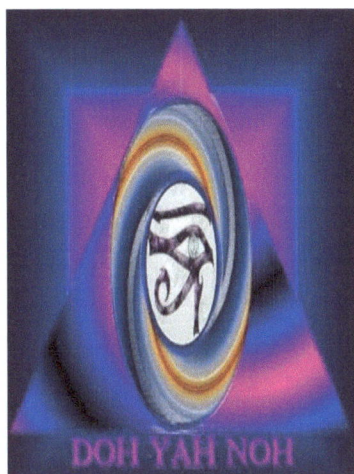

TANRAN SYMBOL ACTIVATION, DETAILS, ATTRIBUTES, AND MEDITATIONS
SYMBOL: DOHYAHNOH
CHAKRA: BINDU
COLOR: MAGENTA
TONAL NOTE: B
RELATED ESSENTIAL OILS: white angelica to increase the aura, or the blend of marjoram, lavender and peppermint to clear ones aura, the Harmony blend also balances the chakras. Forgiveness works wonders for releasing and letting go of old issues.
RELATED STONES: Clear Quartz, Meteorite, Tectonite, Black Opal, Tanzanite, Moldavite, Peacock Quartz Crystal, Kyanite

MUDRA - AAKASH (ETHER)

Begin by facing the direction of the south. Focus for a few moments on circular breathing and relax the body/mind even deeper allowing it to align you more deeply with the element of the wind and the earth. Once you've become relaxed and attuned bring your mental attention to your 8th Chakra (the Bindu) and activate the symbol of Dohyahnoh by visualizing the symbol within your mind or by drawing the symbol in the air. At this point breathe deeply into the belly or abdomen then very slowly vocalize the symbol of Dohyahnoh -preferably in the tonal note of B- allowing the vibration to reverberate deep within your head and chest cavity for as long as you can. By vocalizing the symbol you create a resonance within the chakras that stimulates movement within them which amplifies the movement of life force and increases the influx of Reiki healing energy that the symbol represents. Using the proper tonal note has the added benefits of harmonizing the resonant vibration within the corresponding chakra which makes it an even better receptor of the healing aspects of the symbol. However, whether you vocalize the symbol in the exact tonal note or just vocalize the symbol the healing properties of each symbol will still be received and flow into your chakras at the level of healing integration that you are open and ready to receive. After you've toned the symbol and fixed its image within your inner vision, open yourself up to its energy by either meditating on its geometrical design or by meditating on its soul properties and attributes. As you continue to envision the symbol allowing it to fix in your mind, start the sequence by stepping out into the direction of southeast and inhaling the life force of that direction slowly and deeply.

As you work throughout the 8 directional cipher you may notice that it may take some effort to remain focused on the symbol throughout the entire series. If you should find your mind wandering, just gently bring your focus back to envisioning the symbol and note which direction you were facing at that time. Continue focusing on the symbol throughout the entire first cipher. (refer to pages 78-79 for the 8 directional movement pattern details). If your intention is to send the energy of the symbol out into the surrounding environment or out to others or into the universe exhale as you step out into

115

each direction or each turn, and inhale its energy into yourself as you shift backward in preparation of each turn. If your intention is to draw the energy into yourself from the surrounding earthly and universal life forces than inhale as you step out into each direction and exhale the healing energies downward from your crown chakra into your root chakra or the pelvic floor as you shift backwards in preparation of each turn.

Once you have completed the 8 directional cipher for the 8th chakra and are again facing south, stand up straight and place both hands over your abdomen right below the navel. Again, open yourself up to its energy by either meditating on its geometrical design or by meditating on its soul properties and attributes but this time do so with the intention of allowing the symbol as well as the chakra to channel and reveal to you the messages of divine intelligence and wisdom concerning your past, present, or future and the guidance that your soul has been desiring. Remain in this position until you feel that the communication is complete take mental/visual notes so that you can journal the insights later on, and then inhale all that was communicated to you down from the bindu to your heart and exhale this same communication down from your heart, through the lower chakras and into the earth as a means of grounding what you received into yourself and into this world then give thanks with gratitude and prepare to move onto the next symbol and/or chakra.

SYMBOL ATTRIBUTES:

THE 8TH CHAKRA is an emerging portal into transpersonal awareness and the Seat of the Soul. It is the temple of the Higher Self from which human cleansing and the releasing of karmic patterns that are outdated and lifetimes old takes place. By accessing this chakra, we can identify and release old traumas, fears, and behavioral patterns that are causing us pain or limiting us in some way. As our awareness expands and we shed old fears, we come closer to unity and the Universal Heart. This in turn leads to an increased understanding of the Cosmos, and access to other transpersonal chakras. As our understanding grows, we begin to sense not only *how* the Cosmos is as it is, but perhaps why. *Jude Currivan PhD.*

DOH YAH NOH correlates to the 8th chakra known as "The Seat of the Soul" and is the sentinel that surrounds the aura protecting it from toxic energies and unwanted influences working deeply to protect vulnerable areas within the aura as they heal. It also can be sent to surround the outer layer of Earths auric field to transmute and dissolve negative thought forms or the manifestation of thought forms that no longer serve the highest good of the planet and the human collective by raising the conscious awareness to that contained within the divine blueprint for this planet. DohYahNoh seals the aura by expanding over and around your energy fields encapsulating them within its protective seal. I found during meditations and Reiki sessions that it at times surrounds the aura protecting one from other's negative thoughts and unwanted influences as it works deeply to protect vulnerable areas within one's spiritual, mental, and emotional bodies as one healed until they had learned how to protect themselves. It has the ability to keep negativity out of your energy fields by shifting your thoughts and perceptions to those of a more positive spiritual context. If activated during any type of healing and or personal spiritual work it remains as a seal until the healing or spiritual work has taken root and has become embodied. It also acts as a shield against outside negativity vibrations that bombard one's subtle bodies helping one to become immune to the negative effects the toxicity that our environment radiates.

I use DohYahNoh when creating sacred space around myself or the environment where I am doing Kun Qi Kung. I find that it allows me to remain more highly attuned to the elements of life force within the environment while meditating in movement versus noticing the distractions that people, cars, and the world around me can create. Also, I find that sealing myself within Dohyahanoh whenever I go out into the public domain, helps me to create a subtle yet powerful barrier against the toxic influences helping to naturally divert the attention of others away from me almost as if I become invisible to those whom would disturb the peaceful presence that I choose to reside in.

As a personal exercise, I encourage you to experiment with using Dohyahnoh when creating sacred space around you or the space that you occupy and note the differences that you notice when you do use it and when you do not.

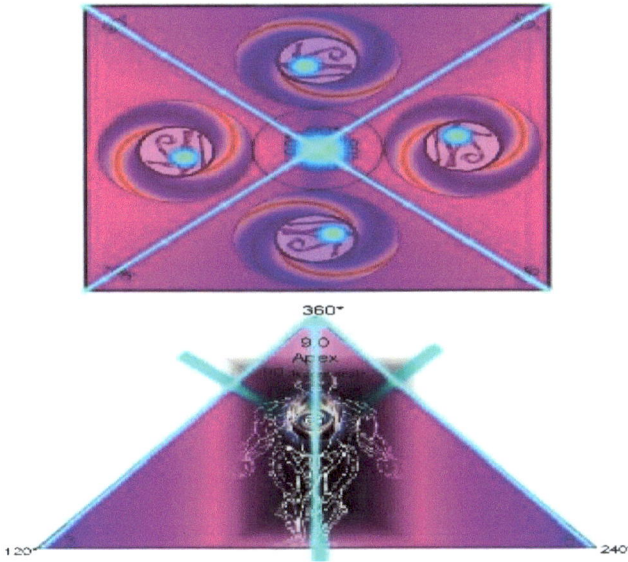

SYMBOL DETAILS:

The eye within the symbol of Dohyahnoh represents the Kemetic all seeing eye of Horus. The Eye of Horus is an ancient Egyptian symbol of protection, royal power and good health. The eye, in its personification, is the Khemetic goddess *Wadjet*.

Within the pupil of the eye is a set of cupped hand holding the symbol of Om. This portion of the symbol represents the sentience and divine intelligence of the healing energy of Reiki to identify the negative energies and to create the protective field around the aura and the mind after separating the energies from the field. Zeegahnah is also used for this purpose but with the added benefit of recycling the negative energies that are being removed rather than having them float around.

The triangle or pyramid that surrounds it reflects the triune aspects of pure wisdom, unconditional love and absolute truth amongst other universal triune associations that we possess.

KUN QI SYMBOL MEDITATIONS:

Sit or stand in a comfortable position that allows your chakras to align vertically. Once comfortable, begin to engage deep slow circular breathing to clear and focus your mind. Bring your inner awareness to the sound of your breath while simultaneously noting any areas of tension in the body. Upon your next inhalation breath into the area of tension and allow it to relax upon exhalation unto you are fully relaxed. Visualize the symbol of Dohyahnoh surrounding you as depicted in the image below. Feel yourself encapsulated within its triangle. Visualize the eye of Horus in front of you, behind you, below you, and to each side of you while sensing its protection and healing energy as you breathe. With each inhalation, breathe more of its loving, healing, protection and with each exhalation send out your love and gratitude, giving thanks for its protection as you heal and its insights of divine wisdom as to how to protect yourself as you implement the guidance given for your healing process. You may perform the 8 directional cipher movement meditation with this symbol for the bindu chakra. Or, if you feel guided, you could do it for each chakra individually as a complete chakra re-attunement to the symbol. You can either inhaling it in or exhaling it out as you move into each direction. Make sure to perform one complete 8 directional cipher per each chakra. Or you may perform this meditation as a seated meditation focusing deeper on the symbol by feeling its around you and meditating on its characteristics, functions and attributes working to heal and protect you within whatever situation comes to mind.

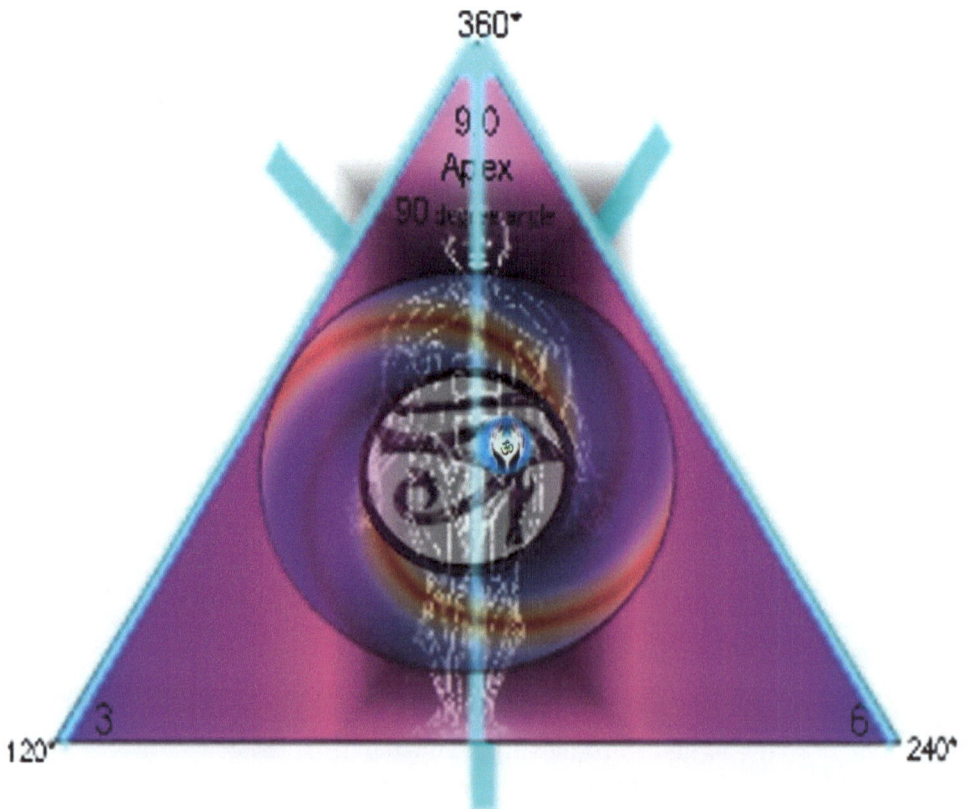

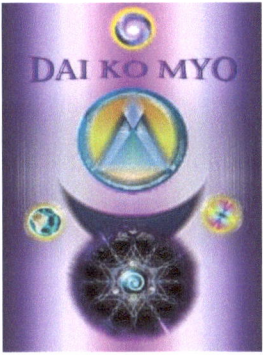

SYMBOL: DAI KO MYO
CHAKRA: CROWN
TONAL NOTE: B
ESSENTIAL OILS: 3 Wise Men, Acceptance, Release, Frankincense And Myrrh.
STONES: Amethyst, Diamond, Alexandrite, Quartz, Selenite.

MUDRA(S) - Gyan

 Apaan

SYMBOL ATTRIBUTES:

It is the Center of spirituality, enlightenment, and reveals the Unity and Higher wisdom of life and to the center of devotion to spiritual and personal matters, dynamic thought, and energy. DAI KO MYO brings the gift of cosmic consciousness and the inward flow of wisdom from the ethers enabling one to see the truth concerning illusory ideals within one's life, materialistic pursuits, self-limiting concepts, and delusion. It allows one to experience continuous self-awareness and conscious detachment from personal emotions, and to have Unconditional love for self, and all sentient beings through humanitarianism, service, spiritual values, and a true sense of oneness.

When out of balance, there will be feelings of disconnection from the Divine, lack of purpose, and inability to see the Light within oneself. When in balance one is able to become One with the Divine; to experience ones connection and sense of purpose with the Divine plan. The anatomy related to this chakra Cerebral Cortex, Pineal Gland, Central Nervous System, Right eye, skin and muscle systems, depression, sensitivity to the environment, energy/exhaustion problems. The tonal note for the Crown Chakra is B and is vocalized with "EEE". The colors associated to the crown chakra are Violet which represents royalty in enlightenment and the search for attainment of the true meaning of spirituality, life, and existence and Golden White which reflects the state of perfection in the body, mind, emotions, and spirituality.

SYMBOL DETAILS:

The components of Daikomyo depicted in the chart reflect the way in which the symbol aligns within the body. The top sphere over the crown ad 1st eye area represents how the connections we have with the cosmic collective and the Divine Source of Intelligence from which knowledge, wisdoms, and innerstandings are communicated to us through our spirits into our minds. The small light sphere in the center reflects the knowledge of our divine blueprint, ancestral and cellular memory that resides within our DNA and is responsive to the sentient healing energy of Daikomyo. The small sphere at the feet represents the way in which we materialize the healing insights, knowledge and information through physical form such as the integration of herbs, certain foods or activities into our daily practice to improve our condition of health and well being. The larger half moon and spiraling sphere reflects the way in which we receive Divine energy and intelligence and the way in which it is circulated through the chakra centers into the organs and body mechanisms that circulate and regulate this information subconsciously.

119

KUN QI SYMBOL MEDITATION:

Bring your attention to your breath drawing it in deeply, slowly, and rhythmically. Once you've relaxed your body through circular breathing bring your minds focus on activating Daikomyo. Again, the symbols can become 4 dimensional especially during meditation so you can also envision them in this way or start with envisioning Daikomyo in front of you, either is fine. See yourself inside the symbol with the cosmic sphere above your crown chakra, the receptive half moon right at the crown or 1st eye, the cellular sphere encompassing both the navel and root chakras, and the earthly sphere below your feet. You may feel the spiral expand to encompass you or you may feel it moving through the chakra and nervous system spiraling in sync with your breath cycling from crown to root, to 1st eye to navel, from navel to throat to solar plexus to heart at which point it radiates outwardly and throughout your body.

Start by envisioning the cosmic sphere above your head above or through your bindu chakra radiating its energy outward. As you sink deeper into the sentience of the symbol see the energy of the cosmic sphere above your head and inhale its radiant light, down towards the receptor at your crown filling the receptor with its intelligence, and wisdom. Exhale its life force intelligence that has gathered and built up within the receptor down from the crown through the center of the spiral into the 2nd sphere that lies over the navel and root chakras. This is where our celestial, cellular and ancestral memory are said to reside within the body. As you focus your inner vision on the cellular sphere centered between the root and navel chakra spend some time focused within this sphere. Next inhale all that was activated up through the spiral into your 1st eye. Once the 1st eye is activated open yourself to the energy within Daikomyo allowing it to activate the cellular memory more visually, even letting it take you on a journey of various celestial, ancestral, and life memories. It may be as if you are watching yourself move through these memories more as an observer yet at the same time the higher purpose and the divine intention of these memories is being revealed in ways that help you to innerstand why and how you had chosen them.

Next exhale slowly and completely down into the navel chakra through the spiral then inhale again up through the spiral into the throat chakra activating its function-ability so that the energy and revelations of Daikomyo may embed into your future thoughts, perceptions, and actions. You may feel guided to also spend some time to allow time to envision yourself interacting and engaging in life and relationship through the divine wisdom and love of Daikomyo as it plays out within your inner vision. When ready, exhale these visions and revelations down into your solar plexus allowing the energy of daikomyo to embed them into your sense of personal power and connection with all within your life then inhale the energy up into the heart chakra letting the feelings of unconditional love, light, and divine intentions to build there then exhale the fullness of this energy and vision out into the universe through your heart.

Continue to repeat this meditation cipher until you feel a sense of completion. Also, this meditation can be performed in sync with the 8 directional cipher movement sequence or it can be done as a seated meditation. Either form will work to create the same results however, combining it with kun qi movements has the added benefit of intensifying the circulation of the energy throughout the body and sending your envisioned intentions outwardly into the universal field.

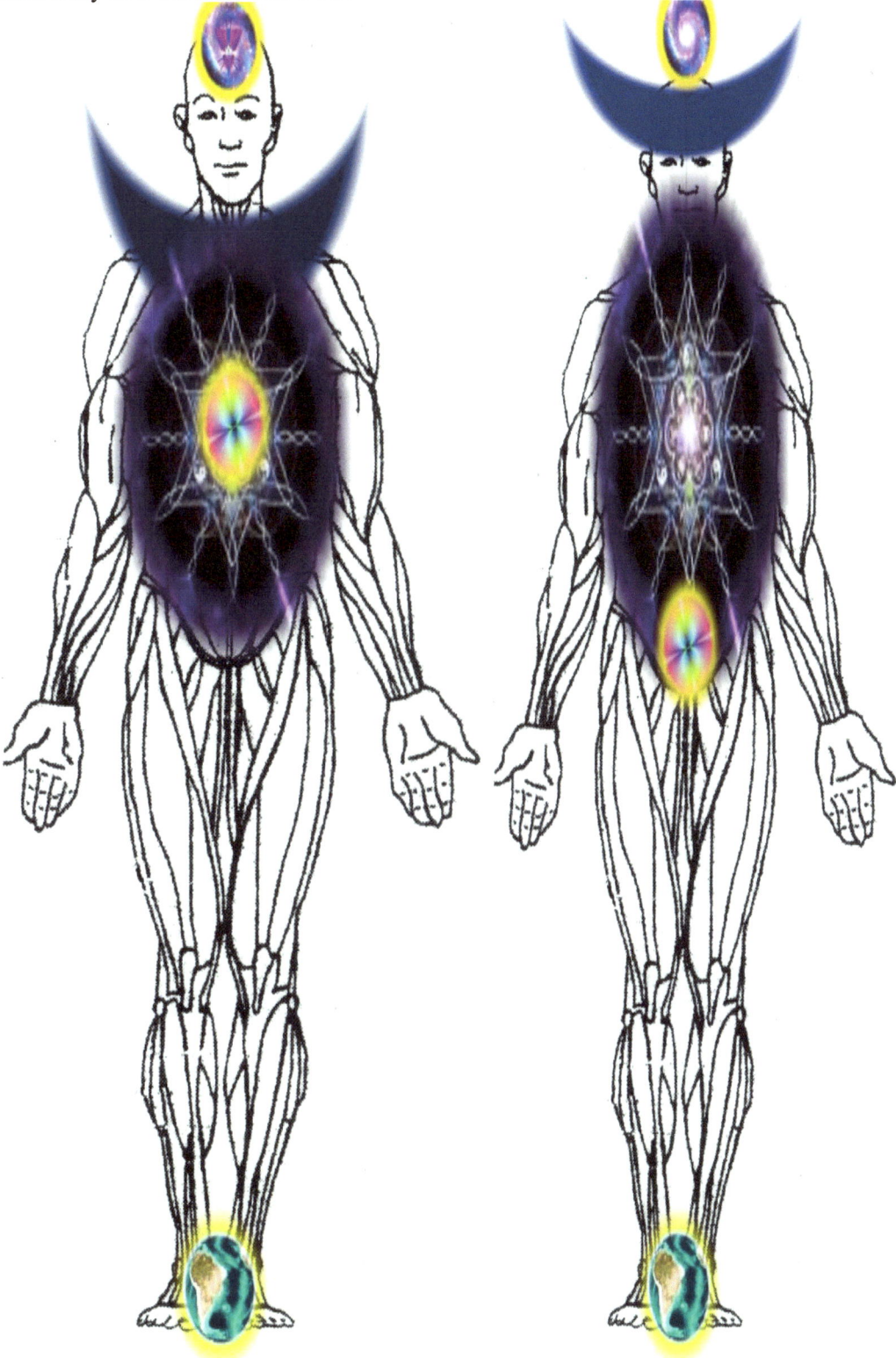

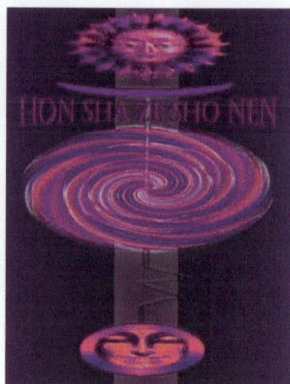

SYMBOL - HON SHA ZE SHO NEN
CHAKRA – 1st Eye
TONAL NOTE: A, A#
ESSENTIAL OILS: 3 Wise Men, Acceptance, Sage, Cedarwood.
3RD EYE CHAKRA STONES: Azurite, Lapis Lazuli, Opal, Sapphire, Sodalite, Topaz.

MUDRA(S): Shunya

Gyan

SYMBOL ATTRIBUTES:

The brow or first eye chakra is the chakra of insight, inner knowingness, and wisdom. Psychic abilities often radiate in this area as well as the heart. This chakra is the center of creativity, intuition, imagination, insight, devotion to spiritual knowledge, and psychic power. It is where higher intuitive information is focused and where wisdom for right intent incubates, where the energies of the spirit, magnetic forces, and light become apparent. The 1st Eye chakra regulates outside guidance and the intuitive "aha", knowledge, intellect, intuitive powers, learning from experience, feeling inadequate, inner wisdom, knowing the higher and lower self as well as self- evaluation, open-mindedness, and the acceptance of oneself and others. It is where the gift of clairvoyance resides where we are able to listen for and see clearly the insights that are being communicated through our senses. When out of balance, there will be denial, and refusing to take responsibility. Quite often when this chakra is blocked there is a lot of confusion. When in balance the ability to see, to own and take responsibility, to be intuitive, and interpret reality clearly.

HON SHA ZE SHO NEN assists in the purification of negative tendencies and in the elimination of selfish attitudes, denial, refusal to take responsibility for one's actions and confusion. HON SHA ZE SHO NEN provides the inner lens to see past the illusion of imperfection in order to relate to all sentient beings from our Godhood with no fear or attachment to what seems to be presenting itself. In truth, we are all Spiritual beings that have chosen differing roles in this play called life on Earth in order to provide us with the opportunities to express the divine love, creativity, and expression of life that we are. Hon Sha Ze Sho Nen also is used as a means to perform remote healings sending our love and healing intentions and prayers to those to whom they are open to receive them. This powerful healing symbol, of many Reiki lineages, aligns us to the Divine within ourselves and to recognize the Divinity in others and within all life itself.

The anatomy related to this chakra Cerebellum, pituitary and pineal glands, liver, gallbladder, nose, ears, left eye, central nervous system, learning problems, spinal problems, hearing problems, tinnitus, and eye problems. The color associated to the 3rd eye is Indigo Blue which represents Attainment, psychic abilities, clairvoyance, the search for spiritual knowledge and insights, and those who search for the spiritual purpose of life.

SYMBOL DETAILS:

The top sphere represent the Higher Self/Mind or Spiritual Self and the divine sentient wisdom and vision that it possesses activating the pineal and pituitary glands. The half moon represent a receptical that the intelligence of the Higher Self funnels down into your conscious awareness through the portal of the 1st eye chakra(s) activating the cerebellum as it prepares to move down into and through the body.

The spiral represents the way in which the healing energy cycles within and through the chakra and nervous systems of the body. As its moves thorugh the chakra, meridians, and organs of the body it simultaneously identifies where outdated thought forms and repressed memories of trauma or disorder reside that one has become ready to address and brings to light the higher truths and purposes for the experiences into one's awareness. Honshazeshonen is used to perform this process, (sometimes along with the soul retrieval symbol of Ehleah). Most of the time it does this on a subconscious level but when it brings the subconscous to the conscious awareness it does so in a way that allows one to observe the internal awakening and transmutation without reliving the emotional scarring that took place with it. The lower sphere represents the lower self or the soul in which the Higher mind directs its wisdom and healing energies in order to impliment its wisdom.

KUN QI SYMBOL MEDITATIONS:

Sit or stand in a comfortable position that allows your chakras to align vertically. Once comfortable, begin to engage deep slow circular breathing to clear and focus your mind. Bring your inner awareness to the sound of your breath while simultaneously noting any areas of tension in the body. Upon your next inhalation breath into the area of tension and allow it to relax upon exhalation unto you are fully relaxed. Visualize the symbol of Honshazeshonen within your mind as it activates inside your 1st eye chakra. Allow it to expand through you until the top sphere is above your head covering your bindu and crown chakras, the half-moon receptor is either at the 1st eye and the spiral is covering your remaining chakras. The lower sphere resides below your feet or within your root chakra. As you continue to breathe envision drawing the divine intelligence, wisdom, insights, visions, knowledge and love of your Higher Self to cycle down through your chakras during inhalation and during exhalation envisioning the energy flowing down into the lower sphere or lower self. Continue to allow the symbol to share its insights and messages with you while encapsulated in its energies until you feel a sense of completion. Make sure to note what came to your awareness so that you don't lose any of the guidance shared. Below is a sample diagram of the ways in which Hon Sha Ze Sho Nen has shown itself to work within each chakra to facilitate the purifiction of the energies within each one. It works in the same flow as depicted. The Wisdom of the Higher Self drops down from the Bindu or 8th Chakra into whichever chakra is in need of purification and re-aligning. The spiral works to transmute all negative or outdated energies into higher consciousness and light which allows one to process the things that are brought to ones awareness in a detached yet unconditionally loving, accepting manner. Thus the lessons and purpose served for what is being released comes to be known without having to relive any of the related trauma or negativity related to what is being released.

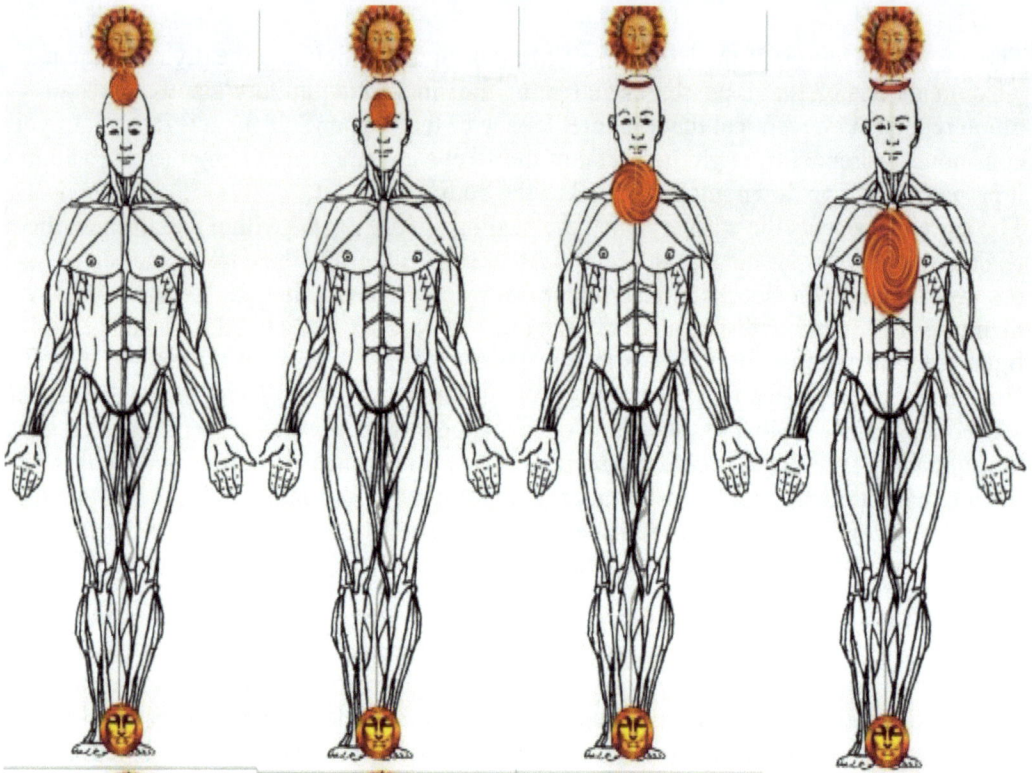

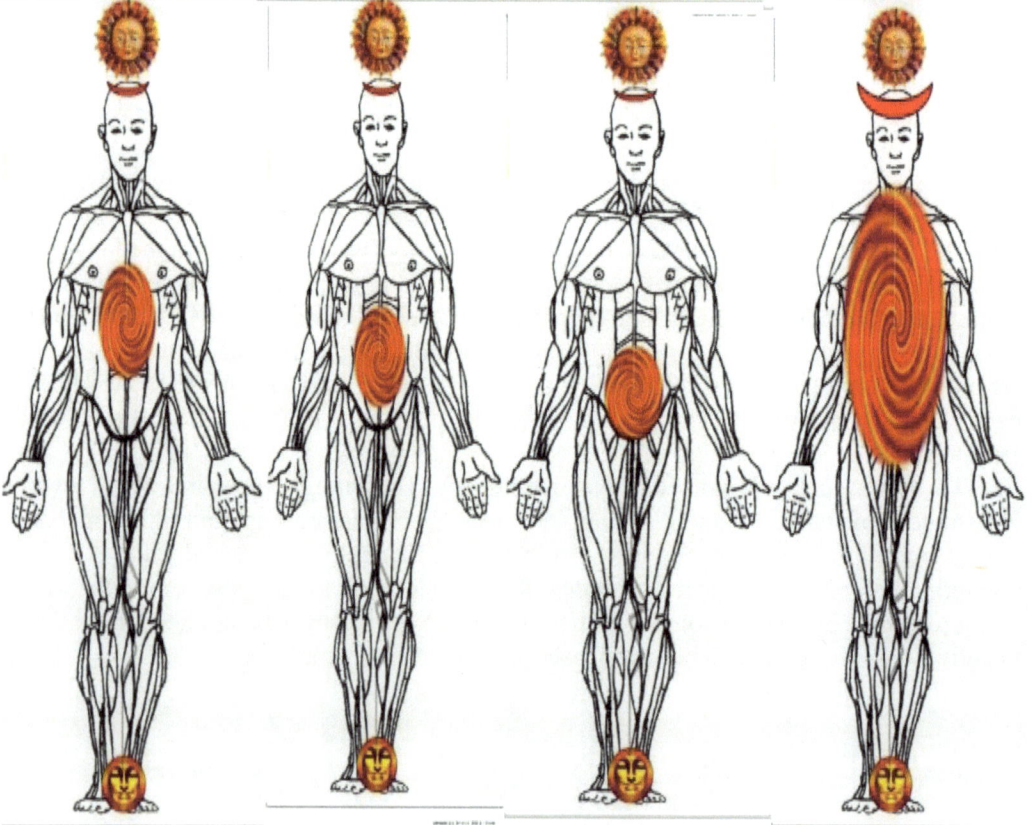

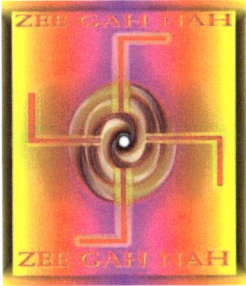

SYMBOL: ZEEGAHNAH
CHAKRA: Throat
TONAL NOTE: G,G#
ESSENTIAL OILS: Sandalwood, Rose, Eucalyptus, Ylang Ylang.
CHAKRA STONES: Aquamarine, Turquoise,

MUDRA(S): Vayu Another Mudra is Ling

SYMBOL ATTRIBUTES:

There are laws that govern transformation, the space between the death of one state of being to the birth of another. These laws apply to each moment throughout eternity and affect emotional energies. Zeegahnah represents these laws as they pertain to the emotions of anger, fear, sorrow and their transmutation into love, faith, peace and joy. The Throat chakra is the chakra of externalization; the center that controls all forms of expression & communication such as speech, dance, artistry, crafting, music, and movement. The inner ability to Express oneself, speak one's truth, follow one's dreams and be true to oneself as well as the drive to act upon addictions, habits, judgment, faith, decisions knowing and being yourself, criticism, will power, doing what you said you would do, knowledge, wisdom, kindness comes from this chakra center. Though it would seem that this would come from either the 1st eye or the heart, the throat is the center from which we speak our thoughts, beliefs and feelings into existence and the center that allows us to take in the Spirit of life (breath) which provides energy in order to act out these things and the understanding of both verbal and mental communication.

When the throat chakra is out of balance, there will be suppression, fear of making mistakes, inhibited self and growth or the opposite of constantly talking and monopolizing conversations, venting of criticisms and judgmentalism. When in balance the ability to communicate, express one's thoughts and passions unhindered and radiate the essence of one's divine sense of self through creative expression will flow consistently into all that one does.

SYMBOL DETAILS:

ZEE GAH NAH's three bands represent holding chambers that transmute our egoic tendency to suppress the emotional dimensions of our physical experiences that relate to anger, fear, and sorrow and the process of transcendence of these three emotions in the following ways. The first or outer band represents our anger. The root of anger relates to control issues of the ego which at its root wants everything in life to go the way it desires for it to go as well as through whom it feels these things should come through. This is the root of what causes conflict between people. When we give up the illusion that we can command, either through aggression or manipulation, the people and things in our lives to do and be what we want them to, and accept those people and things for what they are unconditionally, we are no longer held within this band of death that our anger creates and are able to birth forth ourselves and our lives in a more harmonious way. The second band reflects our sorrows which revolves around having and hold onto the past or the things that we want specifically as we see them versus experiencing and/or envisioning those things that we have had or desire and them letting them go

125

without limiting them by holding onto the details of our inner vision. At the root of sorrow is the essence of hunger, greed and self-esteem issues. When we are able to innerstand that it is our limited beliefs about ourselves and our ability to create what we are wanting out of life that keep us from receiving what we desire. Zeegahnah helps us to transcend the limiting beliefs about ourselves that come from forgetting that we are spiritual in nature and are meant to operate by spiritual truths of our power to experience life as we choose by our actions and responses to it. The third innermost band represents confusion and the feeling of not being able to make a decision concerning a thing. This is the most complex of the three to transcend and become free from thus is why it is the deeper of the bands. The root of confusion is our tendency to identify with the conflict and the conflicting sides of an issue as being outside ourselves and our perspective concerning these things. When we can visualize the issue in its entirety as a whole without feeling the need to control the outcome, then we free ourselves from the perceived issues and confusion then transforms into silence and the peace of not knowing and open to wanting to know without attachment. This transformation enables us to move into the wisdom of the 1st eye and receive illumination.

The central core of all three of these emotions and their conditions is FEAR (False Evidence Appearing Real). Through meditating in movement with ZEEGAHNAH we can transmute these emotions, and our fears of vulnerability or making mistakes into positive externalization of peaceful poise as it guides us through our insights and our ability to visualize and understand the best ways to communicate one's thoughts and feelings in a positive constructive manner. This creates openness and receptivity in others and the world around us. This empowers us to be able to shift from struggling with addictions, habits, judgments, faith, decisions, criticism, etc. sharing our truth of soul, self honor, living our passions, and generating peace and happiness within life.

All aspects of personality are regulated within the throat chakra and purified by ZEE GAH NAH. The anatomy related to this chakra are the vocal cords, throat, mouth and jaw, respiratory system, lungs, large intestine, alimentary canal, thyroid, Neck area, teeth, gums, Esophagus, problems could consist of laryngitis, hiatal hernias, sore throats, choking, gagging, mouth sores, and glandular problems. The colors associated to the throat chakra are Aqua Blue to a deep sky blue which are the colors that reflect knowledge of Oneness and help one to open to Divine guidance, and the clairaudient power we possess to speak our truth.

The images below depict ZeeGahNah working 1st, to bring in positive light filled energy by spinning clockwise, 2nd, spinning counter clockwise to vacuum out and transmute any dark heavy energy one is carrying into light before it is released out of your auric field. And 3rd, to bring Divine spiritual energy into oneself through one's crown and to transmute one's own energy before releasing it into the earth and into the area or environment where one steps. There is a biblical scripture that speaks to how we can draw upon this divine power metaphysically versus in the literal sense that it was used in Deuteronomy 11:24. Our bodies being a conduit of energy and life force are designed to channel energy from and out into the environment. Our feet as well as our hands and mouths are the physical mediums that our bodies use to do so.

126

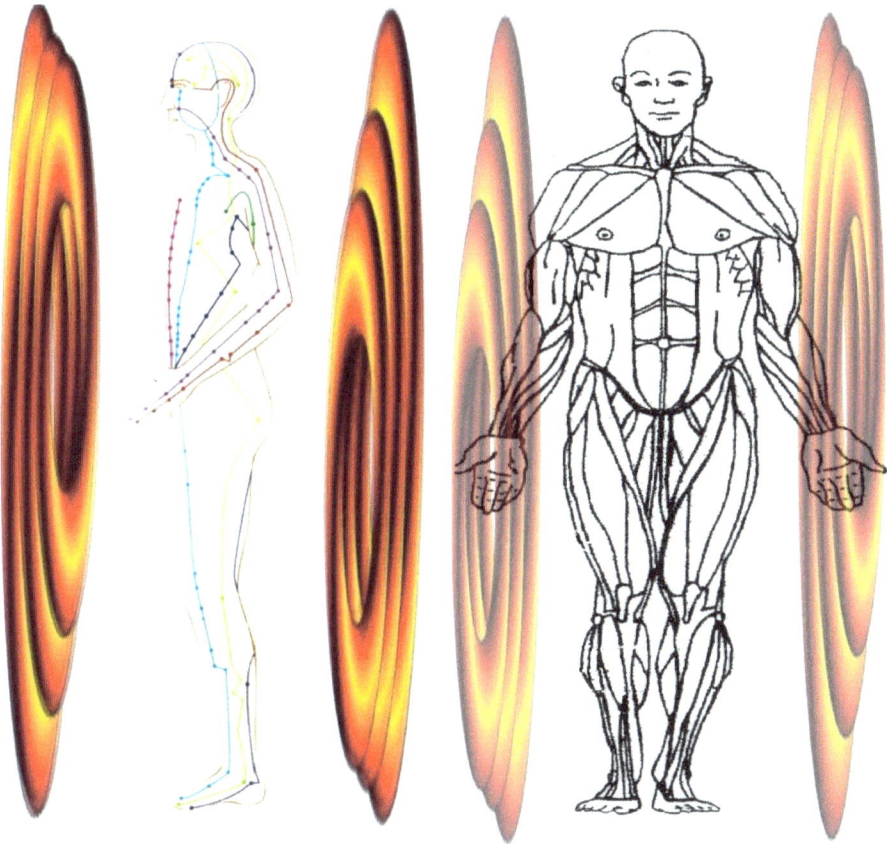

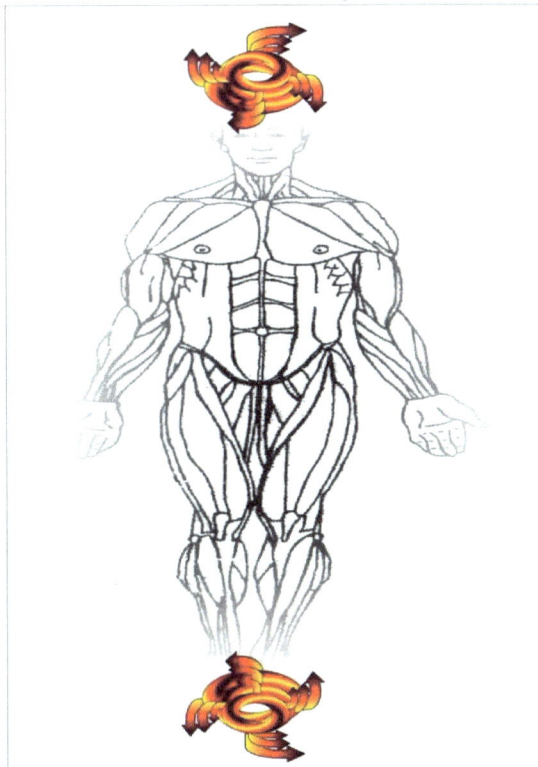

127

KUN QI SYMBOL MEDITATIONS:

Once you've come to relax your body and focus your mind through circular breathing, bring into your minds vision the symbol of Zeegahnah. You may choose to align it within the through chakra or surrounding your body as in the diagrams on the previous page. As with all symbols it may take on a life of its own aligning in the way that is most beneficial for you so allow for it to align in whichever way comes. See within your minds eye which band you find yourself standing within or where you see the bands aligned in respect to your body. Once noted open yourself to is energy and allow it to bring to light any aspects of your life, relationships, or self-view where you are holding anger, sorrow, confusion or fear in relationship to it. When you are clear as to what the energy wants to work on and transform within yourself and your life inhale deeply, the energy of the symbol, step into the direction of southeast and exhale fully as you move into that direction. Continue to work through the 8 directional cipher inhaling the insights, wisdom, and transmutational energy and light within Zeegahnah into your consciousness as you shift backwards or step to turn in another direction and exhale the thoughts, energies, and outdated life forces that no longer serve you, out through the center of the symbol as you move into each of the 8 directions.

You can either continue the 8 directional cipher going through 1 cipher for each chakra and going from crown to root or root to crown. Or you may perform the 8 directional cipher with Zeegahnah until you feel you have transmuted within yourself any negative energies around the situation you are working to clear and can release it with compassionate detachment in peace.

After you have finished the meditation with Zeegahnah, do one more cipher focused on Dohyahnoh in order to seal and protect your auric fields and its energy continues to heal your mind, body, soul, relationships, and life experiences. Below is a diagram depicting some of the ways in which I have used Zeegahnah during meditation and during Tanran Reiki sessions.

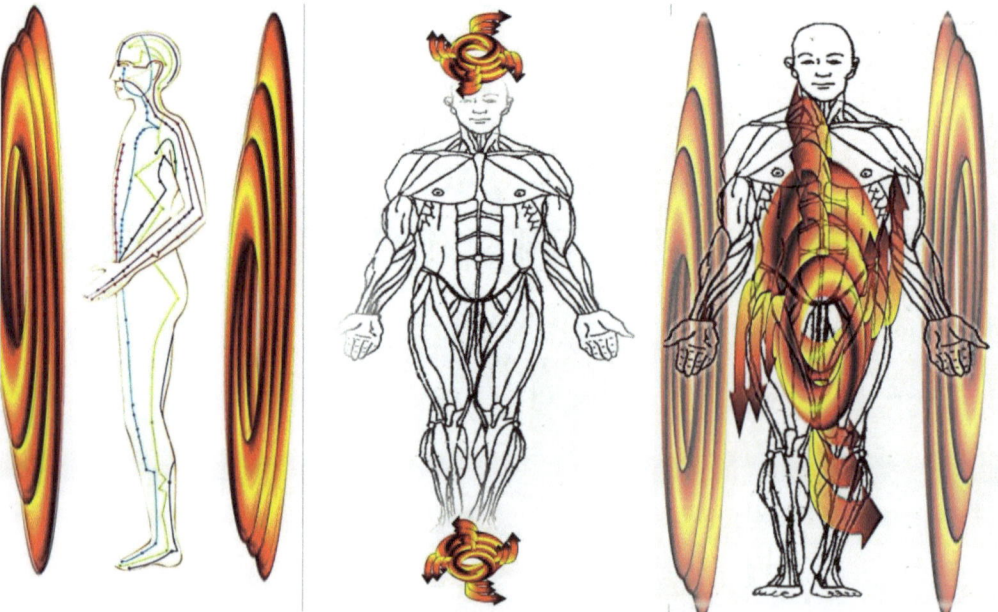

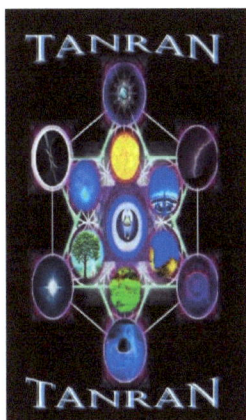

SYMBOL: TANRAN
CHAKRA: Heart
TONAL NOTE: F, F#
ESSENTIAL OILS: Sandalwood, Bergamot, Rose, White Angelica.
CHAKRA STONES: Aventurine, Emerald, Rose Quartz, Moonstone, Peridot, Ruby.

MUDRA(S): Shunya Prana

 Mrit Sanjivini / Apaan Vayu

SYMBOL ATTRIBUTES:

TANRAN aligns within the heart chakra, the center of Divine love, compassion, altruism and acceptance of reality as it is, as well as that of group and universal consciousness within the spirit of unconditional Love. The Heart Chakra is the center of our spiritual connectedness with Divine Source from which we are able to express love without condition and align ourselves with those truths that allow us to resolve for ourselves differences of all types and in all relationships. When the heart chakra is out of balance, the expression of grief is blocked, and there may be feelings of undeserving and grasping for Love. desire for happiness, sadness, anger, hatred, prejudice, loneliness, forgiveness, compassion, hopes, desires, wants, grief, resentments, commitment, trust in your close interpersonal relationships, choices in love and the choice to avoiding Love and commitment even to the self. When in balance, there is indeed compassion and the ability to move into Divine Love, joy and have an ability to give and receive love without fear with the ability to genuinely live in a sense of peace wholeness and abundance.

TANRAN as a vehicle for inter-dimensional travel affects spirit and body simultaneously allowing us to freely access various dimensions of ascended thought during meditation. It helps one to access Divine love, peace, and creativity that resides within our divine Self and ground these qualities into our physical experience.

The anatomy related to this chakra are: Heart, pericardium, lungs, thymus, large intestines, triple warmer, cardiovascular system, blood, cellular structure, involuntary muscles, arms , breathing problems, chest area, breasts, asthma and associated allergies, pneumonia, bronchitis, upper back, shoulder, and arm problems. Light green and pink colors have a soothing, smoothing, healing effect reflecting the softer side of strength, compassion, empathy and loving without condition. They also tend to evoke feelings of ecstasy, exhilaration, joyfulness and fulfilling anticipation.

SYMBOL DETAILS:

The image reflects the sentient life forces as they mirror the elements of life throughout the universe. The inner merkaba represents the elemental life forces of earth that sustain our bodies. These are the components of the earth itself, the mineral kingdom, the plant life, the air, the water, and the heat of the sun. The outer merkaba represents the elements of universal life force that operate within our bodies. The lightning represents the nervous system and its functions. The star is reflective of the light source within our bodies which stores the effects of the sun within the melanin of our skin and represents the cosmic roots within our DNA. The planet Earth at the feet represents the material part of our bodies. The spiral cloud of star dust represents the gaseous air/wind that is generated within our bodies, and the planet of Neptune represents the circulatory movement of blood and nutrients that flow throughout our bodies. The top sphere represents Divine intelligence of the Universe and the Etheric material that all life comes from which reflects the function of the mind as the incubative space from which we generate the thought forms that we materialize into form for our intents and purposes. The center sphere represents sound or vibration which is the tangible link between the earthly and universal elements share in common and that permeate within all form and space. From a spiritual context the upper triangle represents our valuing love, wisdom, and creativity. The lower triangle represents grace, law, and choice. The middle hexagon represents the many sides of our life. Intuition, feeling, thinking, and sensing are the functions which find balance within the symbol. This is where heaven and earth meet in harmony and balance.

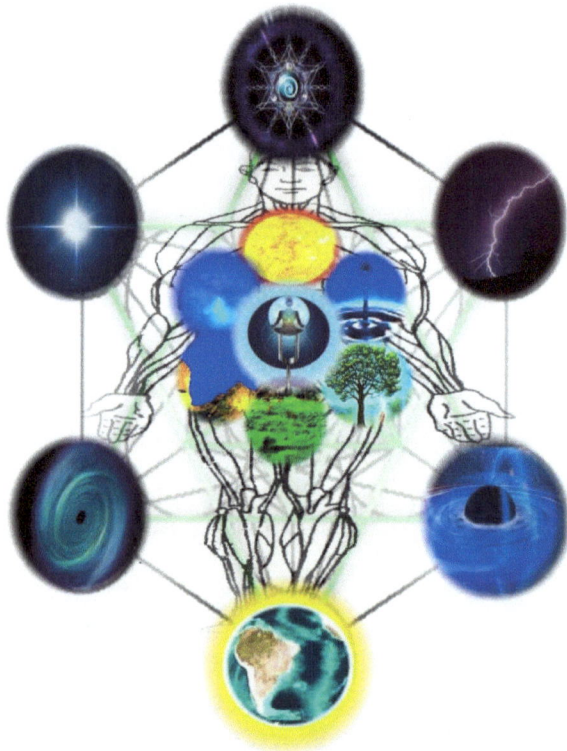

KUN QI SYMBOL MEDITATIONS:

This symbol ca n be meditated on in infinite combinations, on various levels, and in multiple complexities. From divine wisdom, love, and knowledge, to our thoughts, words and deeds; from the elements of the universe to the elements of nature, from past, present, future to spirit, soul, and body the merkabic structure of Tanran is truly a powerful intradimensional medium of spiritual transformation and evolution.

For your first Kun Qi meditation with Tanran we will start by focusing on the elements of nature and/or those of the universe. This meditation helps to awaken ones empathic connection to these elements along with a deeper innerstanding of the sentient intelligence of these elements and how they function within and around us on spirit, soul and body levels. Two of the ways that I have performed the Tanran 8 directional sequence are 1- focusing on one element throughout one 8 directions cipher or 2- attuning the 8 chakras to each element using the 8 directional chakra sequence.

ONE ELEMENT AT A TIME
Begin by activating the Reiki Guides and the Tanran symbol. Once you've become centered in circular breathing bring your attention to one of the elements for instance the Sun. Breathe its essence in through your skin, and/or its embodiment with your eyes as you step out into the direction of southeast. Exhale its essence and energy into the center of your heart to radiate throughout your body as you shift and turn preparing to move into the direction of the northwest. Once facing the northwest again, while breathing in the suns essence and energy, allow it to reveal whatever wisdom or insight comes to mind as you're visualizing and meditating on that element. Then exhale those insights into your heart allowing the suns essence to radiate again throughout your body as you move into the direction of the west. Continue this sun breathing meditation until you've completed the entire 8 directions and are facing the south. Take some time to continue to commune with the sun and the symbol of Tanran until you feel that you have received all that you are meant to receive in insights. Give thanks exhaling your gratitude out into that element through the symbol and prepare to move onto the next cosmic or earthly element within the Tanran symbol.
I find that performing the outer cosmic elements at night and the inner earth elements during the daytime helps deepen one's ability to attune to these corresponding elements and to receive their sentient wisdom and intelligence. However, this Tanran meditation do not require being visible with the physical eye, they can also be performed anytime, anywhere using one's inner vision to visualize and attune to the element.

ELEMENT & CHAKRA ALIGNMENT
This Kun Qi chakra meditation is very similar to the element attunement sequence above however, this Kun Qi sequence attunes the essence of each element to each chakra in ways by which its sentient life force correlates to the characteristics and functions of each chakra.

As with the "One at a Time" element attunement sequence, begin by activating the Reiki Guides and the Tanran symbol. Once you've become centered in circular breathing bring your attention to one of the elements for instance the Sun. Once you feel attuned and enveloped in its energy, breathe its essence, its warmth, and its rays into your Bindu chakra above your head as you step out into the direction of southeast. Allow its essence to ride your breath filling your Bindu chakra, the center of your akashic records with its love, its wisdom, and its warmth. When ready, exhale its essence and energy down into the rest of your physical and subtle bodies allowing it to radiate throughout your body as you shift and turn preparing to move into the direction of the northwest. Once facing the northwest again, while breathing in the suns essence and energy, allow it to reveal whatever wisdom or insight comes to mind as you're visualizing and meditating on the sun and what it represents or speaks to you. Then exhale those insights into the heart of your innerstanding allowing the suns essence to radiate again throughout your body as you move into the direction of the west. Continue this Tanran breathing meditation within your Bindu chakra until you've completed the entire 8 directions and are facing the south. Take some time to continue to commune with the sun and the symbol of Tanran within your Bindu chakra until you feel that you have received all that you are meant to receive in insights. Give thanks exhaling your gratitude out into the sun, the symbol, and the Reiki Guides through your Bindu chakra and prepare to move onto the chakra using the same element until you have done an 8 directional element attunement for all of your chakras sequentially from the Bindu down to the root.

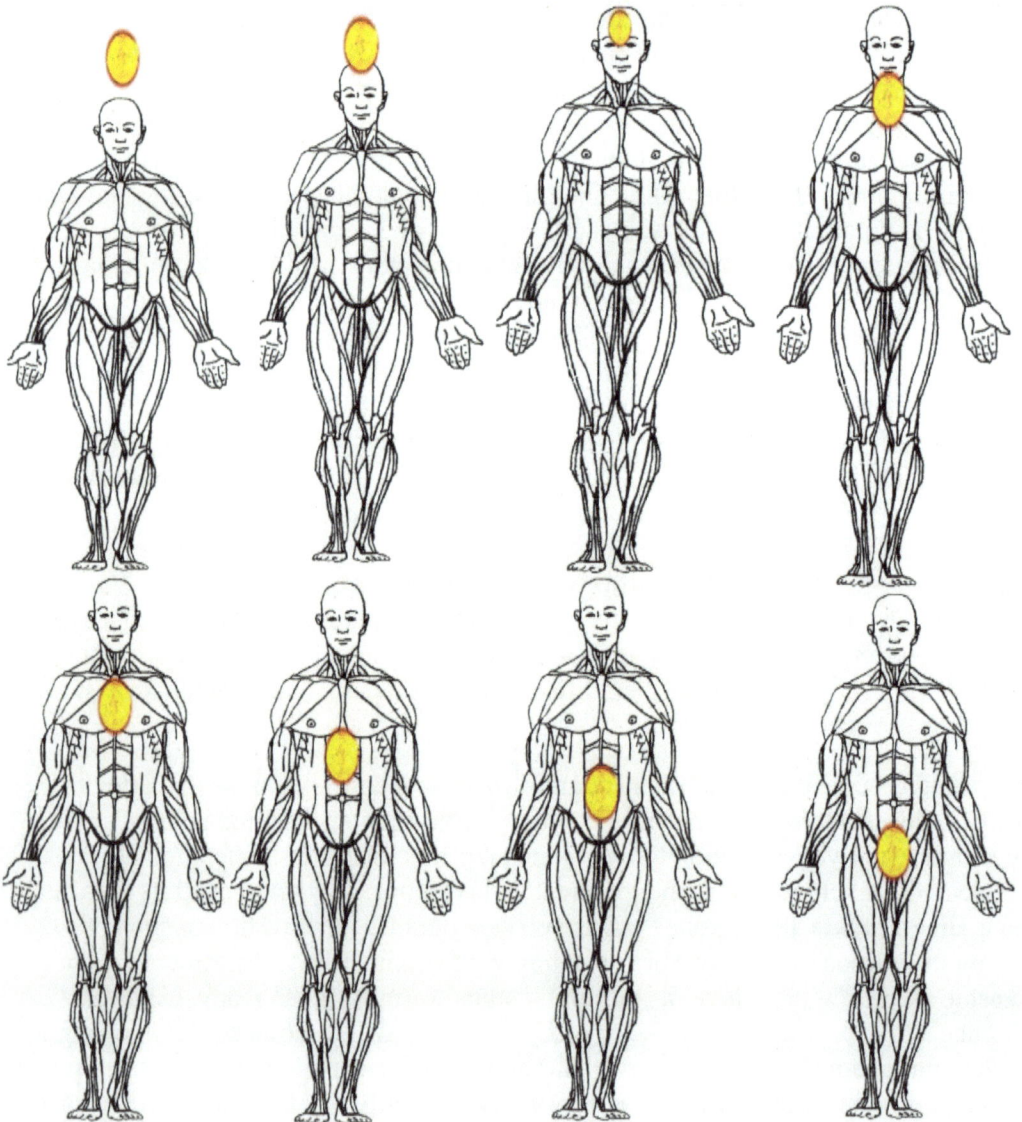

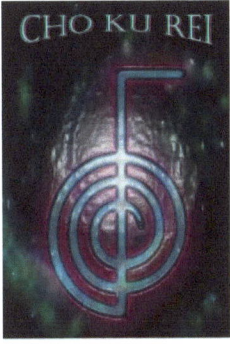

SYMBOL: CHO KU REI

CHAKRA: Solar Plexus
TONAL NOTE: E
ESSENTIAL OILS: Fennel, Cedar Wood, Juniper, Sacred Mountain Blend.
STONES: Agate, Amber, Malachite, And Tigers Eye.

MUDRA(S): 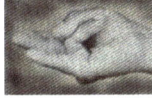 Surya Prithvi

SYMBOL ATTRIBUTES:

CHO KU REI is the basic life force symbol of Reiki and resides within the Solar Plexus chakra the center of personal power, ambition, intellect, astral force, self-respect, willpower, confidence, self-control, physical energy and anger emotionally. Chokurei re-aligns ones sense of personal power to reflect that of their Divine imprint, and is empowered to assist in the healing of our internal and interpersonal views we hold of self and others. It helps one to set appropriate personal boundaries so that one can remain in alignment with their truth energizing and supporting our personal autonomy. It honors our healthy values and burns away what does not serve us ad brings our subjective values into alignment with our objective reality.

Issues with responsibility, caring for others, trust, fear, guilt, career, intimidation, personal honor, victimization feelings, self-concern, self-respect, sensitivity to criticism, self-esteem, self-worth and one's own confidence and courage effect the health and functioning of this chakra. When out of balance, the person may appear to be conceited or have an attacking nature, or prideful and may have either an explosive response or tend to be passive aggressive when it comes to expressing anger. A lot of trust issues are in this chakra, including self-trust. Often childhood issues are stored here, particularly around the navel where birth traumas are stored. Prior to the western medical practice of hospitalization for child birthing, people waited until the umbilical cord had stopped pulsing before it was cut. Now days the umbilical cord is cut immediately after delivery, which does not allow the complete transference of the mother's life force which naturally stopped on its own. This simple act of allowing nature to take its course help greater importance than what the medical field had known. By allowing the umbilical cord to remain attached for an extended period of time was practiced in many indigenous cultures as well as those before modern medicine so that the nutrients within the placenta to be completely transferred to the newborn, and for them to acquire the sense of support and connectedness after such a drastic shift of environments. It can be quite a traumatic experience for newborns to make the transition from the warmth and safety of the womb into a sterile and foreign environment. Also, issues of shame and abuse can tend to get lodge in this area. This is indicated by the way in which we get butterflies, queasiness, or gut feelings in these areas whenever we are feeling emotionally unsafe or uncomfortable with others or with our surroundings. When the solar plexus chakra is in balance, we will have a good sense of self and personal power and have a healthy ego. We are able to respond appropriately to conflict in ways that are constructive and non-aggressive.

Chokurei is used to bring our body to health. The anatomy related to this chakra is the stomach, colon, liver, gallbladder, pancreas, adrenal, immune system, sympathetic nervous system, mid-back, and muscular system. Physical challenges such as diabetes, arthritis, liver problems, eating disorders, indigestion, and any dis-ease related to the associated organs can derive from Solar plexus imbalances. The colors associated to this chakra are yellow or bright gold which reflect meditative analytical thought and intellectual activity as well as power, inner strength and will-power.

SYMBOL DETAILS:

The top "L" shaped hook acts similar to a funneling device with radar capabilities. It pinpoints the energies and insights needed for healing as well as needing healing then draws healthy sentient life force energy down into the lower spiral. The lower spiral acts as a dispensary that spreads love, light, healing life force, and higher consciousness to the areas in need with the support of the universe to create the level of healing that brings about the highest good on all levels simultaneously depending on the level of openness to healing each is. It can be drawn where more life force is needed.

KUN QI SYMBOL MEDITATIONS:

You may find the symbol of Chokurei spinning in various directions, from vertically to horizontally, or circularly from head to toe or moving to specific places within the body as it is the symbol of power, activation and implementation. When spinning vertically with the hook at the top I found that it would create a vortex at the crown drawing divine energy all the way down to the root. This creates a sense of being fully embodied by the higher Self and the sense of operating from one's Divine sense of Self. Spinning with the hook at the feet created a sense of being completely connected with life of Mother Earth, the elements of nature and the life forms within this realm on a deeper sentient level where they were able to share their wisdom, thoughts, and desires for planetary harmony with me telepathically. Insights into the ways that humanity can transform their lifestyles in ways that are more harmonious, respectful, and beneficial to all life forms and ways in which we can reverse the harm we've done as a species to Mother Earth, each other and the environment. When spinning horizontally it created a sense of cleansing the entire subtle and physical body by transmuting unhealthy thought forms and life force into healthy more balances and serene one. I've also witnessed Chokurei moving throughout the body, stopping in various locations of the body to move energy there and to pour light energy into whatever area is needing within both the physical and the subtle bodies with the awareness of what has transpired to create the imbalance it is working on and what one can do to heal whatever condition exists there.

The 8 directional movement meditation with Chokurei, can be performed in the same way as the others; by either envisioning Chokurei cycling within each chakra from crown to root, be envisioning oneself encompassed by the symbol, or by viewing the symbol working in whatever area of the spirit/soul/body that it chooses to work throughout the 8 directional cipher meditation sequence.

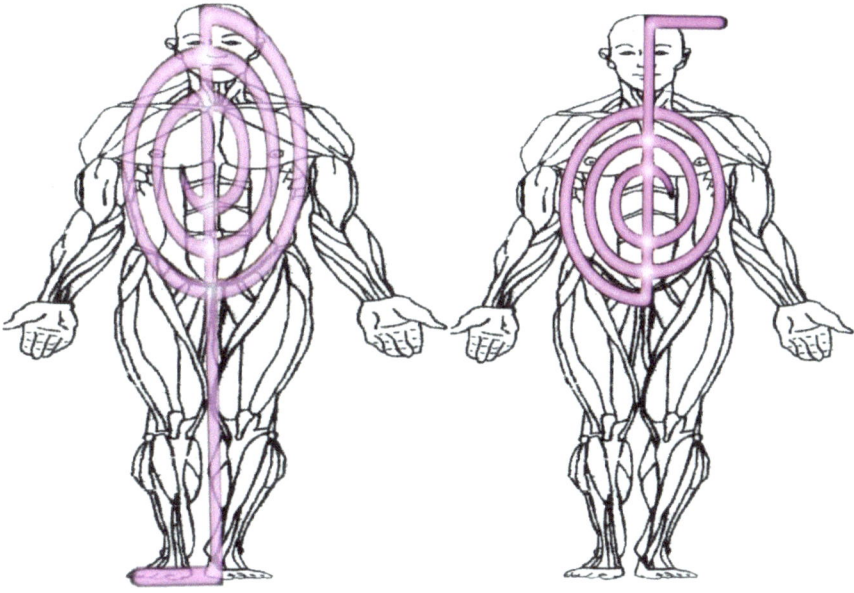

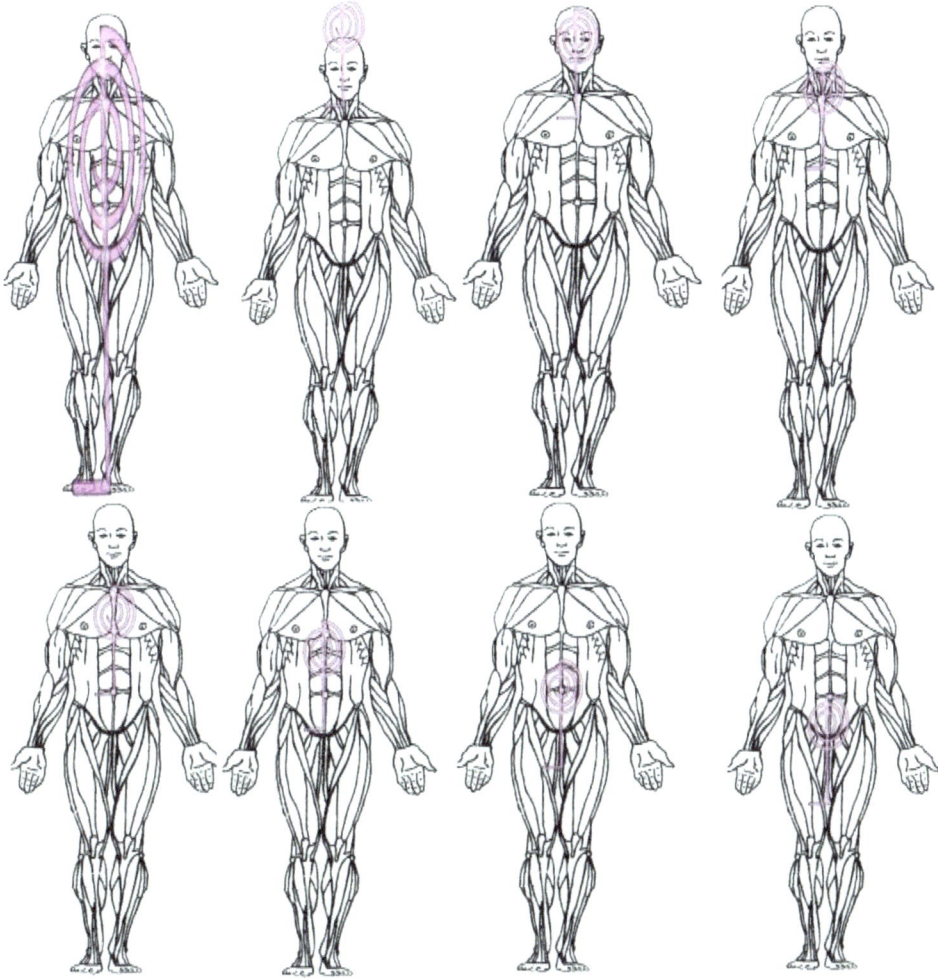

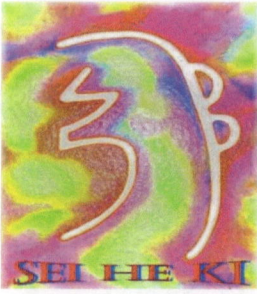

SYMBOL: SEI HE KI
CHAKRA: Navel
TONAL NOTE: D/D#
ESSENTIAL OILS: Sara, Sandalwood, Patchouli, Sage, Acceptance,
STONES: Carnelian, Coral, Yellow Zircon

SEI HE KI

MUDRA(S): Varuna Prana

SYMBOL ATTRIBUTES:

SEI HE KI correlates with the navel chakra, the center of feelings, emotions and their expression, sexuality, desires, creativity and intuition and empathy. Clairsentience is the psychic sense of the 2nd chakra. Power, sexual issues, blame, control, passion, ethics, money, greed, honor in relationship issues, fidelity, feelings of repression or wrongness in sexual matters, reproduction issues and birthing new ideas are all areas of life that associate to this chakra. When out of balance, there will be co-dependency, and inability to freely bond, sometimes even with the self. When more in tune or in balance one will have a sense of belonging, greater tolerance with others and a more balanced and harmonious relationship with the self, others, and our spiritual connection has a more open and fluid interaction. The color associated to the navel chakra is orange, representing wisdom, equity, creativity and benevolence to all life, and Blue/green waters of the Ocean, synthesis of Divine Feminine guidance in the areas of emotional and relationship healing. The anatomy related to this chakra are the ovaries, testicles, prostate, genitals, womb, bladder, digestive system, Gonads, (reproductive hormones) spleen, kidneys, hips, Gluteals, Illiopsoas, and all musculature attached within and around the pelvic girdle. The tonal note that the navel chakra resonates to is D, D# and the vocal sung is "O".

SYMBOL DETAILS:

SEI HE KI assists in the healing of one's emotional past, present, and future perspectives so that one is able to engage in healthy relationships and handle relationship issues that come with compassionate detachment. It pours love into our abandoned child, values our invalidated child and nurtures our deprived child. In the Tanran system Sei He Ki is placed in the belly or navel because this is the chakra center associated with emotional needs and the wanting of emotional support. The external world is based on constant change. We experience gain and loss in each moment as we lose the last moment to gain the next. When we move from one community to another, or one way of life to another we gain new friends and lose old friends. We become healed when we are able to let go of our need for external support, love, and validation, by linking with eternal unconditional love. In eternity, we are all connected together in love. But in space and time, we are limited to one moment at a time. We may cling to old moments inside ourselves, rather than let them go however when we open up to loving ourselves, we begin to attract that which mirrors the love we feel within.

SEI HE KI generates warmth in the belly. It is also a time travel symbol. We can go back to our childhood and our past life issues that we have brought into this life and send love, innerstanding, and healing to places where we did not feel it. We can give ourselves what was not given us then thus heal and transform our sense of self validation, and acceptance. It also is used to heal trauma and imbalances on all levels within the reproductive system.

KUN QI SYMBOL MEITATIONS:

During healing sessions and in meditative movement I at times would witness Sei He Ki enlarge itself to fit the entire body. What I noted was that the inner section of Sei He Ki would align from the head down to the knees with the vertical segment of the inner section connecting between the heart and spleen or the liver and gallbladder. The outer section would align with one of the subtle bodies contracted in or expanded out to align with whichever subtle body was connected to the issue at hand, then it would spin around the entire body at that specific level creating a somewhat centrifugal force around that energetic layer of the body while the inner section seemed to pump in life force from the crown down into the organs from the life force being generated by the outer section. It seemed to me that the work that Sei He Ki was doing was drawing divine life force into the body to dissolve any stagnant emotional debri that had been built up in the organs and to transmute them not only within the organs but the areas within the mental/emotional bodies that they had become lodged as outdated memory triggers. I believe that this action the symbol was making was allowing fresh new space for the persons higher mind to come to innerstand the higher purpose for their past experiences so that they could then use them to help in the healing of others and the positive evolution of their future goals and visions of life.

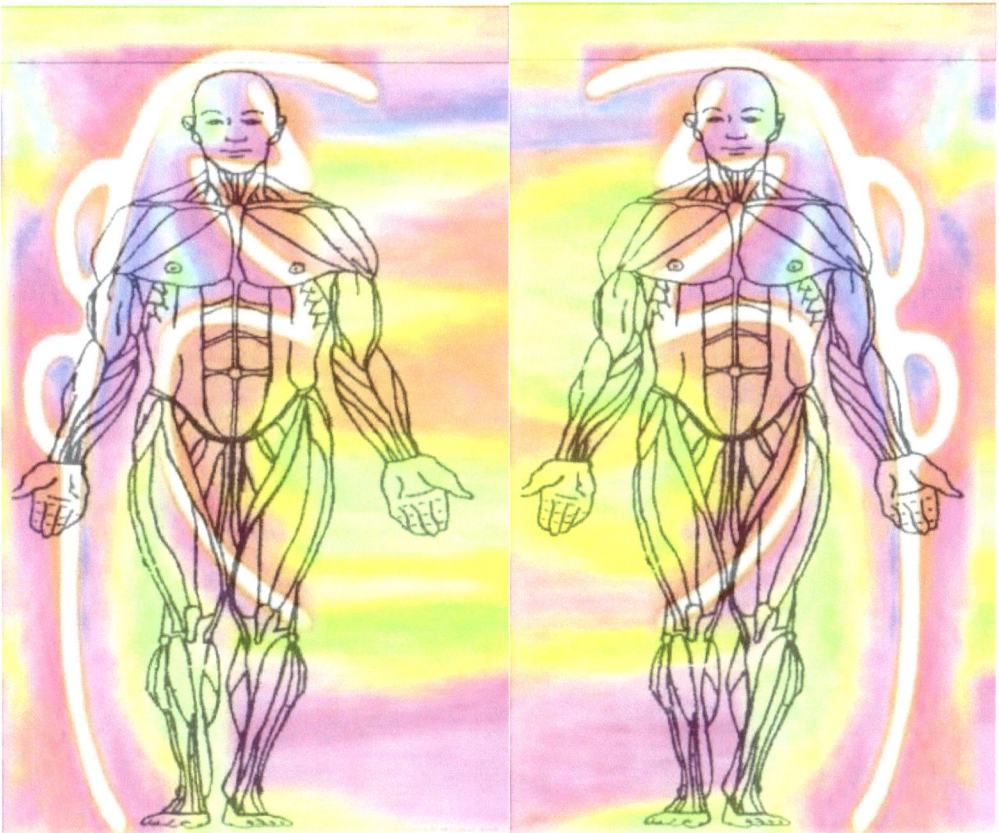

137

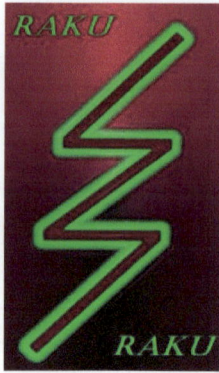

SYMBOL: RAKU
CHAKRA: ROOT
TONAL NOTE: "C/C#"
ESSENTIAL OILS: Western or Canadian Red Cedar Sandalwood, Patchouli, Ylang-Ylang,
STONES: Bloodstone, Chrysocolla, Lodestone, Smoky Quartz. Rutilated Quartz (All) – Aids Development of Personal Potential, Commitment To Others, Connects Past And Future.

MUDRA(S) Gyan Ahamkara

SYMBOL ATTRIBUTES:

RAKU harnesses and grounds our primal life force and animalistic instinct and can empower one to transcend fear-based survival coping mechanisms as we meditate more on the spiritual aspects that it symbolizes. It nourishes our sense of belonging, our connection to family, community and our oneness with life. Raku also stimulates our evolution and positive change to make room for new experiences and regulates the process so that we are not overwhelmed and can transcend outdated ways of living and interacting that no longer serve our best interest or phase of life.

SYMBOL DETAILS:

RAKU correlates with the Root Chakra where the seat of our animalistic survival instincts and programming resides. This symbol relates to primal and past life memories, family, marriage, parenting, correct behavior, society, and our ability to provide basic needs for living. When this chakra is distorted or out of balance, it is due to the traumatic experiences that were repressed in order to cope with the situation at that time. The behavior patterns that were developed as a defense or a protection become imbedded in our subconscious becoming an unconsciously trained response throughout our lives until we are willing and able to look more deeply at our behavioral patterns that are not serving us and find ways to correct them. Fear, timidity, paranoia, anger, anxiety, in general fears of the unknown, and trust issues that derive from past betrayals create a subtle inability to stay present and connected with the flow of life or to be open in relationships. When this chakra is in balance, there will be a feeling of safety, security, stability, desire to maintain or acquire physical health and/or sense of well-being, willingness to connect with others more intimately, and to embrace life's experiences.

The color associated to the root chakra is a deep dark almost blood red reflecting ancestral bloodline; one's genetic roots. This color reflects stability, grounding, security of belonging, and a confidence in one's innate passion for life. The anatomy associated to this chakra are the legs, bones, spinal column, blood, immune system, kidneys, colon, urinary Bladder, and supra adrenal gland. The tonal note that the root chakra resonates to is C, C# and the vocal sung is HU.

KUN QI SYMBOL MEDITATIONS:

While working with Raku in meditation and during healing sessions the symbol became animate and started to align with other symbols in ways that revealed more deeply the way in which the energetic aspects of each symbol align with each other to provide what was needed by the client. Also, the way in which they combined and aligned brought to me a deeper understanding and firsthand experience of how sentient the sacred geometry of the symbols are and the ways in which they work together to provide exactly what is needed at the time.

The following are some ways in which Raku works with other symbols.

1. **Dai Ko Myo & Raku** – removes the learned tendency to over analyze and judge restoring our innate primal ability to trust our first thought and follow it. Restoring the power of our original natural survival and familial instincts.

2. **Raku along the spine** – readjusts physical misalignments along the spine into the sacrum and Illiopsoas helping to posturally readjust imbalances within the pelvic region.

3. **Dai Ko Myo & Raku along the entire body** – when karmic residue was being worked out Raku would align from the Bindu (the temple of human cleansing of outdated patterns of personal consciousness) down through the entire body into the chakras of the feet aligning

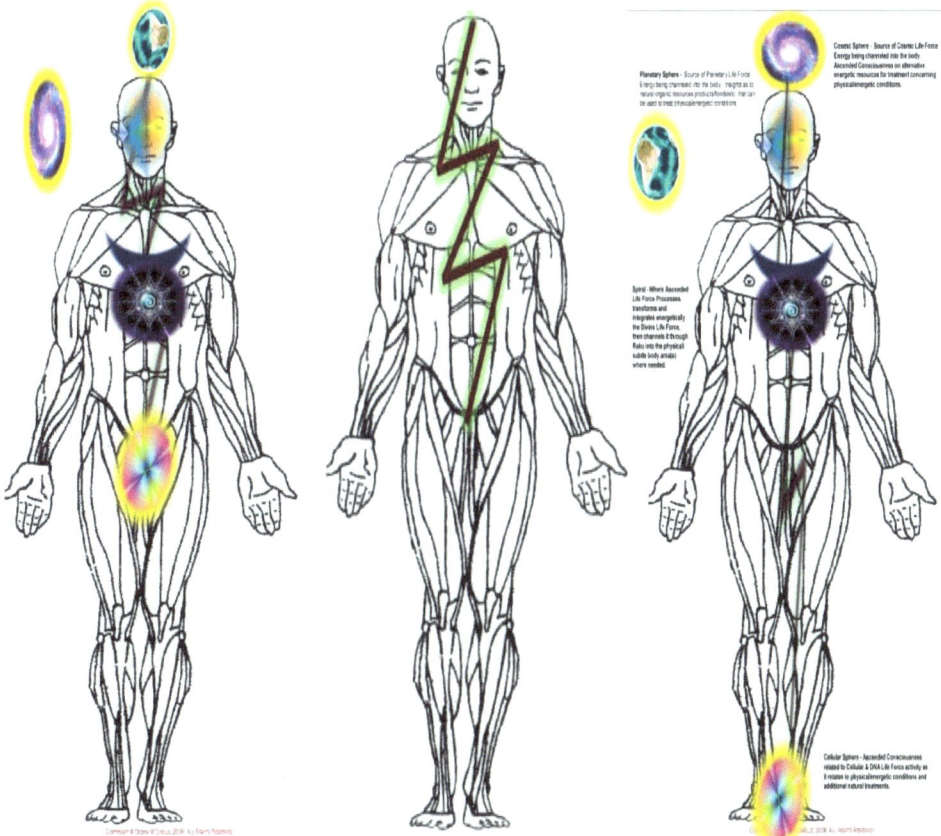

139

SUMMARY

The beginning of this book was designed to introduce you to ways to intentionally heal the body through conscious awareness of the sentient intelligence of Life Force within its various embodiments, our connection to each and the means by which we were originally designed as a combination of their sentient attributes through meditative movement techniques. Some of the meditative movement sequences were designed by Fabien Manman Tama-do Academy of Sound Color & Movement. The intentional meditative aspect of these sequences I have added in order to deepen the healing affects by one conscious intentions, and meditative aspects of these movements and to awaken and restore within you the awareness of our original harmonious alignment with Mother Earth and The Wombniverse.

The second half was designed to introduce you to the ways that Tanran Reiki is used to heal, awaken and increase the embodiment of one's own personal divine blueprint as well as to participate in the healing, awakening and aligning of the same divine blueprint in all sentient life forms on earth. the of within the Kun Qi Kung Series, to deepen the healing effects of the movements internally and externally on the physical, mental, emotional, and spiritual levels of the chakra system and how the two relate. Tanran Reiki can consciously through our desires and intentions, transform our life experiences into more productive pro-active states of being. Tanran Reiki combined with the 8 Directional Cipher movements is a very effective self-healing tool that can help you to accomplish this. The following material will provide you with a deeper innerstanding of what Tanran Reiki is, the process by which one can become attuned to utilize its healing energy and its implementation into the Kun Qi Kung meditative movement series.

These sacred symbols reflect the Divine spiritual healing essences of those that were once commonly used during the Atlantian, Lemurian Era to transmit the Divine Aspects of The Source of all Creation, as part of the daily teachings and spiritual practices within the temple systems that existed then. The essence of these images and the transformative power they possess lies within the vibrations of their sacred geometrical arrangement and the sentient intention of Divine Enlightenment that Reiki radiates through them.

These prints are blessed and attuned to the life force of Tanran Reiki, and the Universal Source. When used as tools of meditation and visualization their energy becomes alive. They possess the power to activate one's divine intentions for healing and enlightenment and to positively restructure one's life to align with one's divine blueprint and purpose as a spiritual being. Many have found the symbols enable them to transcend various limitations in consciousness effortlessly just by setting the intention and without having to direct them. Reiki Artistry is sentient and has the ability to purify the energy within the environment they are displayed in. All one need do is to be open to receiving the miraculous and let go of what no longer serves them.

Prints are made without titles imbedded in them but can be purchase with labels when specifically requested. All prints are available as a limited edition on canvas, acrylic, or metal print that complement the 3 dimensionality of the artistry. Framed glass, glossy prints, calendars, cards and other various healing artistry items are also available in various sizes and can be ordered. To place an order and for customized sizing please visit our website below.

Thank you for your interest and support of this artistry may you find this artistry to be a source of healing, Self-realization, and enjoyment.

VERBAL IMAGERY SPIRITUAL ARTS & PROMOTIONS
www.d-mchelle.artistwebsites.com
dmchelle@gmail.com

Artistry by D'MChelle
Information on Tanran Symbolism by William Bagley & D'MChelle

KUN QI APPENDIX TABLE OF CONTENT

SECTION FOUR – APPENDICES

I.   **APPENDIX A – KUN CHI QI KUNG EXERCISES**
     a.   BREATHING TECHNIQUES & BODY WARM UP   141
     b.   KUN QI MERIDIAN QI CIRCULATION MEDITATION   145
     c.   SEQUENCE I - JOINT ACTIVATION   148
     d.   SEQUENCE II - TAO YIN FA   153
     e.   SEQUENCE III –- SITUATIONAL CLEARING   158
     f.   SEQUENCE IV - CHAKRA ACTIVATION   161

II.   **APPENDIX B – CHARTS & DIAGRAMS**
     a.   UPPER BODY MERIDIAN CHART   162
     b.   LOWER BODY MERIDIAN CHART   163
     c.   ACUPRESSURE POINTS CHART   164
     d.   QI CIRCULATION DIAGRAM   165
     e.   7 PHASE ELEMENNTAL CHAKRA/MERIDIAN CHART   166
     f.   SUBTLE BODY LAYERS DIAGRAM   167
     g.   CHAKRA ANATOMY CHART   168
     h.   CHAKRA ANATOMY DETAILS CHART   169
     i.   PERIODICAL TABLE   172
     j.   HAND REFLEXOLOGY CHART   173
     k.   ELEMENTAL HAND CHART   174
     l.   8 DIRECTIONAL CHART   175
     m.   ORISHA TANRAN ELEMENTAL ASSOCIATION CHART   176
     n.   ORISHA ATTRIBUTES   177

III.   **APPENDIX C – HEALING MUDRAS WITH DETAILS**   180
IV.   **APPENDIX D –**
     a.   **CHAKRA COLORS VOCAL TONATIONS, ESSENTIAL OILS & GEMSTONES**   186

V.   **APPENDIX E – CREATING SACRED SPACE TECHNIQUES**
     a.   INVOKING THE 7 DIRECTIONS SACRED SPACE TECHNIQUES   188
     b.   ANIMAL TOTEM DETAILS   194

VI.   **APPENDIX F – CREATING SACRED SPACE WITH TANRAN REIKI**
     a.   TANRAN REIKI SACRED SPACE INVOCATION   198
     b.   TANRAN ATUN-MENT PRAYER & HEALING SALUTATION   200

APPENDIX A
KUN CHI EXERCISES & TECHNIQUES

BREATHING TECHNIQUES

There are two forms of breath work that are used during the meditative movement sequences and sacred space activation. Each breathing technique has a specific purpose in its application. Circular breathing is used during the body warm up exercise, joint activation sequence, and 8 directional movement sequences. With circular breathing one keeps a deep continual flow of breath <u>without</u> holding the breath at either end of the inhalation or exhalation. In the 8 directions format of meditative movement the direction changes are performed in sync with one's breathing thus allowing for one to create an outer and inner rhythm that unifies conscious and ultra-conscious thought taking one deeper into the altered states of meditation. Circular breathing will also be used during still meditation as it helps keep a continual flow of life force moving through the body unifying visualization with the inner terrain of the meridian and chakra channels while becoming consciously attuned to hear the body's inner wisdom.

SMALL DEATH BREATHWORK
Small death breath work is a form of deep breathing by which one holds the breath at the top and bottom of the inhalation and exhalation for a specific count of 4 to 8 seconds in order to bring life giving properties of the breath deeper into the inner dynamics of the mind/body thus intensifying the calming meditative healing effects of Kun Qi. This form of breath work is performed during the Joint Activation warm-up, and the Tao Yin Fa sequence.

CIRCULAR BREATHWORK
Circular breathing is used during the body warm up exercise, joint activation sequence, and 8 directional movement sequences. With circular breathing one keeps a deep continual flow of breath <u>without</u> holding the breath at either end of the inhalation or exhalation. In the 8 directions format of meditative movement the direction changes are performed in sync with one's breathing thus allowing for one to create an outer and inner rhythm that unifies conscious and ultra-conscious thought taking you deeper into the altered states of meditation. Circular breathing will also be used during still meditation as it helps one to keep a continual flow of life force moving through the body unifying visualization with the inner terrain of the meridian and chakra channels while becoming consciously attuned to hear the body's inner wisdom communicated.

BREATH & BODY WARM-UP

Before starting the movement sequence it's important to settle into a breathing pattern that is comfortable and conducive to the rhythm of the sequence. Start with a 5 - 10 minute intentional walk or run to begin awakening and circulating Qi energy throughout your body. As time goes on, feel free to increase the duration to match your level of fitness. This helps to stimulate movement within the meridian channels increasing the amount of oxygen throughout the body and releasing toxins through the breath. It also increases your ability to consciously direct and regulate the intensity of your workout within the various healing movement sequences. As you become more adept at intentional movement you may find that you will naturally want to increase the circular count of your breathing. This is fine and can be done when you feel ready.

 As you start to walk or run focus your attention on your breath. Start to regulate your breathing by inhaling and exhaling to the count of 3-6 seconds during each. If you find this difficult slow your pace to a level of intensity that's manageable so that you can maintain at least a three-count circular rhythm. This can be done by taking shorter strides or by increasing your stride to match the rhythm. Once it starts to become comfortable and you're able to maintain this pace with ease, start to focus your attention on the muscles that are working as you're moving. By consciously engaging each muscle of the body as you move/walk/run, you help to align the spine, decrease the pressure on the joints during impact, increase the amount of oxygen getting into the lungs, muscle tissue and brain, and improve the circulation of blood, oxygen, and nutrients to the heart and throughout the body while strengthening, tightening, and firming your muscles.

Relax into your breathing, and start to allow yourself to look, with your inner vision, inside and at your body. Become aware of your foot placement and how your legs and arms are moving. If your feet are rotated outward bring your foot placement forward so that your knees and toes are aligned and pointed straight ahead of you. Draw your abdominal wall in toward the spine while tightening or squeezing your glutes holding them tight and firm as you walk. By drawing your abdominal wall towards the spine and engaging your Gluteus Maximus, your spine will automatically align itself and the knees will automatically soften so as not to create any jarring or strain during impact. Engaging the muscles in your glutes and quads versus using the momentum of your stride helps to shape, tone and firm your muscles from the inside out and to align the spine which takes pressure off of the knees, low back, neck and shoulders. By slightly tightening your arm, allowing them to move forward and backward in a relaxed way and intentionally holding the muscles in your legs, gluteus, abs, torso etc. tight, you will soften your body's impact with the ground.

To become consciously in-tuned and present with your bodies rhythm and to learn how to guide it, focus your attention on intentionally using the muscles of your abs, arms, leg, and buttocks to propelling yourself versus using the momentum of your body mass to move you forward. Focus your mind on your inner condition and allow yourself to become familiar with the physical, mental, and emotional sensations and postures that you hold. Notice where you feel tension, looseness, sluggishness, stagnation or over-stimulation, resistance, pain, discomfort and/or stress; notice how your lungs are responding to this activity. Is your breathing labored, is there any burning, is your heart feeling overtaxed or skipping, or is your heart rate beating strong and in a healthy range of the activity?

HOW TO CHECK YOUR HEART RATE: Your maximum heart rate can be determined by subtracting ½ your age from the number 210. This is your maximum heart rate. Your target heart rate should be lower, at approximately 75% of the maximum during movement. If your heart rate is over this range, slow your pace, and focus on decreasing your breath work to a lower more comfortable count. Once you have structured your movement so that your body is actively engaged in intentional propulsion and your heart rate is within healthy limits, allow your focus to go deeper by bringing your awareness to your chakras, tuning into their present state, especially any concerns, or current situations and/or issues that surface. You will be working to clear them with the Level I Situational Clearing using Dai Ko Myo or the Level III & IV Chakra Clearing Series but for now just take note of the sensations, and insights that come up for you.

Bring your attention to your root chakra. Do you feel grounded and center in thought and at peace with your work, family, home, and current life's experiences? If so, move up to the navel chakra. If not, note what concerns or thoughts come to mind then release them before moving to the next chakra; you will be using the information during the Situational Clearing Sequence. Moving up to the navel chakra; are there any emotional situations or feelings that come to mind? If so, note them and the questions, situations, and insights they inspire. Next bring your awareness to the Solar Plexus; your power center. Are you feeling empowered and centered in your sense of self, your boundaries, your spiritual relationship with The Creator, your Self and others? If not, note where you are feeling out of tune or imbalanced, what it is that may be creating the feeling, and whatever comes to mind that challenges your sense of inner peace and oneness with The All and/or with yourself and others. Take note of what comes to the surface, allow yourself to breathe the light of the sun into your solar plexus releasing the tension, noting whatever comes to mind and move onto your heart chakra. Can you sense your love for self, your connection and oneness with life, The Creator and your Divine truth as a spiritual being? Can you envision operating with compassion towards others or are there blocks such as, judgments, anger, resentments, fears or defenses that you are holding? Note what you feel breathing through any negativity that comes to the surface. Allow yourself to own it viewing it objectively without becoming emotionally entangled in mind concerning what comes up by viewing it as something that will be addressed and transcended. Next, move to the throat chakra. Notice any sensations or glitches in communication that may arise that reflect blockages of some sort that aren't allowing you to express your genuine self, your truth, your needs, your desires, etc. Does the air move freely into and out of the lungs? Do you notice any sensations of restriction, soreness, dryness or tension in the throat? Do any communication issues come to mind; things you're having trouble communicating or verbally formulating in thoughts? Again, keep in mind the mental notes taken for clearing during the Situational Clearing sequence. Next bring your attention to your 1st eye and crown chakras. Are you able to remember your dreams? Are you able to envision creative and psychic insights that provide guidance to your goals or life situations? Do you feel connected and in communication receiving insights and direction from your higher self, spiritual guides, etc. note where you feel your level of connectedness to the Divine Realms as far as openness and breathe it in. Allow yourself to move through the chakras gauging your run/walk with the time necessary for you to go through all the chakras.

Once you've finished with this intentional run/walk exercise, take 2-4 minutes to cool down your body rhythms by slowing down your walking pace until you are at a normal breathing pattern for yourself. Check your pulse to determine when you are back to your resting heart rate which can be determined by taking your pulse prior to any activity or upon waking in the morning or lying down to rest at night. Upon returning to your resting heart rate find a place that you would like to start your meditative movement exercises.

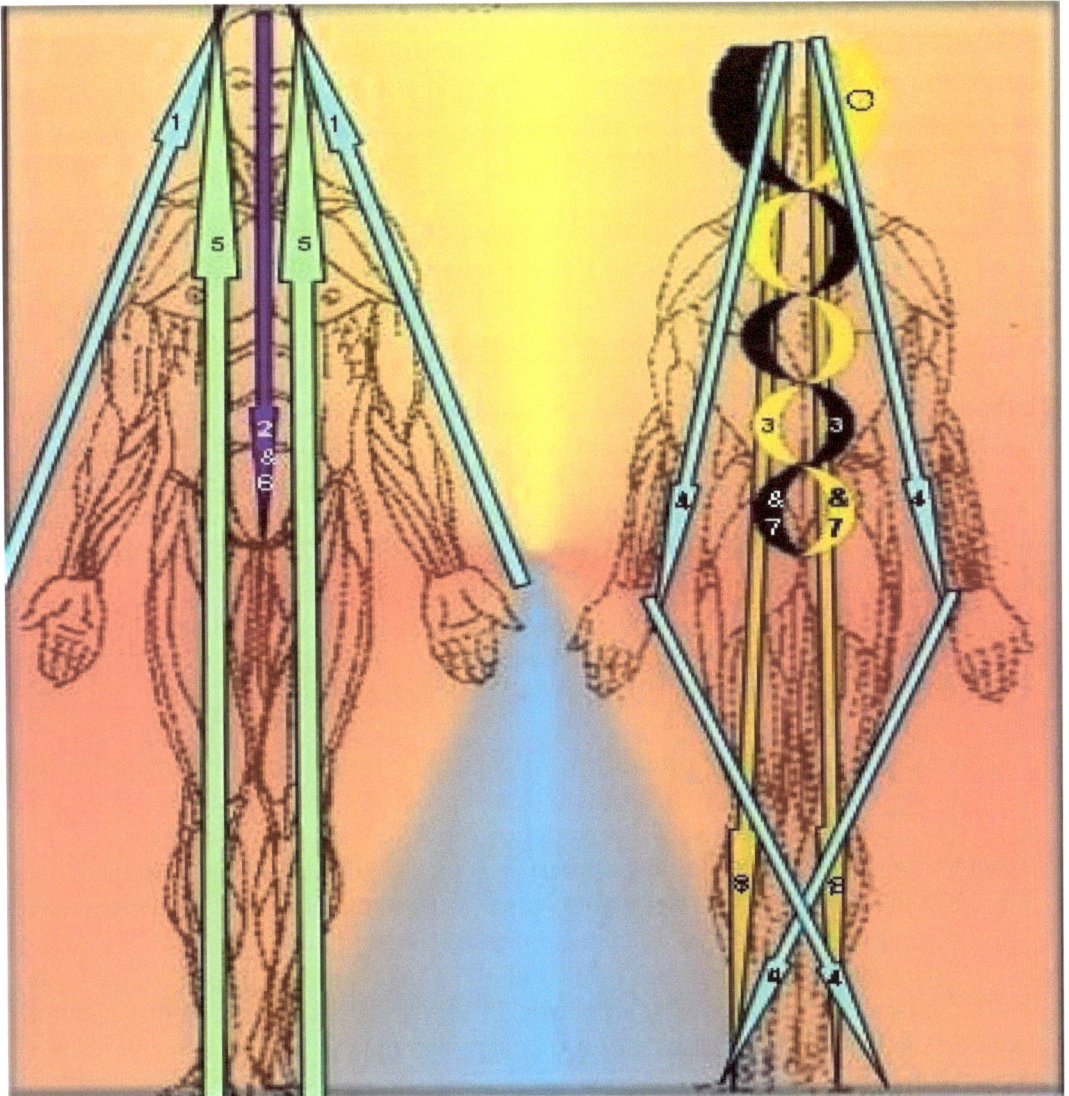

KUN QI MERIDIAN QI CIRCULATION MEDITATION

The purpose of this sequence is to deepen your attunement to the energy channels within your body and for you to learn to not only feel, but to identify and guide the movement of life force throughout your body with your mind and your breath.

To begin, stand with your knees slightly bent gently drawing the abdomen toward the spine allow it to relax and align itself naturally. If done correctly you should feel a sense of weightlessness within the core of the body starting at the pelvis and moving up along your spinal column into the shoulders, upper back and neck. Stretch your arms out in front of you with palms facing in as if you are holding a large beach ball between your arms and your body at a level just below your navel. Keep about 1" of space between the tips of your fingers in order to allow the chi force to flow freely from within the lower Tantien (pronounced dan tien). This is where original qi force processes, out to the hand chakra openings in the hands the organ command points in the fingers. This stimulates their receptivity to cosmic and elemental life-force and creates a strong connection and even flow of energy that is drawn in, out, and throughout the body as it rides the breath. The Qi Circulation Diagram chart is a visual depiction of the flow and order in which the meridian breath work exercise is performed.

Take a few slow relaxing breaths and focus your inner vision and sensory perceptions on connecting and aligning yourself with the Orisha Elementals cosmic and earthly life force. Envision yourself being surrounded by the Iron crystal core of the earth standing within its gravitational pull and its library of recorded earth knowledge. This is where all of the akashic records of the life experience of every entity, life form, or being including mother earth from the beginning of earth's time to now. All earth's experiences have been recorded and stored in the iron core of the earth and flows through the iron within your bloodstream. Therefore, one has access to the history of the planet as well as that of their ancestry through the portal of their blood. For example, when you have a knowing about how the way life was hundreds or thousands of years before your existence that you have no way of knowing, yet still know. Like many renown scientists like Imhotep, Benjamin Banneker, George Washington Carver, Emmett Chappelle and more who have revealed concepts that are now being use scientifically. It is the same with the galactic center of our Universe.

Once centered within these vortexes within yourself envision a portal of light from the galactic center of our universe descending and surrounding you and absorbing into the iron crystal within each blood cell of your body. Inhale envisioning these energies drawing into and merging within your heart chakra. As you exhale envision their combined life force shooting down your spinal column and pooling within the floor of your pelvis igniting your primordial energy (also known as kundalini) that resides there. Inhale again sensing the primordial chi winding up (black and gold spiral in previous image) through the root, navel, solar plexus, heart, throat, and 1st eye stopping there. Hold the chi on either side of your crown chakra holding your breath as you hold it there. Upon exhalation release the flow of qi into the pineal gland at the brain center visualizing it flowing down the spinal column and radiating throughout the nervous system into every cell of your body. Repeat this sequence 2 more times as to fully align and deepen the connection. While doing so, allow yourself to envision these cosmic power centers of energy becoming more aligned and familiar with their presence and their functions.

Now bring your focus to the tips of your fingers. As you slowly draw breath into the belly feel and visualize life force energy from the surrounding vortex of cosmic and earthly elements coming into your fingertips and traveling up your forearms, into your elbows, shoulders, neck and head. Hold the qi and the breath at the top within the center of your crown chakra for a few seconds. Now, while slowly exhaling, envision the life-force energy traveling from the crown chakra, down through the center of the spinal column descending through the chakras then pooling inside the center of the pelvic floor. Again, hold the breath for a few seconds allowing the primordial energy that resides there to awaken recharge, and build.

EARTHLY

Now, to ground and integrate the primordial energy into your present time experiences, inhale again sensing the Qi energy winding up (black and gold spiral in previous image) through the root, navel, solar plexus, heart, throat, and 1st eye stopping there and holding the chi on either side of crown chakra holding it there as you hold your breath. (Refer to kundalini chart on next page for visual details). Then upon exhalation release the flow of chi out from the top of the head down the neck into the front part of the shoulders and down the inner part of the arms into the hands and out the fingertips. At the bottom of the exhale envision the chi energy moving across the body down into the opposite toes. Again, hold the breath a few seconds letting the energy build. Upon inhalation, envision and feel the life force flowing up from the toes into your feet, ankles, the inner and outer legs, hips torso, shoulders, neck and head holding the breath at the top (these are the meridian channels of the stomach, spleen, liver, and gallbladder). Again, exhale all life force down the spinal column into the tantien, hold the breath and allow it to build within the pelvic floor. This time, while inhaling, envision the chi force moving up the anterior core of the body into the acupuncture points on the inside corner ridge of the eyebrows called "drilling bamboo". Hold the breath. You may feel a tingling sensation at these power points as they clear the nasal passage and charge the 1st eye chakra. As you exhale envision the chi energy flowing up over the brow and crown of the head, down the back of the head and neck and continuing down through the bladder meridians to the kidney point at the bottom of the feet allowing all old outdated stagnant energy to release into the earth removing it from the entire body.

Some believe that because of the toxic abuse that Mother Earth has sustained our sending stagnant life force from our bodies back into the Earth is contributing to the toxicity of Mother Earth. Rest easy… this is not the case. The energetic toxins that you are releasing actually feed the Earths molten core vibrationally which fuels and regenerates her power center and the carbon dioxide we exhale provides the Earth's soil and plant life with life force to thrive on.

Performing the Meridian Qi Activation Sequence at least 3 times consecutively in order to deepen your Kun Qi atun-ment helps to awaken and recalibrate the flow of life force through your meridian channels. At this point you should feel relaxed yet with a heightened sense of awareness and vibration in connection to your physical body and the elements around you. You are now ready to start the various meditative movement sequences. Performing these exercises, opens, strengthens and increases the flow of life force to the internal organs and can help regulate and restore their function-ability to that of their natural and optimal state of operating over time with consistent practice. The meridian charts will familiarize you with the meridian channels for each organ, where they are in the body, and the directions that they flow in so that you can more effectively perform the chi activation as well as the Tao Yin Fa series of movements. The meridian charts in "Appendix A" reveal specific acupressure points for each organ and just where each organ meridian channel runs throughout the body. Now that you've attuned to the elemental energies around you and the area you'll be working in, the next step is to create sacred space that acknowledges their sentience and affirms your healing intentions by welcoming higher levels of consciousness to bring greater Self-awareness and personal insights during your meditative movement sessions.

SEQUENCE I - JOINT MOBILIZATION

Begin by standing with your toes facing forward and your legs shoulder width apart with knees slightly bent to relieve pressure from the spine. Draw the lower abdomen in toward the spine and slightly engage your buttocks. This will naturally align your entire spinal column bringing your center of gravity into its most natural alignment. Focus your attention on Kun Chi and begin circular breathing. Inwardly check to see if your lower abs and glutes are engaged then allow your body and mind to relax more deeply into the breath becoming more attuned to the feel of your body from within. At this point you are ready to start the exercise. Follow the Joint Mobilization sequence below making sure that each movement, each rotation, each transition is performed with the muscles that surround the joint fully engaged and activated. The inner tension allows you to properly use the power of the musculature to move the joints instead of the force of momentum through the use of the skeletal. The joint rotation count for each movement starts with 9 rotations in each direction and can be increased up to 18 counts for those who want to increase the intensity level of the exercise.

JOINT MOBILIZATION MOVEMENTS

ANKLES - Lift the left leg up so that the knee is suspended in air at approximately a 90 degree angle. Again, gently tighten the buttocks and the abdomen to naturally align the body inward, balancing the pelvis and spine to create stability and balance of the entire body. Bring your inner attention to the ankle joint and with intent, tighten and use the muscles within the Tibial's (shins) and calves. Very slowly rotate each foot medially (inward) 6 – 9 rotations and then reverse direction rotating laterally (outward) for the same count. Stretch as far in each direction as you can while circling feeling the tension, soreness, and achiness that is generated in the musculature when you use the supporting muscles to move each foot versus momentum. Be sure to go slow paying inner attention to fully feel and identify all the muscles that it actually takes to move the foot at the ankle joint. Remember, the slower you go, the more you use your musculature to move you and the more benefits from the movement that you will achieve.

KNEES - Next move the focus of rotation up to the knee joint of the same leg. Use your quadricep muscles to propel the rotation of the knee for the same amount of rotations as you did for the ankle, medially first and then laterally. You may hear popping or crunching at the joints during rotation which is not uncommon due to nitrogen and synovial fluid buildup in the joint cavity caused by postural misalignments, not having utilized the surrounding muscles properly when moving the joint and lack of consistent stretching and strengthening of the muscles and joints. You can expect this to decrease over time as the synovial fluid starts to evenly distribute and the intentional mobility of the exercise strengthen the surrounding tendons and muscles. Once completed switch legs and repeat the ankle and knee rotations with the other leg. When finished place both feet on the ground with feet facing forward with legs straight.

HIPS – Now, widen your stance to a little beyond shoulder width apart and with intent, rotate the hips in a wide circle first in one direction for 9 rotations then the next. Again, make sure to focus your inner attention on using the muscles of the hips and leg to direct the movement versus momentum. You want to synchronize your breathing to fit in alignment with the positioning of the chest and abdomen. As you bring the pelvis forward in front of you, exhale through the mouth fully. As you move the hips towards the rear, inhale deeply fully filling up the diaphragm and lungs. Complete 9 rotations in each direction then once finished, center yourself and drop the hips by bending the knees a little more deeply. Isolate the pelvis circling the hips alone keeping everything above the waist as well as the legs stationary. This movement is exceptional for releasing energetic and vertebral blockages in the lower back region, especially within the SI joint and in the sciatic nerve area. It's a good exercise to incorporate periodically throughout your day as a treatment for low back pain and stiffness.

CHEST - The next area of rotation is the thoracic cage. While holding the hips stable isolate the chest cavity and shift it to the left. Try to keep the shoulders down focusing on using only the chest cavity in the movement. Be assured, this movement will get easier and smoother with practice. While exhaling, rotate the chest cavity posteriorly letting it sink back, fully compressing all the air out of the chest cavity and diaphragm. Then, while shifting to the right, begin to inhale as you start to rotate the chest cavity forward fully pressing it as far forward as you can. Fully expanding the lungs to maximize the oxygen intake then start to slowly exhale while rotating the chest cavity to the left then back. Rotate 9 times in each direction slowly and with intention focusing on the body parts being moved then reverse directions performing the same number of rotations. Once complete, center the chest and then move onto the cervical joint of the neck.

NECK – While keeping the body faced forward, tighten the neck using its musculature to turn the head fully left than right. Visually look at each shoulder to make sure they are not curving forward on either side. Now, while isolating and holding the neck as tight as you can, use them to push/pull the head to face forward while inhaling. Intentionally focus on using the musculature in the neck to move the head. Circle the head slowly and with intent in front of the body from right to center, exhaling, then from center to left inhaling. Take mental note of where you feel pain or pulling, tightness or discomfort. If you find points of pain or tension, apply pressure with the fingers of the opposite hand breathing deeply at tension points to relieve. Next, slowly circle your head behind the neck 3-6 times exhaling from right to center stopping to inhale at the center and exhaling toward the left. Once completed, bring head back up and rotate head to the right then to the left stretching as far as possible. Make sure that your shoulders are back and aligned. Bring head back to center. As you are performing these movements make sure to ride the breath inhaling during movements that open the wind pipe and exhaling when the wind pipe is being constricted. Next, move onto the eyes.

EYES – With head facing forward, face relaxed and your tongue on the roof of the mouth, look up with your eyeballs moving and stretching them as far up as possible and hold them there for a few seconds. While keeping them stretched tight, roll them as far right as possible until you are able to see the side of the nose and hold. Next circle them downward without moving the head, stretching them as far down as you can. Don't worry if the eyes blur or cross, this is normal. Hold the eyes there for a few seconds then roll them to the left and hold them there for a few seconds, repeat this complete cycle up to 4 times. This helps to improve the vision over time.

EARS & TONGUE – According to Chinese medicine, nerve endings that connect to the internal organs and various parts of the body reside on the ears and tongue. Stretching them out helps to activate them and stimulates and directs life force within the connecting nerves and organs. Gently massage and pull the ears while sticking out your tongue as far as possible and in all directions stretching them both from top to bottom, left to right, and around.

SHOULDERS & ELBOWS – Next, straighten the legs and bring the arms up and out to your sides at shoulder height extending straight out with palms facing down toward the floor. Arms should be extended straight out as if you are forming the letter "T" with your body. Focus and isolate the shoulder blades and shoulder joints using the should blades to draw the shoulders back and the upper part of the deltoids and traps to circle the arms forward and around using the muscles that connect to the shoulder blades and joints only. The forearms and hands should feel weightless and disengaged. Reverse directions circling posteriorly. Next focus on circling just the arms from the shoulder joint disengaging the shoulder blades; you should feel this more in the upper region of the arms. While shoulders and arms are still held straight out from your sides, bend the arms at the elbows allowing the lower region of the arms and hands to go limp and circle the arms around the elbow joint. Perform each of these movement 6-9 times slowly in each direction making sure to focus on engaging the proper musculature and breathing deep and down into the dantien throughout the movements.

BICEPS & TRICEPS – Stretch the arm out in front of you at shoulder height with palms facing inward towards each other. Tighten the arms and press them toward each other while fully extended keeping the elbows bent just enough to feel the biceps and deltoids engage. Begin pressing the arms inwards in slow pulses as if you are pressing against resistance. Exhale as you tighten and press inward, inhale as you tighten the triceps and pull outward. Do sets of 9 and then flip the palms outward facing away from you and repeat. Next are bicep curls. Put one palm squarely over the other with the arm of the bottom hand held next to your side of the body. Perform slow bicep curls using the top hand as resistance, pressing downward while you're pressing upward with the other hand for 9 repetitions; repeat with other arm. Next we work on the triceps. Straighten the arms on either side of you allowing them to hang by your sides. With legs shoulder width apart and knees bent, lean your upper body forward to about a 45 degree angle while at the same time making sure to keep your spine straight. Face palms towards the back of you and with arms straight, press the palms and arms back and up behind the back using the triceps to make the movements. Slowly press upward riding the breath for a count of 18. Once completed bring the arms straight back as far behind you as you can and hold them up. With elbows pointed towards the ceiling, or sky, perform Tricep extensions for a count of 18 squeezing them tightly at each full extension.

WRISTS & HANDS – With fingers extended and stretched as far out as you can, slowly circle your wrists. You should feel stretching and lengthening within the region of the forearms. While doing this movement fan the fingers as well from pointer to pinky bringing them one by one down to the palm and reversing one by one to stretch them out again. Rotate in both directions 6 – 9 times then go in the opposite direction and fan the fingers pinky to pointer fanning them down to the palm and then out again. You will really feel this in the forearms which happen to be one of the most overworked yet neglected areas of the body when it comes to intentional exercise. Next, hyperextend the fingers backwards, away from the palms stretching each finger out successively starting from the pinky until all fingers have been fully extended. You should feel a tight stretch within the hand and along the fingers. Shake hands out and bring palms and fingers together with arms extended straight out in front of the body. Flip one palm over so that the back of the right hand is cradled inside the palm of the left. While pressing the hands together, draw the hands in towards the chest and towards the right bending the elbows outward and keeping the arms shoulder height. Perform 6 – 9 times and repeat on other side then shake arms out once completed.

MERIDIAN ACTIVATION – Extend your arms out in front of your body as if you're holding onto a large beach ball. Using your left hand, make a fist and gently tap the outer side of the right arm from your wrist up to the top of the shoulder the continue tapping downward on the inner side of the arm. Switch arms and repeat on other side. Once completed, use both hands tapping down the inside of the legs down to the ankles then come up the outside of the legs to the hips. Move up to the upper back and tap along the back side of the body down to the floor.

FULL BODY SWING – Stand with legs wide holding body loosely allowing the arms to hang at your sides. Using your hips and legs to move and turn your body first towards the right and then the left like a washing machine letting the arms swing freely as you turn to each side. Perform the full body swing for a count of nine then turn your upper body so that it is facing over either leg having one facing forward and one straddled behind you in a lunge position.

LEG & HIP RELEASE – while facing in the direction chosen, do a set of 9 dips keeping the upper body upright and focusing mainly on using the back leg and quadricep muscles to do the work. Do another set of dips this time going deeper bringing your knees down to a 90 degree angle. Next, with hips facing toward the front leg, lunge your body forward leaning your upper body and hips over your front leg. Do another set of 9 lunges focusing on using your glutes and hamstrings to perform the movement by pressing with your front heal and keeping the glutes tight throughout the movement. Next, straighten the front leg in the lunge position and bend down until you feel the hamstrings stretch with hands on the floor on either side of the front foot or on your lower shin. Breathe deeply a few times allowing your body to move deeper into the stretch with each exhale. Next, move your body into a front straddle position walking your hands around to centerline of the body. Now shift your body to one side aligning it over one leg while keeping the other leg extended at an angle. Bring your body down into a side lunge position allowing the inner thighs of the opposite leg to stretch for a few seconds. You can add to the stretch by pressing the inner thigh of the knee that is bent back with your elbow. Finally, walk your hands back to the centerline while gently lifting your body by straightening the legs. Allow your chest and upper torso to drop down between your legs creating a stretch in the pelvis and low back elongating the spine. Repeat this sequence for the other side then once centered in front again, bring feet together and slowly lower yourself into a sitting lotus position with feet together in front of you.

GLUTE RELEASE – while sitting in lotus position with feet together in front of you, grab your feet with both hands, elongate the spine and gently, while exhaling, draw your chest down towards the floor stretching the lower back, hips and inner thighs. Hold this stretch momentarily, inhale deeply and as you exhale, draw yourself deeper into the stretch. You can add more intensity to the stretch by using your elbows to gently press your knees out and down as you sink your chest and upper body deeper towards the floor with each exhalation. When ready, bring your upper body upright into its proper alignment. Slide your right foot over towards your the left hip until it rests underneath or near it. Place your left foot on the other side of your right knee. If you find this position difficult, you can acchieve the same stretch by stretching your left leg straight out in front of you, then crossing the right foot over to the outer side of the left leg as close to your hip as is comfortable. Once you are in position, wrap your arms around your knee and gently draw it into your chest while elongating your spine. As you do so you will start to feel areas in the glutes that are tight or restricted. Hold each position that you experience tension in, and take 3-4 deep relaxing breaths each time moving a little bit deeper into the tension with each exhalation. When ready switch sides and repeat the same stretch with your other leg.

ABDOMINAL TONING – Now that you have fully stretched and opened up the hip area, lie down on your back and bring your legs into a position where your feet are flat on the floor hip width apart and your knees are pointed towards the ceiling. You will want to draw the lower abdominal wall in toward the spine and tuck the hips slightly in order to keeping your low back flat against the floor. Once positioned, extend your arms between your legs, and perform 9-18 sit-ups curling your upper body in as far as you can while keeping your lower back flush against the floor. When complete bring your arms to the outside of either leg for side crunches and repeat on the other side. If you're feeling up to challenging yourself you can add a set or two of lower leg raises to tighten your lower abdomen specifically.

Once completed, lie flat on your back, extend your legs out straight along the floor while bringing your arms straight up over your head and arch your back. This will help to gently release any tension or cramping in your abdominal wall. Refocus your attention on your breathing allowing your mind and body to fully relax into a peaceful yet vibrant state before returning yourself to a standing position.

LU/LI

"ssseeeeee"

G

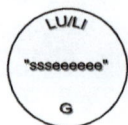

LUNG/LARGE INTESTINE

Create an "L" by stretching the thumb and forefinger out as far as you can while curling the remaining fingers of the hand into the palm. This opens the meridians of the Lung & Large Intestine. This movement aligns directly with the breath in that the lungs are responsible for inhaling or taking in new life force (oxygen) and the large intestine is responsible for eliminating old life force (waste) from the body. While Inhaling extend the hand out in front of the body and move it in an upward curve until it is extended over and outward along the sagittal plane stopping at head level along the frontal plane. When you reach this point of the movement, stretch the arm as far away from the body as possible, then turn palm outward completely keeping the wrist flexed. In this position the life force is being optimally stimulated within the meridian channel. Inhale deeply then hold the position and the breath while imagining the color white filling the LU/LI meridians and organs, flooding them with life force energy. At this point, start to circle the hand downwards envision the color white taken into the organ and meridian being released into the universe while making the sound "seeeee" (like the sound of steam escaping from a pressure cooker) in the note of G. Repeat 3 times with each hand individually and 3 times with hands simultaneously.

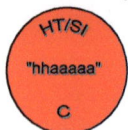

HT/SI

"hhaaaaa"

C

HEART/SMALL INTESTINE

This mudra stimulates the Heart & Small Intestine meridians with the element, fire. Begin the movement with the arm stretched out in front of you. Create a closed circle with the thumb and forefinger while extending the other three fingers of the hand. On the inhale envision the energy being drawn into the body with the hand at waist level. Move the hand back out away from the body in a figure eight movement bringing it up until it is aligned with the frontal plane of the body. At the top of the movement hold the breath while tightening the fingers and stretch the arm as far away from the body as possible. Imagine the color red filling the meridians and organs of the HT/SI with energy. As you start to bring the hand downward, envision releasing all toxicity and stagnation from the organs and meridians thru the breath into the universe while making the sound "haaaaa" in the note of C. The shift from one arm to the other is accomplished as you bring energy down from the top of the movement. In one continuous movement, transfer the energy to the left hand and continue on that side. End the movement with both hands in front of the hara (just below the navel) bringing the energy into the hara and then around and up to the top of the movement with both hands. Pause at the top to visualize the color red and then exhale as you bring the arms down with the sound "ha."

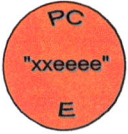

CIRCULATORY/REPRODUCTIVE

The hand mudra for this meridian is performed by drawing the pinky and forefinger of each hand into the palm while fully extending the two middle fingers with palm open flat. THS MOVEMENT IS DONE WITH BOTH HANDS AT THE SAME TIME. With hand palm facing up at waist level in front of you, simultaneously draw a circle moving fingers away from the center and around. As fingers come back to the center turn the palms facing each other yet not touching and move both arms up until they are extended overhead. Once overhead fan the arms out until they are fully extended to your sides at shoulder height flexing the wrists downward so that palms are facing outward and away from the body. This movement scoops the energy up from the root to the crown chakra. Once arms are fully extended above your crown, open the arms out to your sides while still fully extended to receive cosmic energies and pause holding the breath and visualizing the color crimson filling the pericardium meridian with vital energy. Breathe out with the sound "Xeeeee" on the note E as you bring the energy down, arms out to the side. When arms are parallel to the ground turn palms downward and continue lowering towards the earth. At the level of the kidneys, gently turn the hands and bring the energy across the back to the kidneys. Caress the kidney with the back of the hands. Do not break the circular flow as you bring the hands across the sides of the body waist height and to the front.

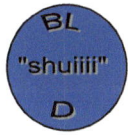

URINARY BLADDER

The bladder, as well as the following meridians, travels through up the body from the feet. Invert the foot inward towards the body so that the lateral edge of the foot and toes are touching the ground in order to stretch the bladder meridian. The bladder meridian also runs along the spine so remember to elongate fully to stretch the meridians. As you breathe in, the hand and opposite foot, begin moving at the same time synchronized throughout the movement. The foot reaches back at the same time the hand reaches up over the head. Open the hand with palm facing inward toward the head, hold the breath, pause, and visualize the color dark blue traveling up the meridian to the organ. Make sure to stretch extend the body to its furthest point. Slowly bring the hand and feet forward back to their starting position while breathing out with the sound "shuiiiii" in the note of D.

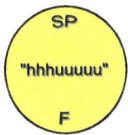

SPLEEN

The Spleen is stimulated by everting the foot fully outward so the instep of the foot is facing forward. Breathe in moving the hand and opposite foot up and back begin moving at the same time synchronized throughout the movement. Move the hand up with palm away from the body while swinging the foot out and behind you in a half circle, keeping the instep facing inward. Hold the breath, pause, visualize the color yellow running through the meridian to the organ, then slowly breathe out with the sound "Hhhuuuuu" on the note F as you return the hand and foot to its original position.

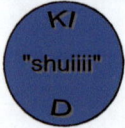

KIDNEY

The next two movements are performed moving both hands simultaneously along with the foot. Flexing the foot upward with toes pointed up towards the head with the back of the heel on the ground. The leg should be extended out in front of the body. Keeping the foot flexed move it in a half circle ending behind you with foot flat on the ground. Leg should be fully extended so that the hamstrings and calves are stretched. This allows the meridian to remain stimulated throughout the movement. Hold the breath, pause, visualize the color dark blue running through the meridian to the organ, then slowly breathe out with the sound "shuiiiii" in the note D as you return the hand and foot to its original position. Both hands move up simultaneously with palms facing inward toward the head.

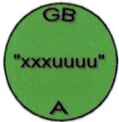

LIVER/GALLBLADDER

This movement stretches the gall bladder meridian by pointing the tip of the big toe down towards the earth as you extend the leg out in front of you. Open the hands so the palms are facing forward in a position of receiving. The movement is again a synchronized sweeping of the foot and arms yet this time the palms are turned outward at the top of the movement stretching the arm as high as comfortable. Move the foot around in a half circle from front to back keeping the toe pointed throughout the movement. When the toe reaches the back, it should still be pointed with the same tension that you started with. At the top of the movement, hold your breath, pause, visualize the color green bringing energy through the gall bladder meridian into the organ as you turn your hands outward. Slowly breathe out with the sound "xxxuuuuu" in the note A as you return the hand and foot to its original position.

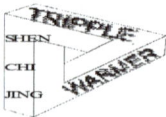

TRIPPLE WARMER

The triple warmer movement is the only movement where you will be traveling across the ground. It harmonizes the first seven movements to ground the energy and stimulate the three heaters that govern the energy of the total body. The triple warmer consists of the upper warmer = lungs & heart, mid warmer = stomach, spleen, pancreas, liver, gall bladder and lower warmer = small intestine, large intestine, kidneys and bladder. Begin this movement by touching each of the Three Heaters and then cupping the energy and bringing it into the hara or Tantien and around again to the front and up. You will have the experience of your arms encircling the energy like a cup. Here you should have finished your first step. As you shift your weight onto the foot which has taken the step,

156

take the Grail energy in your cupped hands and cross them at the wrists with palms facing away from the body giving the energy back to the earth and the universe. This completes the movement and you have returned to the original posture and are ready to begin the movement with your other foot. Gently touch the energies of the three heaters, bring the energy back to the hara as you start a new step... and continue from here. Perform 3-4 steps of this (each foot) working in a forward movement after which you will continue moving backwards with the same movements.

TAO YIN FA AFFIRMATIONS

Affirmations can be internally or externally vocalized in conjunction with visualization while performing the corresponding movements to expand the effects of the movements into the subtle bodies consciously strengthening and increasing their healing abilities.

LUNG: "I breathe in new life visions, new ideas, new insights to self, and new experiences of unconditional love. By this I transmute all negative outdated mentalities that do not reflect my vision of living the divine life and of being in alignment with my divine truth. As I exhale, I eliminate the old outdated patterns of though, disappointments, insecurities concerning my future vision of divine health and any fear of being unconditionally loved and provided for. I breathe in self-love, the pure essence of peace, the sentient beauty of Nature's elements, and the pure essence of divine knowledge and wisdom that surround and embody me. I allow life's elements to reveal their insights to my connection with all life inhaling their life force while exhaling and eliminating any and all past pain, low self-esteem, self-doubt, self-judgments, and/or self-loathing from past lives lived as well as from ancestral memory that may reside within."

LIVER/GALL BLADDER: "I allow divine life force to filter through my, divine ideas, divine insight to Self, and healthier, happier intentions for unconditional experiences of love that sustains me through its life blood and substance feeding my thoughts, words and deeds. I allow these divine thoughts to become a part of my essence expressing its divine influences through me which inspires spiritual healing in those that I come into contact with."

STOMACH/SPLEEN: "I take in divine life force, divine ideas, divine insights to self and divine experiences of love, allowing these things to assimilate and integrate into my consciousness so that they may circulate throughout my life reproducing new healthy thought forms, experiences, and creative expressions that produce greater levels of joy and peace in my life. I allow these new insights, ideas, and experiences of love to dissolve toxic energy from past conditioning and to transmute them into that of divine health, divine wealth, and knowledge of Divine Self through divine evolution (love-u-tion)."

SMALL INTESTINE/LARGE INTESTINE: "I ingest divine life force, divine ideas, divine insights and divine visions of myself living in divine health, divine wealth, and embodiment of divine Self, the ancestors, and my celestial roots. I allow these insights to digest, assimilate within my mind's meditations, and permeate into my conscious way of thinking, speaking and acting so that these new insights transmute outdated patterns of self that do not reflect the image of the life I want to experience. As these meditations circulate throughout my life, they reproduce better experiences, better outcomes, and greater joy & peace in my life."

HEART/REPRODUCTIVE/CIRCULATORY SYSTEMS: "I embody unconditional love and allow divine life force, divine ideas, divine insights to Self and divine experiences of love, to break down any and all existing barriers to healing and creating healthy relationships and experiences. I release what no longer serves my divine vision of personal fulfillment of my divine desires and higher intentions. I activate & unlock my potential to live in optimal alignment with the ancestors, Divine God/Goddess/The Elementals/The Universal Consciousness. I express a healthy attitude towards My body, my spirit, my surroundings, my family & community and my divine purpose breathing out all blockages and allow myself to flow with the blessings and infinite potential for personal and spiritual ascension that living the life I desire to live presents unhindered."

'I stand strong in my resolve to embrace the love that will generate the healing of my body, my mind, my soul, my relationships, my community and the planet."

TRIPPLE WARMER: "I am spirit housed in this body of flesh of which I choose to sustain in divine health that it may assist me in the fulfillment of my purpose, desires, and dreams. I breathe in divine life force, divine ideas, divine insights to self and divine experiences of love, while exhaling the past with each exhalation knowing that within my cellular memory resides the blueprint of my spiritual and ancestral roots. These roots guide, direct, and assimilate the wisdom from the knowledge of our past story from the beginning of time and before and inspires me to live and share the truth of our original life in order to transmute the misrepresentation and subjugation into right-us-ness and harmony of living as one with the land. And each time I embrace and breathe in this truth, I become immune to limitation, lack, fear and all forms of dis-ease instantaneously and as I exhale focused on the fulfillment of my purpose, desires, and dreams, they become manifest as my life. "

URINARY BLADDER/KIDNEY: "I choose to float along the streams of divine consciousness that surround me, bathing in divine ideas, divine insights to self and divine experiences of love. I allow these things to filter through my consciousness and to flush out any and all harmful or outdated thought forms, memories, or ways of being to eliminate them from my thought of the future, my speech and my actions creating new vibrant healthy relationships and experiences of Self-fulfillment."

The following charts depict the meridian channels to each of the organs within the Tao Yin Fa Sequence. These can also be used to familiarize yourself with the organ meridians as a visualization tool should you choose to direct life force through the meridians as an optional meditation. This type of meditation works well in combination with the affirmations as the combination of these two will amplify the healing and soul evolutionary effects that one is intending to achieve.

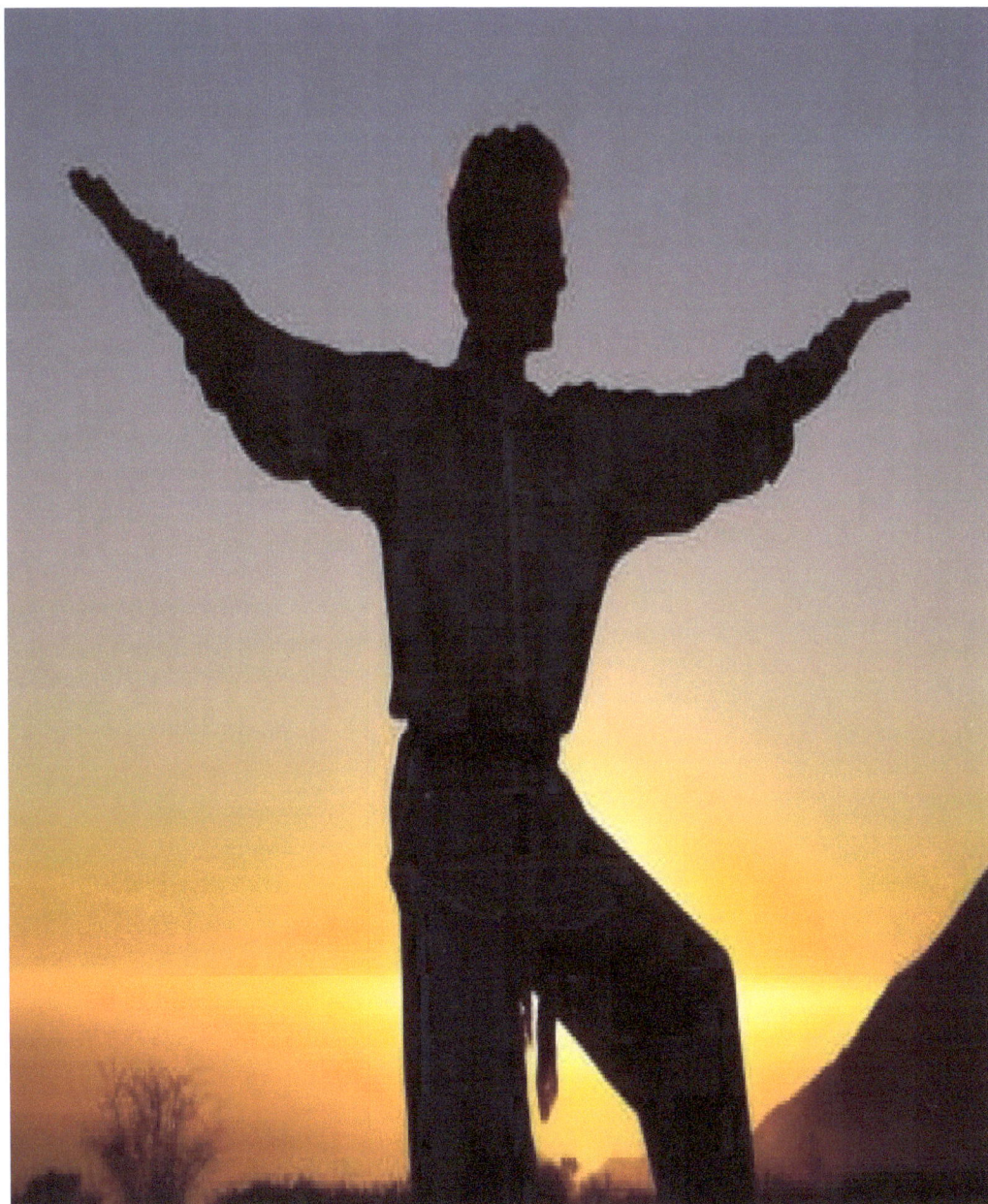

SEQUENCE III - SITUATIONAL CLEARING

The steps for the situational clearing sequence do not require much movement across distance, and are somewhat contained within a small space thus, circular breathing works best. It also will assist you in achieving a meditative state as it combines movement with visualization. Exhaling as you lunge into each direction allows you to send the creative power of your visualizations out with greater life giving force and power of manifestation. It also sends more carbon dioxide out to feed the environment. Inhalation as you rock back and as you make the turns allows you to draw in the life force from the elements into your subtle and physical body fields aligning their life giving energies with your chakras which we will go into more detail later.

THE 8 DIRECTIONAL CIPHER SEQUENCE:

Start by standing facing in the direction of the south. Place your hands palms inward over the dantien and begin circular breathing. Using the inverted heart mudra works well also in creating a healing loving energy to work in.

Bring to mind a situation or circumstance that you would like to gain clarity on, resolve, and/or improve. Spend a moment visualizing the situation as it is then when you feel ready shift your focus to what you would like to have happen or how you would like to see things become. Once you're able to visualize your desired outcome and hold it in mind, start to rotate the hands around each other in front of you. This will start to generate and build the chi, between the palms. While rotating the hand in front of you, inhale deep into your belly and step out in the direction of southeast leading with the left foot. Step forward in that direction pivoting the front of your body in that direction so that your left knee is leaning directly over its big toe. Upon inhalation, rock back shifting your weight to the right leg. While the right leg is holding your weight, turn the left foot in towards your body about 120 degrees then turn your right leg 90 degrees, this should have you facing in the direction of the northwest. Exhale while lunging forward in that direction. This time as you rock back on the left foot inhaling you will then rock forward again onto the right so that the left foot is free to move. At this time lift the left foot and shift your body so that you are facing in the 3rd direction of southwest. Repeat the same sequence of movements moving from southwest to north east then moving into the direction of the east to west and then again for the north to south.

During the rhythmic movements of each directional ciphers envision the highest most positive outcome that you would like to experience with the situation that you are considering. Then with your intentions send loving vibrations to the situation from your heart out through your breath into the environment in each direction allowing yourself to feel the way you would want to feel were everything resolved and everyone or everything involved being aligned with the most positive and productive outcome for all. You will continue this circular movement pattern throughout the entire meditation until you feel that your situation has become cleared within yourself and you are able to see and feel it resolved with the most positive outcome imaginable. Perform one last complete rotation to seal the healing intention and to send it peace, faith, and acceptance, then end the sequence facing where you started, in the direction of the south giving thanks. Repeat this sequence a many times as you feel the need to in order to feel release and resolution with the situation you are wanting to clear.

ADVANCED MOVEMENT FOR 8 DIRECTIONAL CIPHER SEQUENCE

This advance section can be integrated into the 8 directional movement cipher to tone the musculature and increase one's fitness levels. While rotating the hand in front of you, inhale deep into your belly then upon exhalation step out in the direction of southeast leading with the left foot. Lunge forward in that direction pivoting the front of your body in that direction so that your left knee is lunging directly over its big toe. While in this forward lunged position go deeper into the lunge by doing 3 pulsing lunges with that left leg. During inhalation, rock back shifting your weight to the right leg. In this position do 3 pulsations during exhalation sinking into and pressing forward with your right quad. Sink back as far as your quad will hold you then, press forward slightly using the heel and the quad of your right leg as if doing a reverse lunge. Now, while the right leg is holding your weight, turn the left foot in towards your body 90 degrees then turn your right leg 90 degrees, this should have the front of your body facing in the direction of the southwest. In this position, shift your weight to your right leg sinking down into it like a squat while allowing your left leg to straighten. This is called a half sided squat. Exhale slowly while you do 3 squatting pulsations to the right then shift your weight to the left and do the same squatting pulsation while slowly and deeply inhaling. With your left leg holding your weight, shift your right foot another 90 degrees away from your body and allow your entire body to follow until you are facing Northwest corner directly. Exhale while lunging forward in that direction. This time as you rock back on the left foot doing the 3 pulsations and inhaling you will then rock forward fully onto the right so that you are standing on your right leg and your left leg is free to move. At this time lift the left foot and step your left foot in towards your body then move into a lunging position with the left foot into the 3rd direction of southwest. Repeat the same sequence of movements moving from southwest to north east then moving into the direction of the east to west and then again for the north to south, continuing this circular movement pattern throughout the entire meditation until you've moved through the 8 directions. End the sequence facing where you started, in the direction of the south. while standing in this direction become aware of your breath taking some time to center in your breathing and allow your mind to open up to any insights and higher awareness' that come. Take note of them when done by journaling them down once you've completed the entire series, or when you feel guided. I've received many profound insight and messages when I've allowed myself this time to sit at the end of each rotation especially when doing the 8 directional cipher for the chakras.

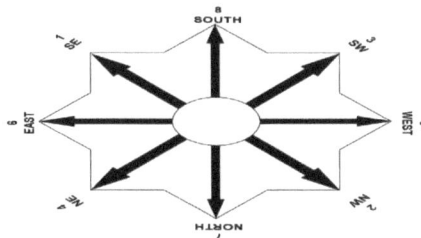

SEQUENCE IV - CHAKRA ACTIVATION USING THE 8 DIRECTIONS

This sequence combines visualization of the color spectrum of the gamma rays from the sun along with the chakras using the 8 directional movement sequence, and circular breathing as a means of clearing and aligning one's chakras. By refocusing the movements, visualization, and breath work, from the organs and their meridian system to the chakra system we combine the physical with the subtle bodies starting with the Bindu and going down to the root. It's important to create sacred space around you and to align with the elementals as it is this which will recharge and rejuvenate your chakras and the electrical circuitry of the nervous system that connects to the physical anatomy that they regulate.

Once you've created sacred space, begin by facing the direction of the south. Focus for a few moments on circular breathing and relax the body/mind even deeper allowing it to align you more deeply with the element of air and wind. Once you've become relaxed, focus inwardly bringing your inner attention to your Bindu or 8th Chakra above and slightly behind your head. Visualize its color, (Magenta) streaming down from the sun into this chakra to fill and activate it. Once you feel ready, begin your 1st cipher of the 8 directional movement by moving the left foot into the direction of Southeast. Continue the 8 directional cipher in each direction inhaling as you lunge outward in each direction and exhaling as you rock back and pivot into the next direction. If you are performing the advance movements then you will adjust the breath work to align with the extra middle movement. Once you've completed the sequence for the Bindu or 8th Chakra move your focus down to the Crown chakra envision the color of Violet flowing down into your Crown chakra and repeat the 8 directional cipher. Perform the same for the following chakras using the following colors and ending/beginning each cipher facing the direction of the south allowing yourself time to open up to any new insights and awareness' that you may receive.

- Aakash - Bindu – Magenta

- Gyan - Crown – Violet or Purple

- Sunya/Gyan - 1st Eye – Indigo

- Vayu - Throat – Aqua Blue

- Mrit Sanjivini Apaan Vayu - Heart – light Green

- Surya - Solar Plexus – Yellow or gold

- Varuna/Prana - Navel – Orange

- Prithvi/Apaan - Root – Red or Black

162

APPENDIX B

CHART & DIAGRAM INFORMATION

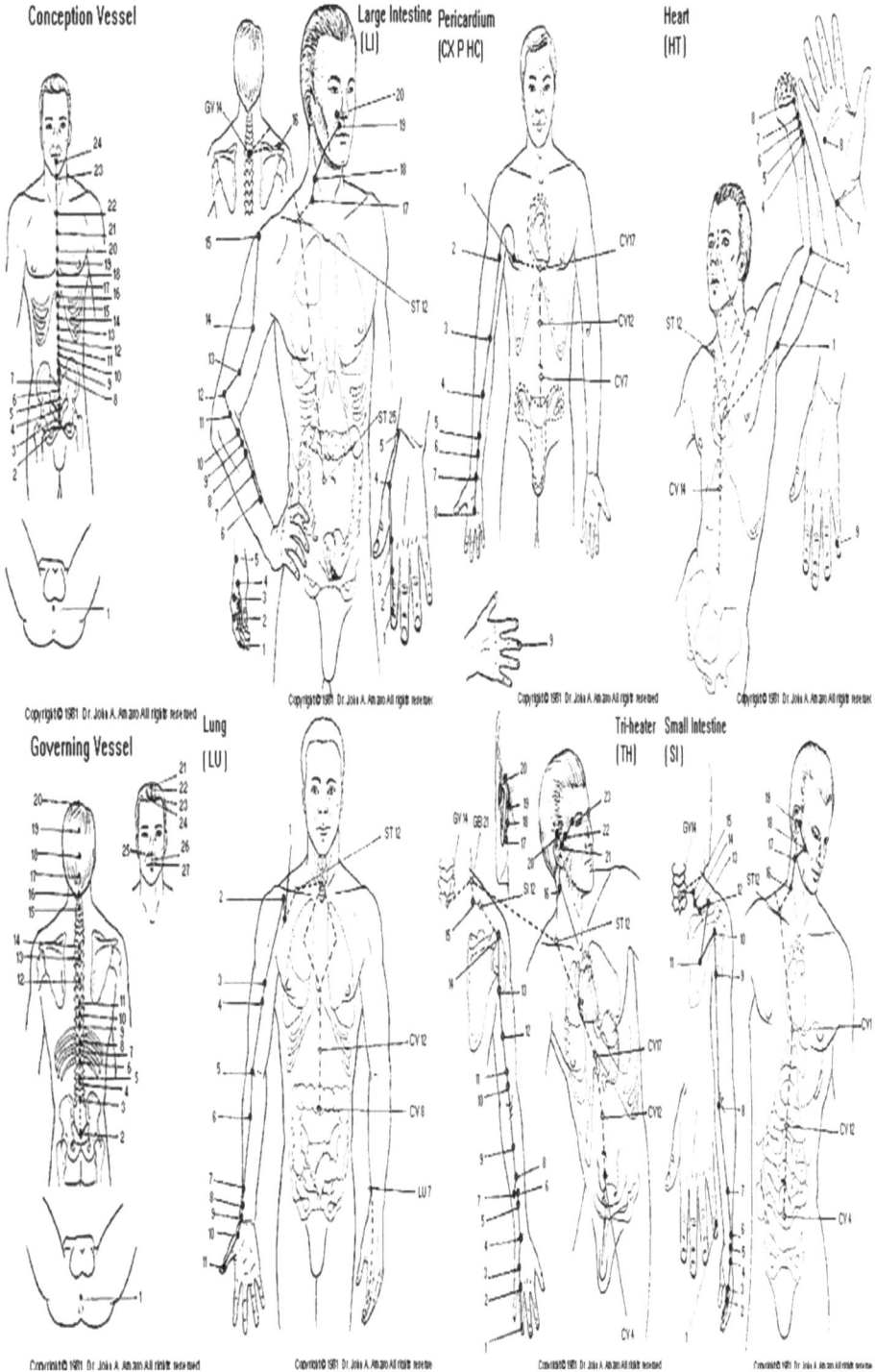

UPPER BODY MERIDIANS CHART

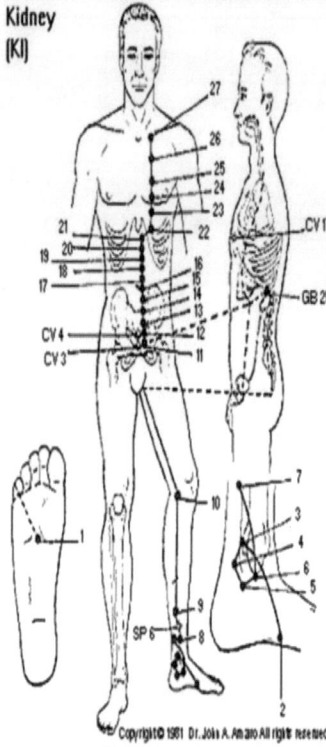

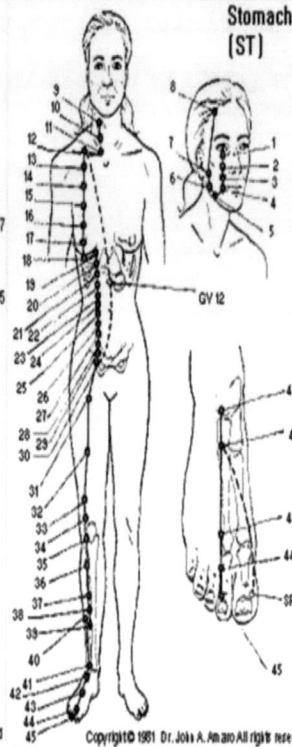

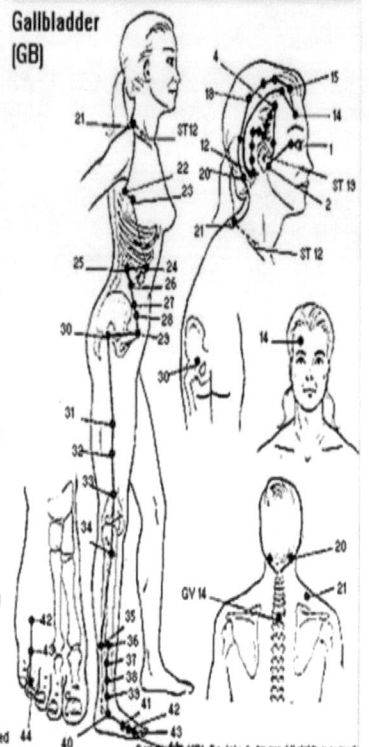

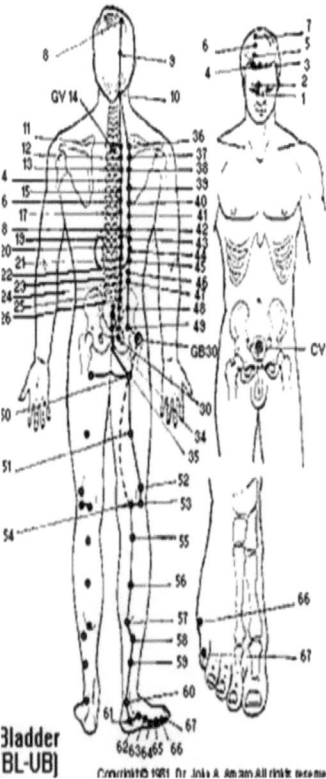

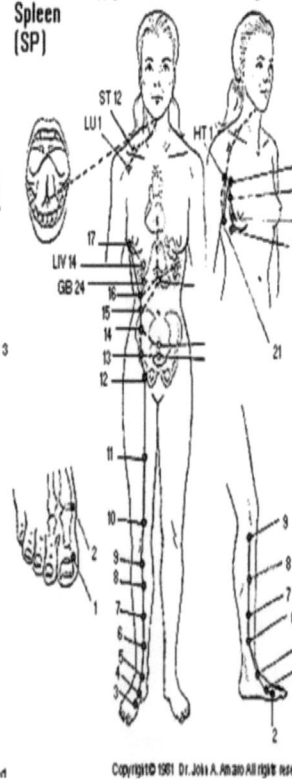

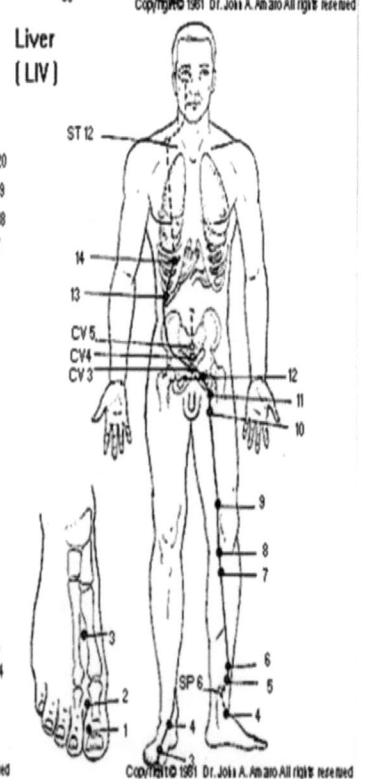

LOWER BODY MERIDIANS CHART

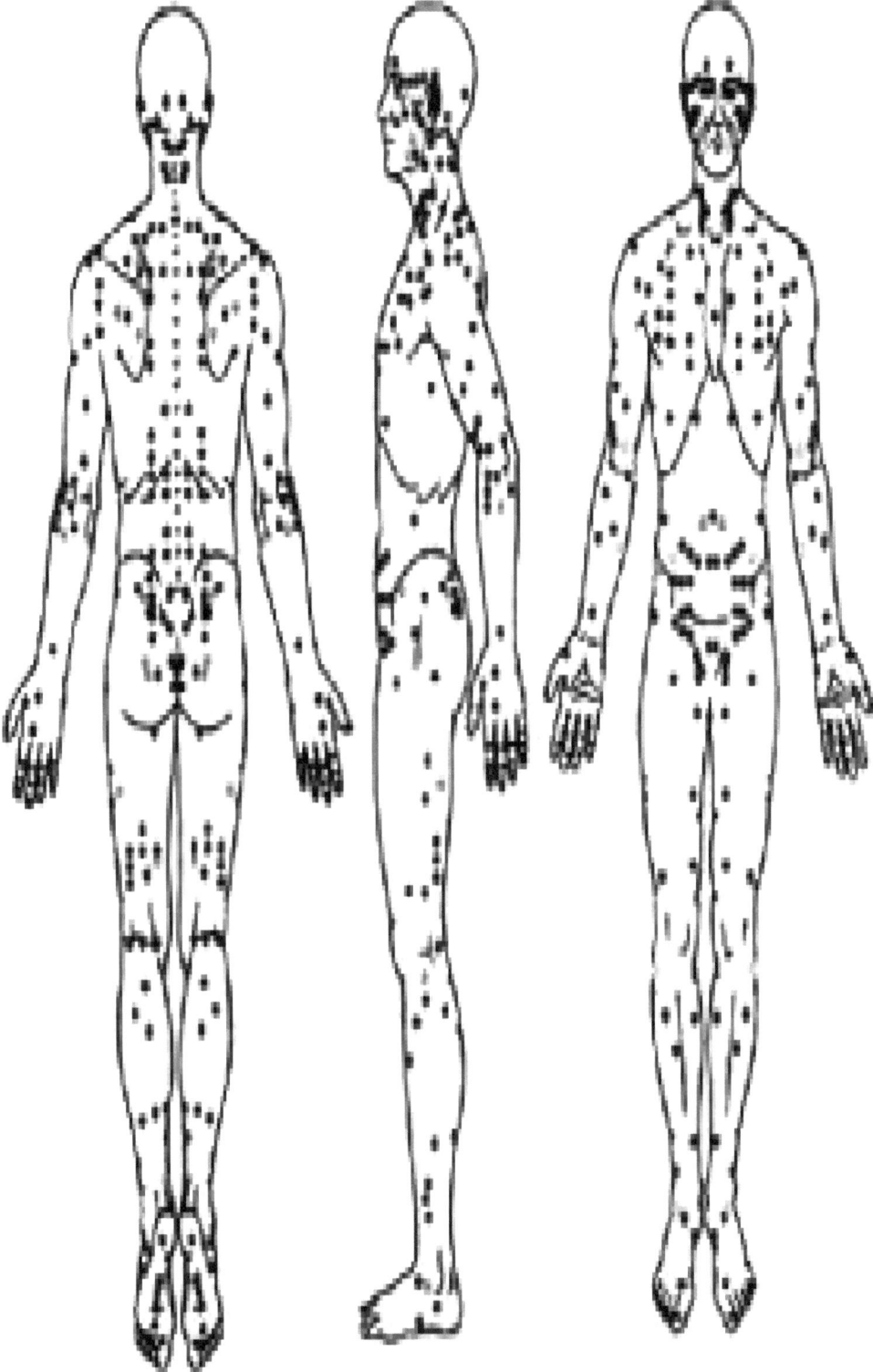

ACUPUNCTURE POINTS CHART

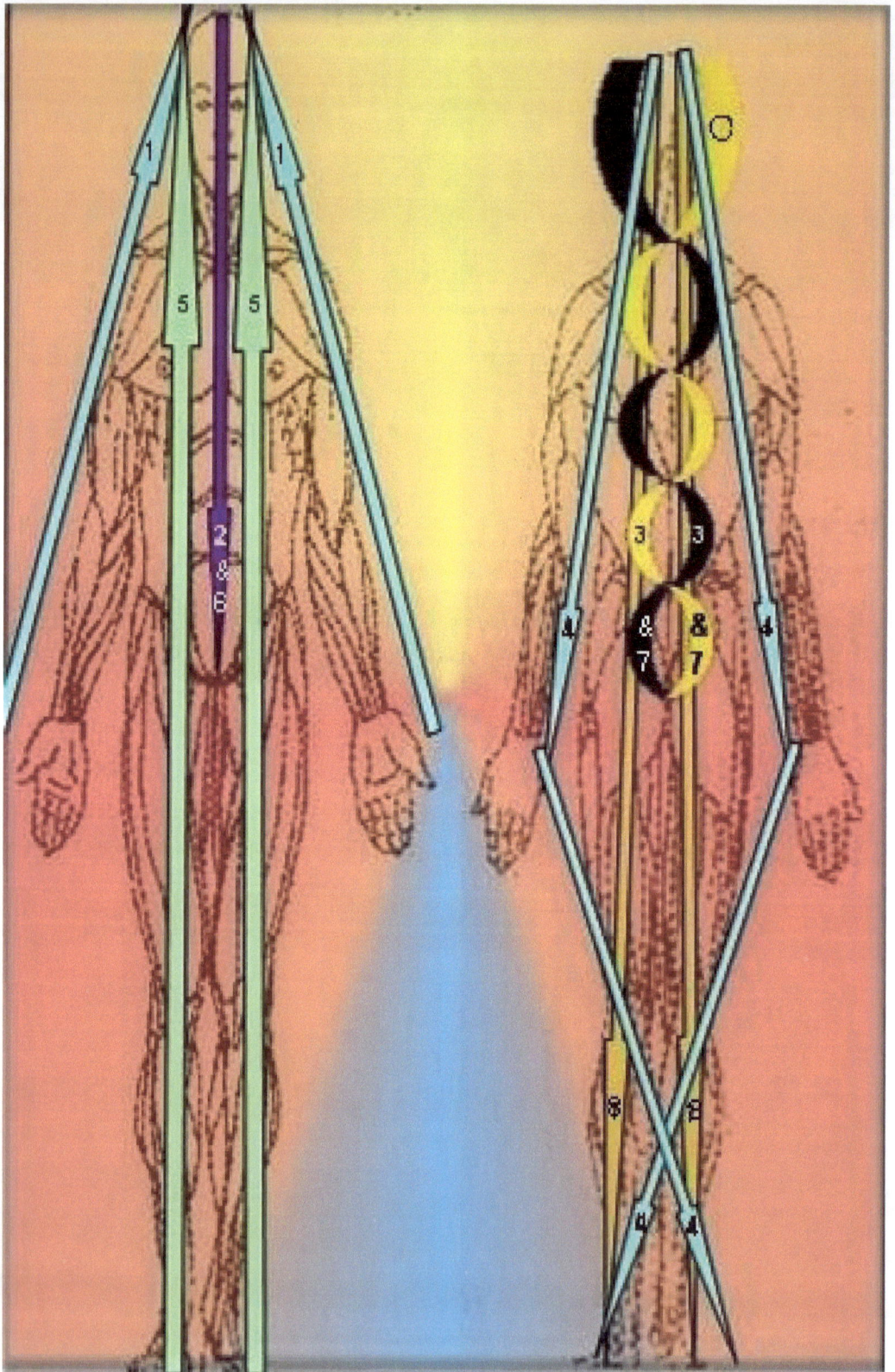

QI CIRCULATION DIAGRAM

7 PHASE ELEMENTAL CHAKRA MERIDIAN CHART

YIN (SOLID) ORGANS

(- HT) HEART
(- PC) PERICARDIUM
(- SP) SPLEEN
(- LU) LUNGS
(- KI) KIDNEY
(- LV) LIVER
(GV) GOVERNING VESSEL

YANG (HOLLOW) ORGANS

SMALL INTESTINE(+ SI)
TRIPPLE WARMER (+ TW)
STOMACH (+ ST)
LARGE INTESTINE (+ LI)
URINARY BLADDER (+
GALL BLADDER (+ GB)
CONCEPTION VESSEL (CV)

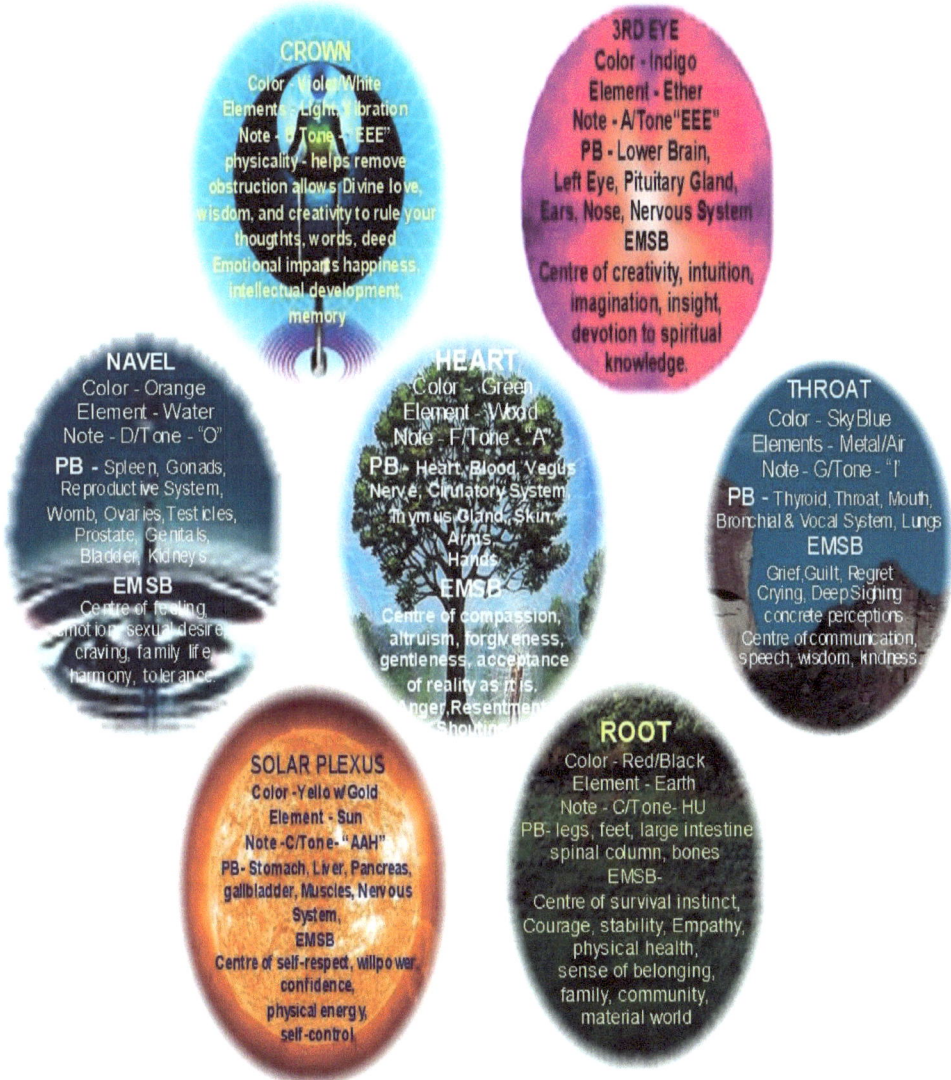

CROWN
Color - Violet/White
Elements - Light, Vibration
Note - B Tone - "EEE"
physicality - helps remove
obstruction allows Divine love,
wisdom, and creativity to rule your
thougthts, words, deed
Emotional imparts happiness,
intellectual development,
memory

3RD EYE
Color - Indigo
Element - Ether
Note - A/Tone"EEE"
PB - Lower Brain,
Left Eye, Pituitary Gland,
Ears, Nose, Nervous System
EMSB
Centre of creativity, intuition,
imagination, insight,
devotion to spiritual
knowledge.

NAVEL
Color - Orange
Element - Water
Note - D/Tone - "O"
PB - Spleen, Gonads,
Reproductive System,
Womb, Ovaries,Testicles,
Prostate, Genitals,
Bladder, Kidneys
EMSB
Centre of feeling
emotion, sexual desire,
craving, family life,
harmony, tolerance

HEART
Color - Green
Element - Wood
Note - F/Tone - "A"
PB - Heart, Blood, Vagus
Nerve, Circulatory System,
thymus Gland, Skin,
Arms
Hands
EMSB
Centre of compassion,
altruism, forgiveness,
gentleness, acceptance
of reality as it is.
Anger,Resentment
Shouting

THROAT
Color - Sky Blue
Elements - Metal/Air
Note - G/Tone - "I"
PB - Thyroid, Throat, Mouth,
Bronchial & Vocal System, Lungs
EMSB
Grief,Guilt, Regret
Crying, Deep Sighing
concrete perceptions
Centre of communication,
speech, wisdom, kindness

SOLAR PLEXUS
Color -Yellow Gold
Element - Sun
Note -C/Tone - "AAH"
PB - Stomach, Liver, Pancreas,
gallbladder, Muscles, Nervous
System,
EMSB
Centre of self-respect, willpower,
confidence,
physical energy,
self-control

ROOT
Color - Red/Black
Element - Earth
Note - C/Tone - HU
PB - legs, feet, large intestine
spinal column, bones
EMSB-
Centre of survival instinct,
Courage, stability, Empathy,
physical health,
sense of belonging,
family, community,
material world

7 PHASE ELEMENTAL MERIDIAN CHART

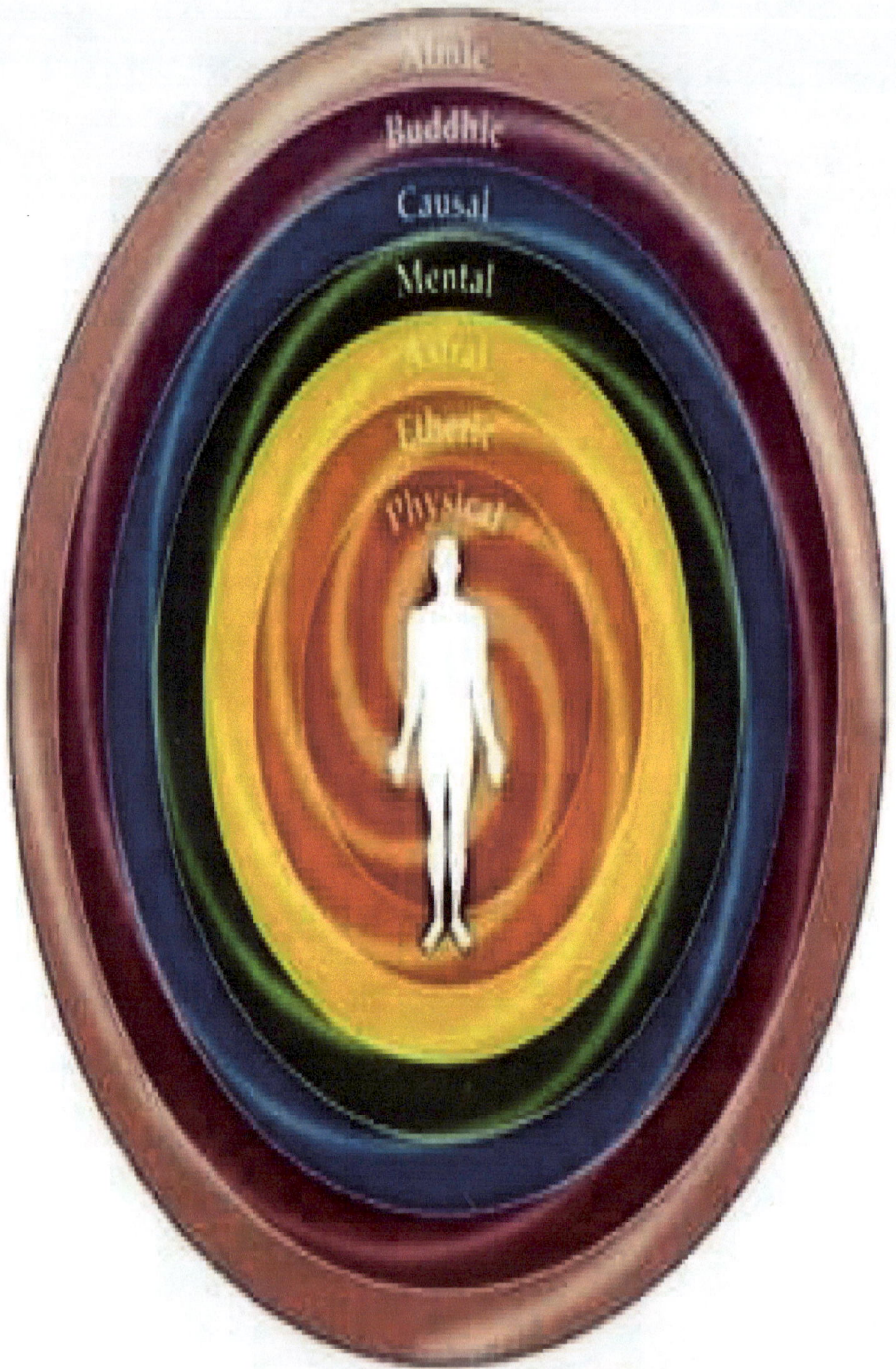

SUBTLE BODY LAYERS CHART

Chakras

Crown
Sahasrara

Thrid Eye
Ajna

Seat of
Consciousness
Bindu

Throat
Vishuddah

Heart
Anahata

Solar Plexus
Manipura

Tantien
Swadistana

Root
Maludhara

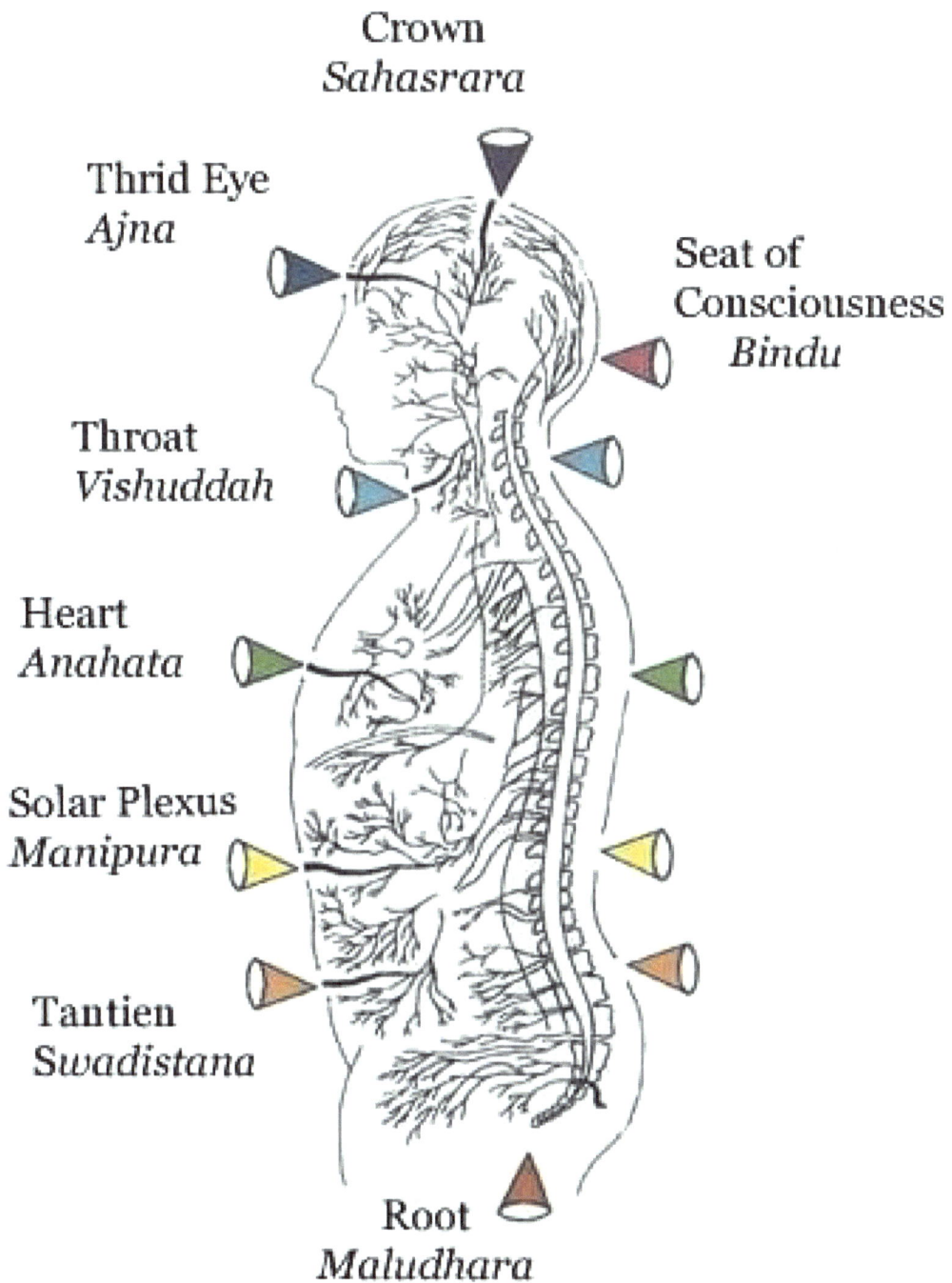

CHAKRA ANATOMY CHART

CHAKRA ANATOMY DETAILS CHART

CHAKRA DETAILS	PHYSICAL BODY DETAILS	EMOTIONAL, MENTAL & SPIRITUAL BODY DETAILS
ROOT CHAKRA: • Color - Red/Black, • Element - Earth, Fire • Resonant Frequency C – 91 hz - 104 hz • Intonation – HU	**Location:** L5 – Coccyx – Gastrocnemius, Soleus, Peroneus, ankles, feet, descending colon, spinal column, bones, hip bones, buttocks, Rectum, Anus, blood, immune system. **Affects:** Rectal and colon problems, immune system disorders, base of spine/lower back problems, varicose veins, feet and leg problems, cramping in legs, tightness in Glutes, quads, IT Bands, Tensor Fascia Late and hamstring musculature.	Survival, tribal associations, instinct, past life memories, family, marriage, parenting, correct behavior, society, ability to provide basic needs for living. Following the establishment of or what family rules. Doing what your family/spouse wants. Trying to fit in. Compromises to these issues, depression, problems with decision making.
NAVEL CHAKRA: • Color - Orange • Element – Water/Earth • Resonant Frequency D – 107 hz - 116 hz • Intonation – "O"	**Location:** T10 – L4 Reproductive organs, Kidneys, urinary bladder, small intestines, lymph circulation, inguinal rings, appendix, rectus, oblique & transverse abdominals, Quadratus Lumborum, quads, hamstrings, glutes, sacral spinalis, Peroneus, Anterior/posterior Tibials, Illiacus/Psoas, hips and knees, prostate gland, lower back muscles, sciatic nerve. **Affects:** menstrual cycle problems, cancers in this area, impotency. Pelvic and lower back pains, urinary and bladder problems, chronic tiredness, gas pains, sterility, difficult breathing, varicose veins, constipation, colitis, diarrhea, hernias, Sciatica, lumbago, hip problems.	Power, creativity, sexual matters, blame, control, passion, ethics, money, greed, honor in relationship matters, fidelity, feelings of repression or wrongness in sexual matters. Reproduction issues. Birthing new ideas.
SOLAR PLEXUS CHAKRA: • Color – Yellow/Gold • Element – Sun/air • Resonant Frequency E – 118 hz - 124 hz • Intonation – "AAH"	**Location:** T4 – T9 – gallbladder, liver, solar plexus, circulation, stomach, pancreas, duodenum, spleen, adrenal and suprarenal glands, Latissimus Dorsi, Erector Spinae, upper Quadratus Lumborum, Rib Cage. **Affects:** gallstones, jaundice, shingles, arthritis, circulation problems, ulcers, heartburn, indigestion, gastric reflux, duodenal ulcers, gastritis, lowered resistance to infection, anemia, allergies,	Responsibility issues, caring for others, trust, fear, guilt, career, intimidation, personal honor, victimization feelings, and courage. Self concern issues; self- respect, sensitivity to criticism, self-esteem, self-worth and own confidence, independence, reliability, decision making.

	hives, skin conditions, exzema, Indigestion, stomach, intestinal, and colon problems. Eating disorders. Diabetes, adrenal, pancreas, liver dysfunctions, gall bladder, kidneys, and ulcers. Spleen and middle of back problems.	
HEART CHAKRA: • Color - Green • Element – Wood/Earth • Resonant Frequency F – 129 hz – 139 hz • Intonation – Hu "A"	**Location:** C7 – T3 – Thyroid/parathyroid glands, shoulders, trapezius, rhomboids, rotator cuff, Pectoralis Major/minor, Upper Latissimus Dorsi region, subscapularis, elbows, muscles of the arms, hands, wrists, and fingers, esophagus, trachea, heart, valves, coronary arteries, lungs, chest, and breasts. **Affects:** Bursitis, colds, thyroid conditions, asthma, pneumonia, bronchitis, upper back/shoulder/arm weakness and structural misalignments, difficulty breathing, pain in lower arms and hands, heart conditions, chest conditions, circulatory system conditions, Bronchitis, pleurisy, pneumonia, congestion, influenza,	Love, happiness, desire for happiness, sadness, anger, hatred, prejudice, loneliness, forgiveness, compassion, hopes, desires, wants, grief, resentments, inability or resistance to reach out to others, commitment, trust in your close interpersonal relationships. Choices in love.
THROAT CHAKRA: • Color – Turquoise/Sky Blue • Element – Metal/Air • Resonant Frequency G – 142 hz - 149hz • Intonation – "I"(eye)	**Location:** C4 - C6 – Nose, Nasal Cavity, lips, jaw, mouth, Tongue, Eustachian tube, Vocal cords, neck glands, Neck Muscles, shoulders, tonsils, Larynx. **Affects:** Hay fever, runny nose, hearing loss, tooth aches, deterioration of the teeth and gums, canker sores, herpes of the mouth, laryngitis, hoarseness, sore throat, thyroid and gland problems, hiatal hernias, choking, gagging, chronic neck problems, subluxation in cervical vertebrae, stiff neck, pain in upper arms, carpal tunnel, chronic cough, winged scapula, upper back pain, atrophying of the PMC low oxygenation to the brain and head.	Communication, expressing yourself, telling truth, following your dreams and being true to yourself. Addictions, habits, judgment, faith, making decisions, knowing and being yourself, criticism, will power, doing what you said you would do. All forms of expression & communication.

THIRD EYE CHAKRA: • Color - Indigo • Element - Ether • Vibratory Frequency A A – 159 hz – 175 hz • Intonation – "EEE"	**Location:** C2 - C3 – eyes, optic nerves, auditory nerves, sinuses, jaw bones, cheeks, outer ear, face, teeth, facial nerves. **Affects:** sinus problems, allergies, pain around the eyes, fainting spells, crossed eyes, deafness, eye weakness, earaches, Tinnitus, ringing in the ears, pressure on brain stem, nervous system, full spinal problems, learning problems, Bell's Palsy, acne or pimples, eczema.	Truth, knowledge, intellect, intuitive powers, learning from experience, feeling inadequate, inner wisdom, knowing yourself and self-evaluation, open-mindedness, accepting yourself and others. Listening and seeing openly.
CROWN CHAKRA: • Color – Violet/White • Element – Light/Vibration • Vibratory Frequency B/B~ 180 hz – 244 hz • Intonation – "EEE"	**Location:** C1 – Head, Pituitary Gland, bones of the face, inner/middle ear, brain. **Affects:** Headaches, migraines, nervousness, insomnia, head colds, high blood pressure, dizziness, memory loss, energy/exhaustion problems, increased dysfunction of mental/emotional faculties, skin and muscles systems.	Spirituality, devotion to spiritual and personal matters. Unconditional love to self, the earth, and to others. Empathy, humanitarianism, selflessness, values, and ethics. Connection with ULEK™, ability to go with the flow of life and to see the larger picture, inspiration without wants. The Higher Self. Mystical depression, searching feelings, sensitivity to the environmental elements, (sun, light, sound)
BINDU CHAKRA: • Color - Magenta • Element – Magnetism/Electricity • Vibratory Frequency High C –254 hz + • Intonation – "AUM"	Brain, nervous system Pineal Gland.	Knowledge of past lives, akashic records of past lives, Divine design and higher purpose Seat of the soul, center where we communicate with our ancestors who have left physicality. Higher Self

Periodic Table by Article Value

December 2008

	Quality		
	High	Mid	Low
High	Showcase		Blemish
Views **Mid**			
Low	Treasure		Under the Rug

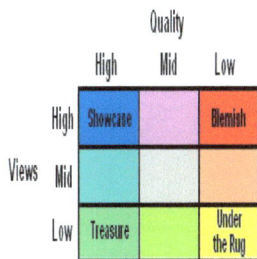

1 H Hydrogen																	2 He Helium
3 Li Lithium	4 Be Beryllium											5 B Boron	6 C Carbon	7 N Nitrogen	8 O Oxygen	9 F Fluorine	10 Ne Neon
11 Na Sodium	12 Mg Magnesium											13 Al Aluminum	14 Si Silicon	15 P Phosphorus	16 S Sulfur	17 Cl Chlorine	18 Ar Argon
19 K Potassium	20 Ca Calcium	21 Sc Scandium	22 Ti Titanium	23 V Vanadium	24 Cr Chromium	25 Mn Manganese	26 Fe Iron	27 Co Cobalt	28 Ni Nickel	29 Cu Copper	30 Zn Zinc	31 Ga Gallium	32 Ge Germanium	33 As Arsenic	34 Se Selenium	35 Br Bromine	36 Kr Krypton
37 Rb Rubidium	38 Sr Strontium	39 Y Yttrium	40 Zr Zirconium	41 Nb Niobium	42 Mo Molybdenum	43 Tc Technetium	44 Ru Ruthenium	45 Rh Rhodium	46 Pd Palladium	47 Ag Silver	48 Cd Cadmium	49 In Indium	50 Sn Tin	51 Sb Antimony	52 Te Tellurium	53 I Iodine	54 Xe Xenon
55 Cs Caesium	56 Ba Barium	57 * La Lanthanum	72 Hf Hafnium	73 Ta Tantalum	74 W Tungsten	75 Re Rhenium	76 Os Osmium	77 Ir Iridium	78 Pt Platinum	79 Au Gold	80 Hg Mercury	81 Tl Thallium	82 Pb Lead	83 Bi Bismuth	84 Po Polonium	85 At Astatine	86 Rn Radon
87 Fr Francium	88 Ra Radium	89 ** Ac Actinium	104 Rf Rutherfordium	105 Db Dubnium	106 Sg Seaborgium	107 Bh Bohrium	108 Hs Hassium	109 Mt Meitnerium	110 Ds Darmstadtium	111 Rg Roentgenium	112 Uub Ununbium	113 Uut Ununtrium	114 Uuq Ununquadium	115 Uup Ununpentium	116 Uuh Ununhexium	117 Uus Ununseptium	118 Uuo Ununoctium

*	58 Ce Cerium	59 Pr Praseodymium	60 Nd Neodymium	61 Pm Promethium	62 Sm Samarium	63 Eu Europium	64 Gd Gadolinium	65 Tb Terbium	66 Dy Dysprosium	67 Ho Holmium	68 Er Erbium	69 Tm Thulium	70 Yb Ytterbium	71 Lu Lutetium
**	90 Th Thorium	91 Pa Protactinium	92 U Uranium	93 Np Neptunium	94 Pu Plutonium	95 Am Americium	96 Cm Curium	97 Bk Berkelium	98 Cf Californium	99 Es Einsteinium	100 Fm Fermium	101 Md Mendelevium	102 No Nobelium	103 Lr Lawrencium

PERIODIC TABLE

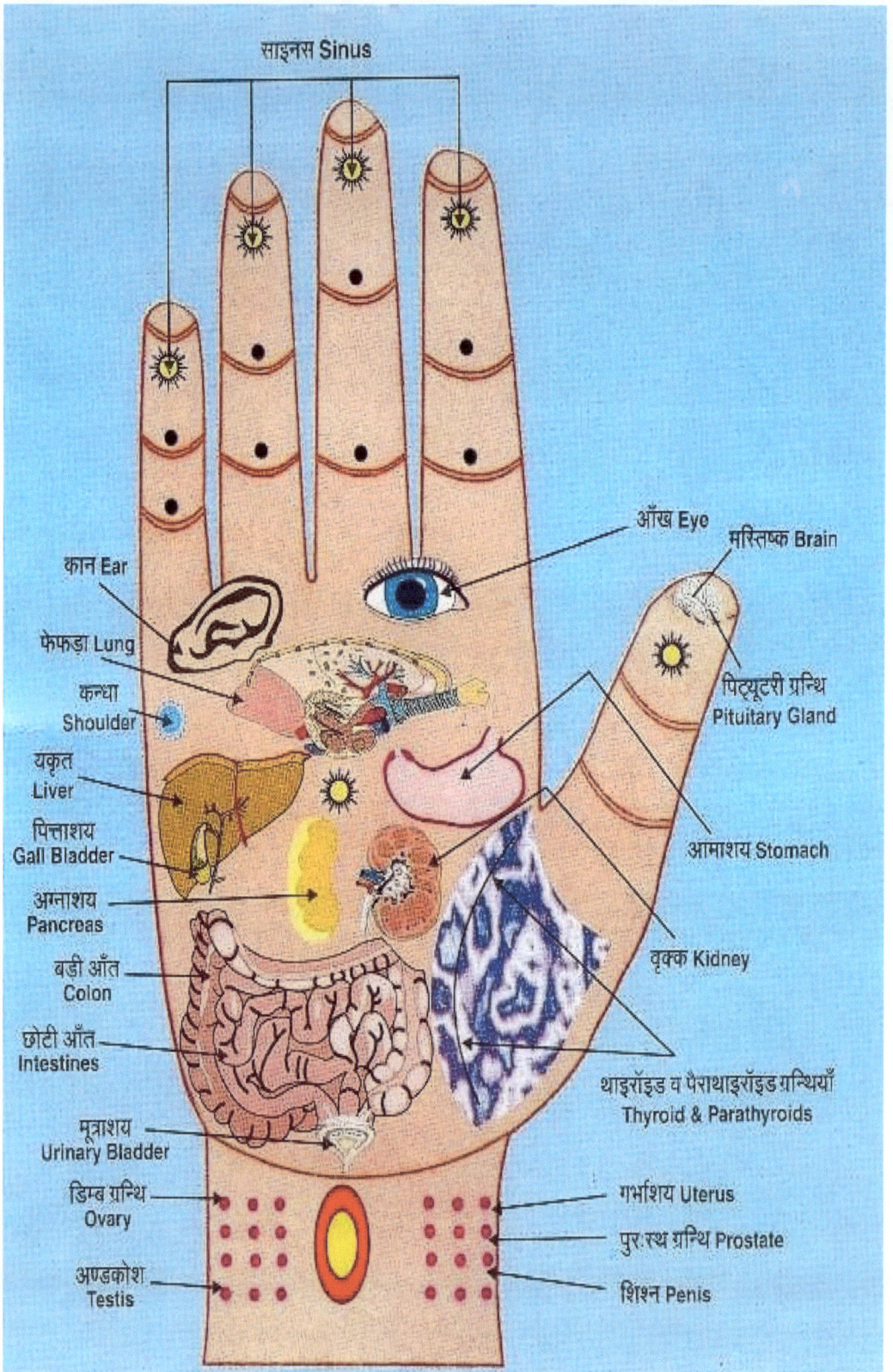

HAND REFLEXOLOGY CHART

174

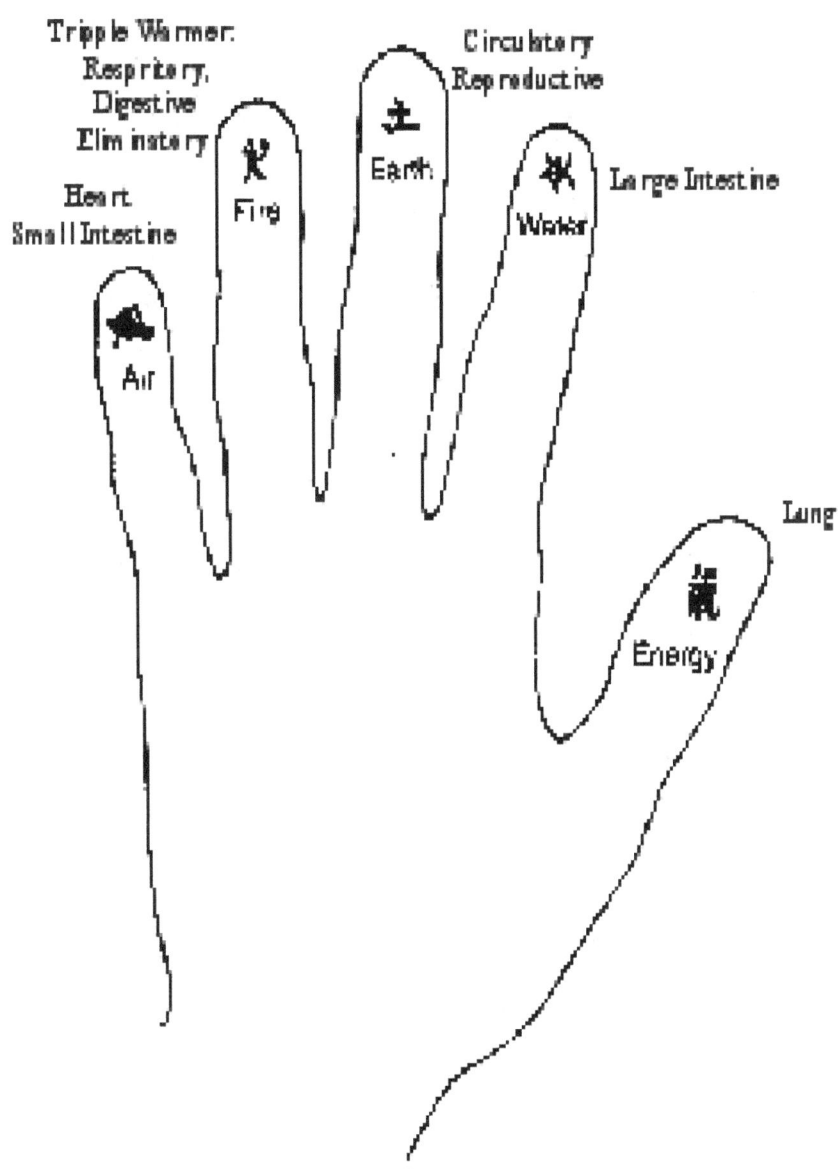

Triple Warmer:
Respritory,
Digestive
Eliminatory

Heart
Small Intestine

Fire

Air

Earth

Circulatory
Reproductive

Water

Large Intestine

Lung

Energy

Elements corresponding to the fingers and thumb
according to Chinese palmistry: little finger with air;
ring finger with fire; middle finger with earth,
forefinger with water, and thumb with chi. From
Chinese Hand Analysis

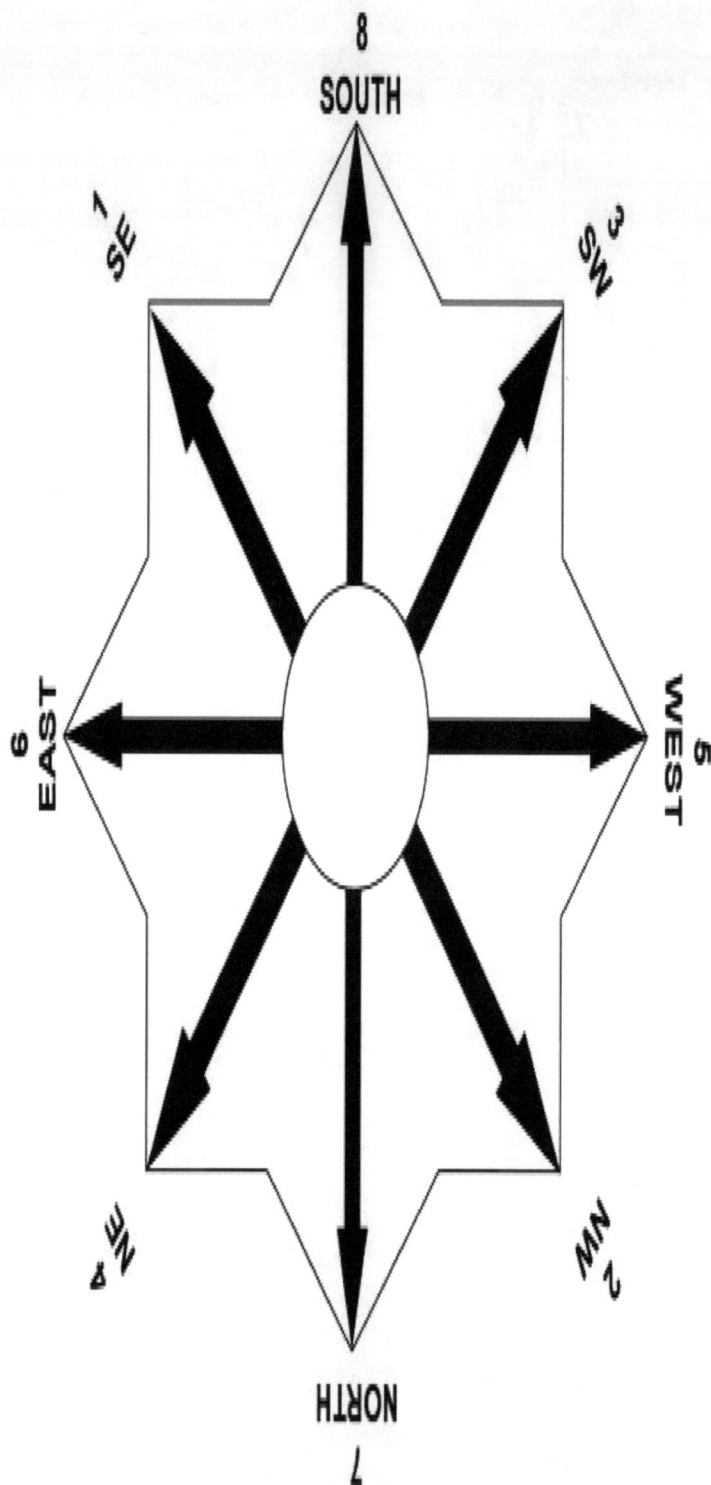

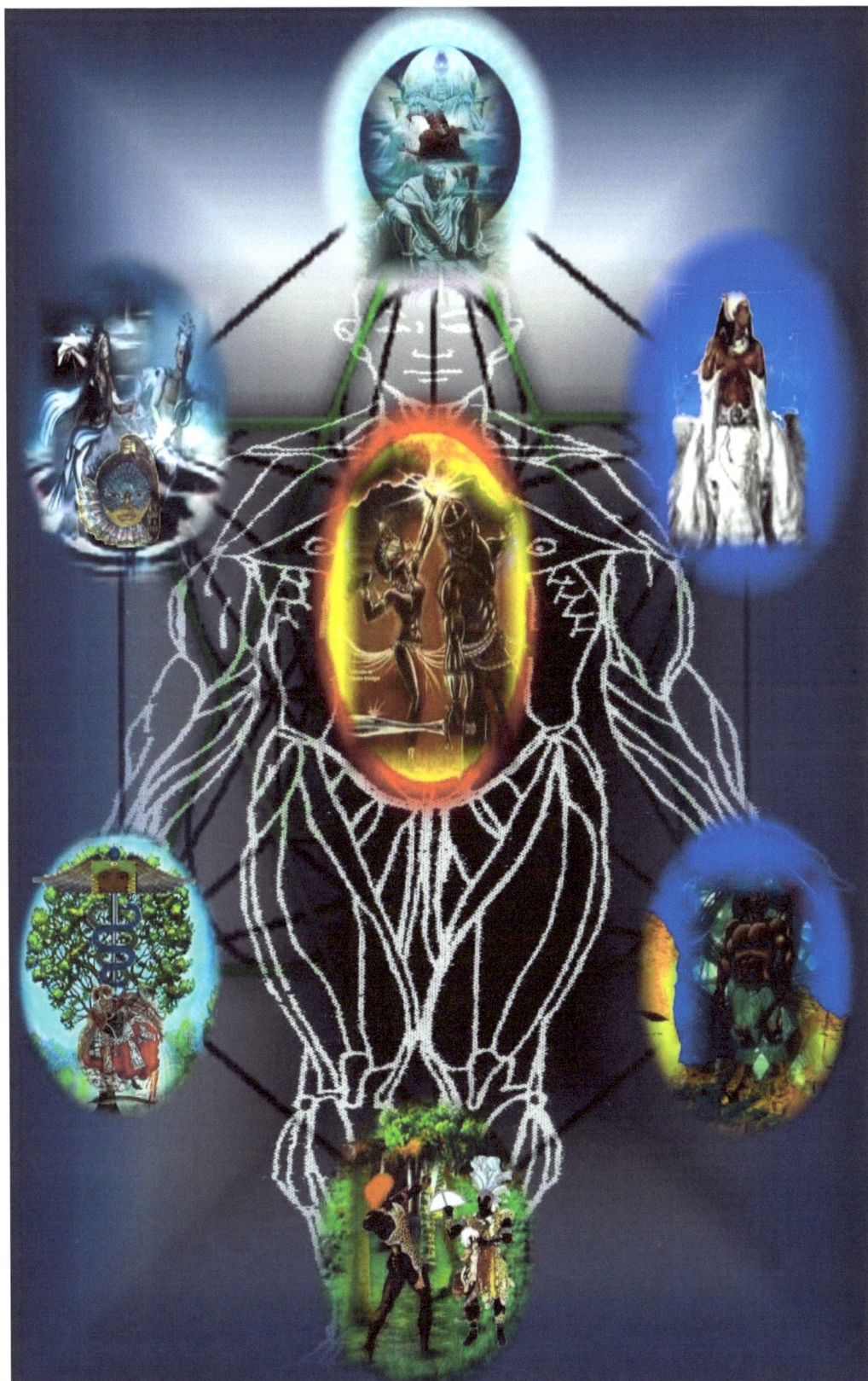

ORISHA TANRAN ELEMENTAL ASSOCIATION CHART
ORISHA ATTRIBUTES

<u>**HEAVENLY ORISHA**</u>

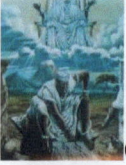

OLORUN (OLDUMARE) - Creator of the Universe /Divine Life Force of Nature and All of Creation

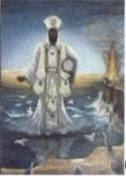

ORUMILA – The One Mind/Orisha of Divine Wisdom, Divine Knowledge, and divination, psychic gifts (Holy Spirit of God) – The Pineal Gland/The Brain allowed to witness creation of the Universe by Olorun

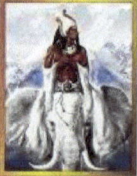

OBATALA – Father of The Orisha & Human Kind/Creator of the World of Humanity, Source of all that's pure, wise, peaceful and compassionate. Divine Justice and Reason, Rules Court cases, karmic justice,

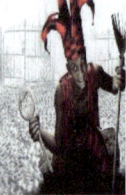

ELEGGUA – Spirit/The Cross Roads – Spirit/Soul Intelligence behind the bodies operations, functions, etc.

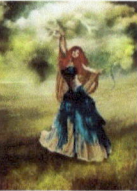

AYAO – Air – breath, the calm of the storm

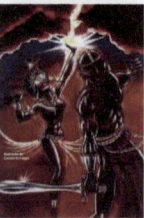

OYA – Whirl Winds/Tornadoes/ Transitional Change – nervous system signals (neurotransmitters), gas, facilitates connection with ancestral memory and Celestial communication with Ancestors.

Shango - Fire, lightning, drums – internal heat, nervous system, internal physical and subtle body rhythms, Heart

HEAVENLY/EARTHLY ORISHA

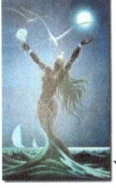

YEMONJA – Water – bodily fluids, sweat, The Womb or incubative space within the body & mind

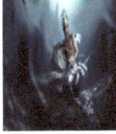

OLOKUN – Deep Waters - Subconscious physical and subtle body functions and operations

EARTHLY ORISHA

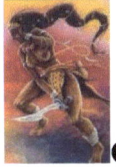

OBA – Turbulent Waters – digestive imbalances, fertility

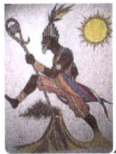

AGANJU – Volcanoes/fire - internal body heat, digestion, heart, skin perspiration (the desert)

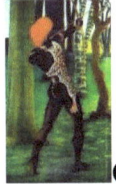

OCHOSSI – Warrior – instinct, ability for fight or flight, internal justice, breakdown of meat based foods

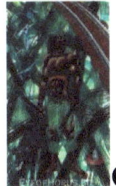

OGUN – Material and technological operations and manifestation – Iron and mineral absorption and distribution of plant based foods

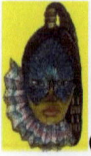

OSHUN – Fresh Waters – emotional healing/2nd chakra, balance, regulates the digestive and meridian channels of the organs throughout the body – distribution of liquids

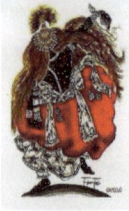

BABALOU AYE – Orisha of healing & knowledge of all plant & mineral life force properties digestion and nutritional distribution of plant life nutrients

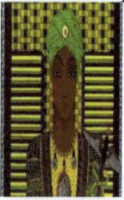

ERINLE – Healer and patron of gay people/Guardian of plant life, its assimilation, absorption, distribution, and elimination processes in the body along.

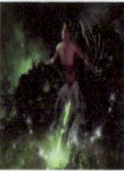

OKO – Harvest and fertility of land

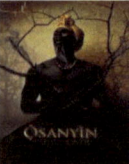

OSAIN – Rules the secret knowledge of Herbs and naturopathic medicine, the immune system and the body's ability to heal itself when supported by natural non-chemically treated nutrients

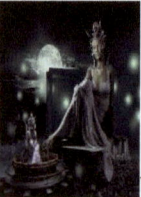

YEGUA' - Orisha of cellular/physical decomposition – cellular decomposition & the dying process

APPENDIX C
HEALING MUDRAS WITH DETAILS

The following mudras are used in conjunction with Kun Qi Kung in order to enhance and amplify the healing effects of the movement. Each chosen mudra has direct associative purposes to the chakras, the link between the physical and the Ka body. These mudras are used specifically with the 8 Directional Series as direct energy channels to both internal and subtle body systems designed to increase the flow of life force to these systems.

Try first to give the body a chance to heal itself before giving it invasive medicines and drugs, which must and will have some side effects. The use of Mudras works best as a preventative measure for improving and sustaining good health. If one has been diagnosed with a physically debilitating condition, first give the body a chance to heal itself before giving it invasive medicines and drugs, which will have some side effects. If one has been prescribed medications as treatment, then mudras can be used in conjunction with the prescribed treatment as ones condition improves.

BINDU

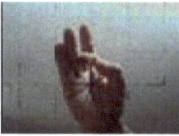

AAKASH (ETHER): aligns with the Bindu (8th) Chakra. The use of this mudra helps to remove weakness of bones and hearing deficiencies. **Caution:** This Mudra should not be done while walking. This mudra helps to stabilize the chakra of the universe within you.

CROWN –

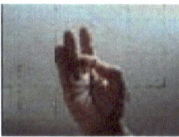

AAKASH (ETHER): aligns with the Bindu (8th) Chakra. The use of this mudra helps to remove weakness of bones and hearing deficiencies. **Caution:** This Mudra should not be done while walking. This mudra helps to stabilize the chakra of the universe within you.

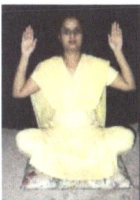

SINGHAKRANTA MUDRA Helps to regain the lost halo due to abuse of the body.

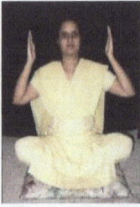

MAHAKRANTA MUDRA Helps to regain the lost halo due to abuse of the body.

1ˢᵀ EYE –

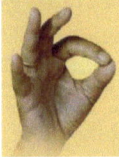

GYAN (DIVINE LIFEFORCE KNOWLEDGE), is a mudra of knowledge, which enhances ones access to Divine Inspiration. The tip of the thumb is the hand center of the pituitary and endocrine glands. When we press these centers by index finger the two glands work actively. The benefits of this mudra are many. It increases concentration, mental peace, sharpens memory, enriches spirituality, and has been used for treating insomnia, mental disorders, stress, depression, anger issues and drowsiness. It helps in the development of telepathic, clairvoyant, and extra-sensory abilities as well. This mudra is good for: stresses and strains, insomnia, emotional instability, indecisiveness, excessive anger, idleness, laziness, indolence, and is a great help in increasing memory and I.Q. It can help cure sleeplessness and get one off sleeping pills where these are being taken.

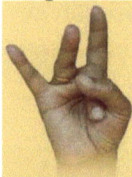

SHUNYA (SOUND/ETHER, EMPTINESS, or the VOID) represents the deep dark quiet stillness of the night and the inner chamber or creative space of the mind where thoughts are formed and ideas built upon through our imagination. In the body, Sunya represents the brain, the mind, the inner chamber of head and nervous system. Shunya reduces numbness in the body, relieves an earache within 4 or 5 minutes It is useful for the deaf and mentally challenged, but not for inborn ones. This helps those with impaired hearing. If there is no physical defect, the mudra, if practiced regularly, can restore the hearing power. Remarkably, it helps in getting rid of earaches within minutes. It takes no more than 2 to 3 minutes to get rid of most earaches. It helps in relieving the nausea and vomiting sensations felt while driving on winding hilly curves or while taking off or landing in aircrafts. It helps in many problems of vertigo. The mudra should not be continued after the problem has been removed.

THROAT –

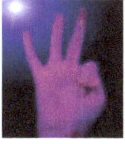

VAYU (AIR/WIND), represents things that grow, expand, and enjoy freedom of movement. Aside from air, smoke, and the like Vayu can in some ways be best represented by the human mind. As we grow physically, we learn and expand mentally as well, in terms of our knowledge, our experiences, and our personalities. *Vayu* represents breathing, and the internal processes associated with respiration. Mentally and emotionally, it represents an "open-minded" attitude and carefree feeling. It can be associated with will, elusiveness, evasiveness, benevolence, compassion, wisdom, and electricity. It prevents all diseases that occur due to the imbalances of the air. It cures Rheumatism, Sciatica, Arthritis, Gout, Parkinson's disease and paralysis without any medicine. It is useful for Cervical Spondilytis, paralysis to face and catching of nerve in neck and corrects the disorder of gas in the stomach. This finger position is unbeatable in quickly and effectively removing the accumulated wind in the stomach. Depending on one's physiology, it may take anywhere from 1 minute to 15 minutes or so to effectively expel all accumulated wind in the stomach without the use of anti-flatulants. Mudra should be stopped when the trouble abates. It also helps in alleviating all wind based aches and pains. Considering that almost 80 % of the body's aches and pains are due to wind, the practice of this Mudra is a must, before taking recourse to any other treatment. It is very effective in Parkinson's disease (an ailment of the nerves where the patients body, head and limbs shake uncontrollably).

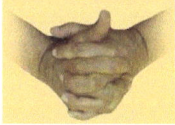

LING, generates heat in the body. It destroys phlegm and helps in problems of colds, catarrh and coughs. It is excellent when the body is cold due to shortage of cover in inimical weather. This mudra must be performed under supervision or with full knowledge.

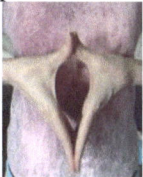

YONI MUDRA Helps to overcome loss of virility, loss of pure qualities and stimulates the lungs and large intestines.

HEART –

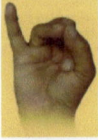

MRIT SANJIVINI MUDRA / APAAN VAYU
In the case of severe heart attack, this life giving divine Mudra provides instant relief within a few seconds. They are a helping hand for Cardiac's and first aid for heart problems. They strengthen the heart, emergency first aid for severe heart attack if administered within 2 seconds. It also improves self-confidence, normalizes blood pressure, and has been used to help treat menstruation related problems. Mrit Sanjuivini and Apaan Vayu can be used as tools for purification of the entire body. This finger position works like an injection in cases of a heart attack. Regular practice is an insurance in preventing heart attacks, tacho-cardia, palpitations, depressions, sinking feeling of the heart. Also known as the Mritsanjivani Mudra for arresting heart attack.

SOLAR PLEXUS –

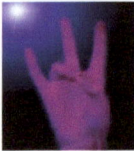

SURYA (SUN or FIRE) represents the energetic, forceful, moving things in the world. Animals, particularly predators, capable of movement and full of forceful energy, are primary examples of *fire* objects. Bodily, *fire* represents our metabolism and body heat, and in the mental and emotional realms, it represents drive and passion. *Fire* can be associated with motivation, desire, intention, and an outgoing spirit. This Mudra sharpens the center in the thyroid gland. It reduces cholesterol and the accumulated fat in the body helping to reduce weight. It reduces anxiety and corrects indigestion problems.

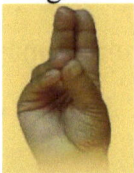

PRANA (METAL/LIFE FORCE), As it is the mudra of life, integrates the power of life-force at a cellular level. Weak people become strong. It reduces the clamps in blood vessels. If one practices it regularly, it can restore one's energy bank; improving vitality of the body physically, and psychologically. It improves immunity, inner vision and the power of the eyes plus reduces eye related diseases. Prana treats dizziness, improve s circulation, brings clarity in thought improving concentration, helps to lower blood pressure, breathing, helps to control eating habits, and helps to open blocked veins. It has been said to remove vitamin deficiency and fatigue. This finger position is an all time useful Mudra and can be done for any length of time, any time, any place and will only help in adding to the benefits. This is the mudra which, along with the Apan Mudra, precedes any efforts at higher meditation by the Yogis and saints. The mudra helps to increase the Pran Shakti or the "Life force". It increases one's self confidence. It helps the body in increasing it's vitality and sustenance when deprived of food and water. It helps in improving weak eyesight and quiescence (motionlessness) of the eyes. It supports any other treatment where the patient is short on confidence.

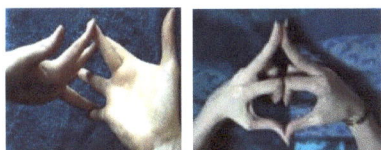

SURABHI MUDRAS This mudra helps to cure and eliminate diseases related to bile. It helps in curing diseases related to urine and assists easy passage. By increasing the ethereal vacuity, it helps the sadhak to increase the hearing power manifold. it helps to eliminate all ailments resulting from the increase of wind in the system. These mudras can help to cure all ailments of the stomach generated due to defects in the digestive system and are especially effective for people with chronic digestive ailments.

NAVEL –

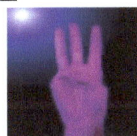

VARUNA (WATER) represents the fluid, flowing, formless things in the world. Outside of the obvious example of rivers and the like, plants are also categorized under *water*, as they adapt to their environment, growing and changing according to the direction of the sun and the changing seasons. Blood and other bodily fluids are represented by *Varuna* as are mental or emotional tendencies towards adaptation and change. Varuna helps to retain purity in the blood by balancing the water content in the body. It helps prevent the pains of Gastroenteritis and Muscle Shrinkage. *Varuna* can be associated with defensiveness, adaptability, flexibility, suppleness, and magnetism. It is used to enhance beauty, remove impurities from the blood, restore moisture to skin, relieves painful cramps, treat diarrhea and

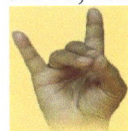

APAAN (VEGETATION/EMBODIMENT) plays an important role in our health as it regulates the excretory system. It has been used by some to regulate diabetes. It cures constipation and piles and helps regulate normal regular waste excretion. Apaan can help provide relief in urinary problems, as it facilitates discharge of waste material from the body. Apaan can be used to assist in the Cleansing & purifying of the liver and gall

185

bladder improving their function ability, helps remove toxic waste products from the body, regulate bladder problems, and balances the mind increasing one self-confidence, patience, sense of serenity and inner harmony. Helps in purification of the body, urinary problems, easy secretion of excreta, regulating menstruation and painless discharge, easy child delivery, Piles, Diabetes and kidney disorders.

ROOT –

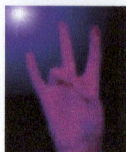

PRITHVI (EARTH)

Prithvi or "Earth", represents the hard, solid objects of the world. In people, the bones, muscles and tissues are represented by *earth*. Mentally it is confidence; *earth* is predominantly associated with stubbornness, stability, physicality, and gravity. Emotionally it is a desire to have things remain as they are; a resistance to change. When under the influence of this mode or "mood", we are aware of our own physicality and sureness of action. This mudra helps to reduce all physical weaknesses. It improves the complexion of skin and makes the skin to glow. It makes the body active by keeping it healthy. It improves ones sense of Inner stability, Self-Assurance, calms the stomach, Strengthens the body and mind and Increases ones energy. **Prithvi Mudra**: Increases solidity in the body. Removes weakness and lack of body solidity and helps gain for those underweight, chronic fatigue and weakness

APPENDIX D
CHAKRA COLORS, VOCAL TONATIONS, ESSENTIAL OILS, AND GEM STONES

BINDU (AURIC SEAL) CHAKRA:
- **TONAL NOTE**: B
- **VOCAL TONE**: AUM/OM
- **RELATED ESSENTIAL OILS**: lavender, abundance, white angelica to increase the aura, or the blend of marjoram, lavender and peppermint to clear ones aura, harmony also balances the chakras. Forgiveness works wonders for releasing and letting go of old issues.
- **RELATED STONES**: Clear Quartz, Meteorite, Tectonite, Black Opal, Tanzanite, Moldavite, Peacock Quartz Crystal, Kyanite
- **MUDRA** – AAKASH (DIVINE ETHER)

CROWN CHAKRA:
- **TONAL NOTE**: B/B#
- **VOCAL TONATION**: "EEE"
- **ESSENTIAL OILS**: 3 Wise Men, Acceptance, Release, Frankincense and Myrrh.
- **STONES**: Amethyst, Diamond, Alexandrite, Quartz, Selenite
- **MUDRA(S)**: GYAN/APAAN (DIVINE LIFE FORCE/KNOWLEDGE)

1ST EYE CHAKRA:
- **TONAL NOTE**: A/ A#
- **VOCAL TONATION**: EEE
- **ESSENTIAL OILS**: 3 Wise Men, Acceptance, Sage, Cedarwood.
- **1ST EYE CHAKRA STONES**: Azurite, Lapis Lazuli, Opal, Sapphire, Sodalite, Topaz.
- **MUDRA(S)**: GYAN/SHUNYA (DIVINE LIFE FORCE/ETHERIC VIBRATION, EMPTINESS)

THROAT CHAKRA:
- **TONAL NOTE**: G, G#
- **VOCAL TONATION**: "I"
- **ESSENTIAL OILS**: Sandalwood, Rose, Eucalyptus, Ylang Ylang.
- **CHAKRA STONES**: Aquamarine, Turquoise,
- **MUDRA(S)**: VAYU (AIR)

HEART CHAKRA:
- **TONAL NOTE**: E
- **VOCAL TONATION**: AAY
- **ESSENTIAL OILS**: Sandalwood, Bergamot, Rose, White Angelica.
- **CHAKRA STONES**: Aventurine, Emerald, Rose Quartz, Moonstone, Peridot, Ruby.
- **MUDRA(S)**: MRIT SANJIVINI MUDRA

SOLAR PLEXUS CHAKRA:
- **TONAL NOTE**: E
- **VOCAL TONATION**: "AAAH"
- **RELATED ESSENTIAL OILS**: Fennel, Cedar wood, Juniper, Sacred Mountain Blend.
- **RELATED STONES**: Agate, Amber, Malachite, and Tigers Eye.
- **MUDRA(S)**: SURYA/PRITHVI (SOLAR POWER or INTERNAL FIRE/GROUNDING TO THE EARTH)

NAVEL CHAKRA:
- **TONAL NOTE**: D, D#
- **VOCAL TONATION**: "O"
- **RELATED ESSENTIAL OILS**: SARA, Sandalwood, Patchouli, Sage, Acceptance,

- **RELATED STONES**: Carnelian, Coral, Yellow Zircon
- **MUDRA(S):** VARUNA (FLOW OF WATER

ROOT CHAKRA:
- **TONAL NOTE**: C, C#
- **VOCAL TONATION**: HU/OOOH
- **RELATED ESSENTIAL OILS**: Western or Canadian Red Cedar Sandalwood, Patchouli, Ylang-Ylang,
- **CHAKRA STONES**: Bloodstone, Chrysocolla, Lodestone, Smoky Quartz. Rutilated Quartz (All) – Aids development of personal potential, commitment to others, connects past and future.
- **MUDRA(S):** GYAN/PRITHVI (EARTH KNOWLEDGE)

APPENDIX E
CREATING SACRED SPACE TECHNIQUES

INVOCATION OF THE 7 WINDS

I often use this invocation of sacred space when doing movement as I find that it feels more attuning and in sync with my personal style of sacred communion and honoring The Creator, my ancestors, and all our relations.

Invoking the Winds is a Native American ritual that acknowledges the spirit totems associated to the 7 cardinal directions. (South, West, North, East, Above, Below, and Within.) It is meant to invite these spiritual guardians that assist, protect and provide us with the wisdom and divine sentience within the nature of each totem and how they are reflected within our own essential being. There is a fluid movement sequences that can be performed along with the salutation that allows us to align energetically through the sacred tone of welcoming, with those who are of higher dimensional frequencies that help us to manifest our intentions of going deeper into our journey of Divine Self-awareness, self-healing and self-mastery.

This method of creating sacred space is one that is performed as a means of honoring the indigenous life forms of earth and of the spirit that give life to all things based on the beliefs and practices of the Original ancestors of the America's. The wisdom within the cyclical and energetic patterns of nature and various animal and universal totems were honored and esteemed for their influences and guidance as to the natural flow of life and how to live in sync with it peacefully. These symbols of nature when recognized and acknowledged, are still very powerful sources of life force energy and wisdom as to our oneness with them and how we were originally designed to operate in alignment with them as part of the whole of nature itself.

TOTEMS

Totems have been used since the recorded history of humankind in many cultures from all over the world as messengers of our oneness with nature and the animal kingdom. A totem is a being, object, or symbol (such as a God, the Sun, planets, stars, animals, plants and Mother Earth herself) that represent the life forces that sustain us our bodies and their beauty that sustains our souls. These serve as an emblem for a group of people, (Such as a family, clan, group, lineage, or tribe) that reminds them of their kinship, ancestry or mythic connection. By inviting these spiritual totems or guides and their sentient energies we come to recognize their wisdom within us and our Oneness with them.

The following invocation is used to help one re-attune with the sentience of nature and to deepen our innerstanding of its Divine purpose and the deeper relationship we share within ourselves. I have found that when performing the movements while repeating the salutation of the 7 directions I have felt a deep opening of my heart and spirit that reveal the characteristics of Divine Source, the transcended and ascended ancestors, animal spirits, and cosmic counsel that are honored by it. They reveal to me their characteristics and insights that are being called upon and addressed in my life at the time. In other words, how they speak of and reveal their nature and the wisdom of their life experienced within me to guide me through the phases of my life as I pay attention to their subtle messages that come to my attention in everyday life.

OPENING THE DOORS TO EACH DIRECTION

To begin this opening meditation, fix your gaze in front of you (or close your eyes) and move your hands into a prayer pose in front of your heart. While holding this pose, in sacred meditation, draw in your breath deeply and slowly, focusing your inner awareness to that of your spiritual heart allowing a sense of calm and peace to embody your consciousness. Maintain this sense of centered energy as you slowly exhale, moving hands upwards with great intentionality reaching up past your forehead so that your palms are together above your head at your eighth charka, "The seat of the soul". As you inhale, envision the suns radiance enveloping your entire body as you drop your arms until they are shoulder height, and parallel to ground. With palms upward, start to bend your elbows drawing your hands in toward the body as if balancing two birds on your palms. Bring them in until your arms are close to your body. While hands are in this position, rotate them in front at the level of your heart and extend your arms fully forward in front of you offering your love and acknowledgement as gifts from your heart towards the direction of the wind you are facing.

With arms stretched out in front of you fan your arms out to your sides again, in welcoming the presence of the elementals into the space. Once your arms are out to your sides again turn the palms over so that they are facing down towards the earth. Bring your arms down towards the earth as if drawing a half circle from the outer edges to the middle gathering energy between them from Mother Earth until your hands are back together in front of you, then as you bring your palms together, return them to prayer pose and bring them back up in front of your heart. This sequence is performed in each direction in accompaniment with each invocation of the 7 winds.

The following salutation can be used to invoke the energies of each direction either verbally or from within yourself while performing the accompanying movements or upon completing the movement for each direction whichever feels most comfortable for you. Start by facing south. speak the associated invocation and allow yourself to connect and attune to its message and the presence of the totem that it associates to. When ready to move onto the next direction turn ¼ turn to the right (west) and speak the invocation for each direction while allowing yourself to connect to the presence of each of the cardinal directions until you are facing south again. The last three invocations (above, below, and within), can be done facing south or in any direction that you feel led to begin them.

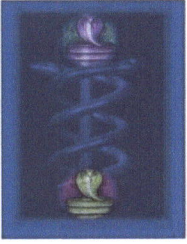

To the Winds of the South - Great Kundalini Serpent & Caterpillar

"Spirit of Knowledge, sexuality and the healing powers of nature; awaken your kundalini light within me. Fill me with your wisdom and innerstanding of the flow of Divine life and how to remain one with it. Help me shed what no longer serves my highest good, in the same way that you shed your skin, releasing the old paradigms of this world while embracing the new visions of living as one with divine life, innerstanding and embodying what it is to live as my divine Self. Thank you for teaching me to move silently on this earth plane, with the eyes to recognize the purpose and beauty of all things with appreciation for the lessons learned, the truth revealed, and the freedom to choose anew. Aho!"

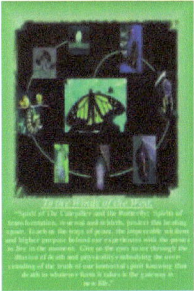

To the Winds of the West - The Butterfly

"Spirit of Transformation create in me the peaceful acceptance and ability to embrace without fear, the endless cycles of death, metamorphosis, renewal and rebirth. Protect me during the times of transformation. Provide for me the safe space and self-time for the healing, metamorphosis and renewal of my spirit, soul, body, and mind that I need in order to embody fully Your Divine Nature within me that I am designed to reflect. Thank you for teaching me the ways of peace and the impeccable wisdom and higher purpose behind my experiences with the power to live fully present in the moment with no attachments to what was, is, and shall be. I thank you for giving me the eyes to see through the illusion of death and physicality embodying the over-standing of the truth of my immortal spirit knowing that death, in whatever form it takes, is a gateway to a new higher life. Aho!"

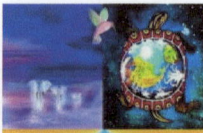

To the Winds of the North - The Elephant and The Tortoise

"Spirits of my extraterrestrial, celestial, and terrestrial ancestors, Ancient ones, come... commune with me in this time of personal and universal transformation and ascension and whisper your wisdom in the winds of my mind. So much honor and gratitude to all of you who have come before me, and all who will come after... unto the children of my children's children. Reveal to me the meaning behind the lessons within your life's experiences, the wisdom gained and the akashic knowledge of creation so that I can come to inner-stand and fulfill the purpose behind my own with your guidance to creating the future that your wisdom contains for the healing of our people and harmonizing of all life forms on this earth plane and throughout the universe, eternity and beyond. Aho!"

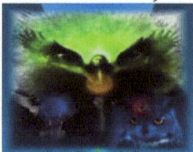

To the Winds of the East - "Amun Re, Atum Re, Atun Re"

The Eagle, The Owl, and The Seagull

May your spirits provide me with the ability to rise above the concerns of this life and transcend the limitations of the psychological and material constructs within the manmade world. Come to me from The Most High... from the place of the Triple suns... Keep me under your wings of protection and the light of your wisdom as you show me how to navigate through the rivers of life unscathed and the path of consciousness that leads to the Divine destination within my dreams. Thank you for teaching me how to live, love, heal and create as One, free in Your Great Spirit."

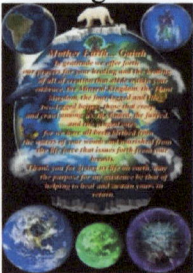

To Mother Earth, Earth Elementals and All My Relations... Gaiah

"In gratitude I offer forth my prayers for your healing and the healing and harmonizing of all of creation that abides within your embrace, the Mineral Kingdom, the Plant kingdom, the four-legged and the two-legged beings, those that creep and crawl among us, the finned, the furred, and the winged ones, for we have all been birthed from the waters of your womb and are nourished from the life force that issues forth from your breasts. Thank you, Mother Earth, for giving us life here. May the purpose for my embodiment be that of helping to heal and sustain yours in return as well as all of my relations for you have revealed to me the wisdom within nature and taught me to respect its beauty and simplicity as my own. "

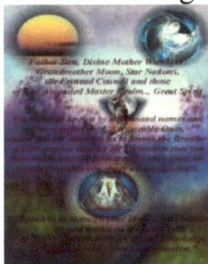

To Father Sun, Divine Mother Wombyin, Grandmother Moon, Star Nations, The Orisha, Elohim, Reiki Guides and Those of the Ascended Master Realm...

"You who are known by a thousand names and You who are the Un-nameable Ones, thank you for allowing me to breathe the Breath of Life for another day, for all of the loving creations that You have made, and the beauty that comes from the creative insights You share within my soul. Surround me with your presence, Speak to me through Your Divinity within me and guide me along the path of Right-Us-Ness through Divine knowledge, order, and healthy creative expression."

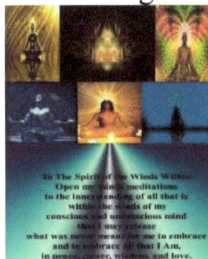

To The Spirit of the Winds Within

"Open my minds meditations to the innerstanding of all that is within the winds of my conscious and unconscious mind. Thank you for allowing me to release what was never meant for me to embrace and to embrace all that I Am in You in spirit, soul, body, and mind with peace, power, wisdom, and love abundantly. Inspire me to take action on the insights that you awaken in me and reveal from On High so that I may live in complete alignment with my Divine Purpose as my Divine Self."

In gratitude I speak this prayer to the Spirits in the directions of the north, south, east, west, above, below... and within...
Ashe', Ashe', Ashe'

"To the Winds of the North,
Grandfather Elephant/Grandmother Tortoise and Hummingbird... spirits of our terrestrial and celestial ancestor, Ancient ones, come and sit with us in this time of personal and universal healing and whisper your wisdom in the wind. As we honor those who have come before us, and those who will come after us, unto the children of our children's children, reveal to us the meaning behind the lessons within your life's experiences so that we can come to over-stand the purpose behind our own."

Father Sun, Divine Mother Wombhyili, Grandmother Moon, Star Nations, the Ennead Council and those of the Ascended Master Realm... Great Spirit.

You who are known by a thousand names and you who are the Unnameable Ones, thank you for allowing us to breath the Breathe of Life another day, for all the creation that you have made, and the beauty that comes from the creative insights you plant within our souls.

"To the Winds of the East,
Atum Re, Atun Re, & Aman Re, Great Eagle, Great Owl, Great Seagull; spirit that provides us with the ability to rise above the concerns of this life and transcend the limitations of the material constructs within this world. Come to us from the place of the tripple suns bearing messages from The Most High. Keep us under your wings of protection as you show us how to navigate through the rivers of life unscathed and the path of consciousness that leads to the Divine destination within our dreams. Teach us to live, love and create as One with Your Great Spirit."

To The Spirit of the Winds Within Open my minds meditations to the innerstanding of all that is within the winds of my conscious and unconscious mind that I may release what was never meant for me to embrace and to embrace all that I Am, in peace, power, wisdom, and love.

Mother Earth... Gaiah
In gratitude we offer forth our prayers for your healing and the healing of all of creation that abide within your embrace, the Mineral Kingdom, the Plant Kingdom, the four-legged and the two-legged beings, those that creep and crawl among us, the finned, the furred, and the winged ones, for we have all been birthed from the waters of your womb and nourished from the life force that issues forth from your breasts. Thank you for giving us life on earth, may the purpose for my existence be that of helping to heal and sustain yours in return.

To the Winds of the West,
"Spirit of The Caterpiller and the Butterfly; Spirits of transformation, renewal and rebirth, protect this healing space. Teach us the ways of peace, the impeccable wisdom and higher purpose behind our experiences with the power to live in the moment. Give us the eyes to see through the illusion of death and physicality embodying the over-standing of the truth of our immortal spirit knowing that death in whatever form it takes is the gateway to new life."

194

ANIMAL TOTEMS DETAILS FOR SENTIENT LIFE FORCE INVOCATION

The following is a description of the spiritual characteristics, qualities, and energies of the animal totems referred to in the invocation.

- **THE SERPENT/SNAKE** The caduceus Symbol that is used in the medical profession is one of the most ancient symbols of the snake. It symbolizes the center of our DNA's design where "The Mind of God" & "The Mind of Man" connect, commune, and create. The two snakes intertwined around a staff, represent the communication network of the central nervous system and that of our DNA that intertwines throughout the spinal column and the DNA of our cells. The wings represent the left and right hemispheres of the brain, with the circle representing the pineal gland which is the seat of the soul or psychic center of our being also referred to as the 1st or 3rd eye. This image of the serpent/snake also symbolizes kundalini, the corporeal energy responsible for the awakening and evolution of our spiritual Self, our sexuality and the healing powers of nature. Its qualities are that of rebirth, wisdom, fluidity, wholeness, transmutations, and sexuality, transitions, changes and new opportunities. Creative forces are awakening with heightened intuition. The nature of snakes can teach us many things such as the shedding of what is outdated within our perceptions, attitudes, and ideals, the way in which energy moves, how to access vitality, ambitions and dreams along with intellect and personal power. Consider the things that are surfacing in your life that are inspiring you to strike out and take advantage of. Perhaps there is something in your life that has you mesmerized or hypnotized… or maybe it's time to reflect on things within your life and your world. Listen to your intuition and visions at this time. Contemplate the colors, striking ability and activity of the snake to further understand the message that it wants to reveal.

- **THE CATERPILLER'S** infant stage prior to transformation, teaches patience that all things will come to fruition in nature's time and not before its perfect timing thus, the value of patience and living in the moment. Caterpillars represent the time of growth and harvesting, the preparation and storing up period where life is clearing the way, preparing you for your next venture. Notice the areas in your life that are moving like the caterpillar; inching along, resting, slowly moving, while pausing now and then. Caterpillar qualities will show how one should move for the moment while preparing yourself for what's ahead, how to focus your time and you're actions so that you are ready for what's to come and the greater good of the transformation that will be arriving so that you are ready when it arrives. Consuming energy that will be needed during the stage of metamorphosis from one phase of your life into the next.

- **THE BUTTERFLY** represents Major transformations and transmutations taking place within oneself. Or the unknown and unpredictable outcome of the ways in which your dreams, visions, and expectations take a twist turning out different yet better than what you may have expected. Butterflies are a symbol of joy, color, beauty, gentleness, lightness, and change in life. The way in which they dance on the winds seemingly without a care… the epitome of a peacefully carefree, harmonious divine life. The message they aspire to teach us is that growth doesn't have to be painful, it's meant to inspire us to discover the important issues in life for conscious transformation. Consider if you have taken the time to contemplate on and discern what is important for you right now. Are you sweating the small stuff or are you being peacefully joyful and unattached to the whims of the world that drive one to seek the material or external gratifications versus being able to recognize the blessings and the gifts that exist in your life in the moment such as your health and the areas in life where your needs have been met. They remind us of our ability to see things in a better light, the power we possess to recognize the personal message, to innerstand the lesson in our experiences in life, what they are trying to teach us, and our ability to be thankful for the blessings that reside within the simple things of life.

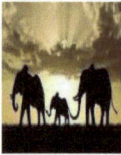

- **THE ELEPHANT** – represents strength, power, affection, loyalty, royalty, and wisdom. They are powerful warrior yet maternal and nurturing. They are known for having excellent memory, yet poor eyesight, thus relying on smell (higher form of discrimination) which can be an indication that aroma therapy may help to clear ailments and ease tensions. The Elephant represent family ideals and strong family connection they shows how to care for the young and the elderly. Ask yourself if you are applying your wisdom to help others at this time? Are you discerning and aware? Would a family gathering help to ease the tensions and stresses of everyday life? The Elephant teaches us the importance of having a balance between Self, family and occupation.

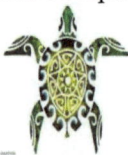

- **THE TORTOISE** teaches grounding and patience and represents longevity, wisdom and the illuminating guidance that comes from the moon. They demonstrate how to shield and protect what is important in life from feelings and emotions from work and family. Tortoise also shows the importance of contemplation and discernment before taking action and can provide insights on how to maneuver in the physical with patience and tenacity reflecting what it takes during long lasting time period which will require patience and reflective innerstanding of the purpose for delays. Tortoise is about grounding with the earth and keeping your feet on the ground, remembering and applying the wisdom shared by those who have crossed your path in past times. Tortoise also represents the life sustaining nourishing powers of the sea.

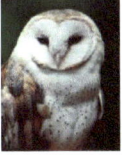

- **OWL** – is the Mystery of silent wisdom, heightened vision and hearing and the ability to pinpoint subtleties of motives, actions and people. He teaches the power of silence and contemplation and the balance of waiting and acting. When action is taken it is swift and exacting. Owl teaches the ability to extract secrets from within, so listen carefully. He also aids in clearing the deception of appearances and the hidden deceptions within oneself and/or others. Question… are you trusting your instincts about people? Are you listening to your surroundings? Do you have patience? Owl has much wisdom in teaching how to see and sense the world around you along with determination and patience in waiting for the opportune moment. The Owl is the symbol of wisdom, knowledge, and unique vision, the feminine, the moon and the night. The owl is the symbol of magic and darkness, of prophesy and clairvoyance. The Owl totem gives you the power to extract secrets. Owls are associated with mediums, psychics, clairaudience, clairvoyance, and vision quests/journeying. Owl people are usually very psychic and in tune with or able to communicate with different dimensions and experience alternate realities. They don't fear death and darkness and tend to embrace it as part of the continual cycle of life. Listen to its voice inside you and you will hear what is not being said by others, that which is hidden. You can detect subtleties of voice that others cannot. People cannot deceive those whose totem is the owl. Most Owl people are clairvoyant and can see into the darkness of other people's souls. This can be scary at times for the both parties as it comes unbidden and one is not necessarily informed as to how to use the information shown. Learn to trust your instincts about people and let your Owl totem guide you. When owl comes to visit you it is because you are being challenged to open your "inner eyes and ears" and expand your perceptions of "reality". Owl people are often inclined towards metaphysical careers, philosophy, and new thought. Owls are usually heard calling at dusk and at dawn. People with owl totem also embody this twilight aspect, with the unique ability to pick up on realities that others often don't perceive themselves. Owl people are considered to be "walkers between worlds".

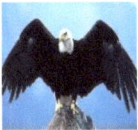

- **EAGLES – in** many indigenous cultures represents Divine Spirit, sacrifice, The Connection to The Creator Intelligence, renewal, courage, illumination of spirit, healing, creation, freedom, and risk-taking. It represents Creation, mental-spiritual-emotional swiftness, healing, dignity, strength, courage, wisdom, healing and insights, awareness of surrounding, aids in seeing hidden spiritual truths and higher balances, illumination of spirit. Eagles are strong and quick in action, are responsible for surveying and protecting and providing for those within their territory. They are a messenger of the ways in which we are meant to connect with intuition and higher spiritual truths. Are you willing to soar to new heights at this time? Are you ready to be involved with your creation and

197

manifestations? Eagle teaches that you can achieve balance and intuit the winds of change while remaining connected and grounded.

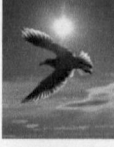

- **SEAGULL** – Seagulls are spiritual messengers that demonstrate that a higher communication of Divine guidance is taking place. They show us how to see above situations with a higher clarity and teach us that there are many perspectives to consider. Seagull shows a sense friendship and community and the cooperation that is needed for the whole to operate successfully. They are teachers of how to ride the currents of the mental, emotional and physical worlds peacefully by respecting and accepting the truth of one's own nature and that of others. Are you going with the flow or fighting it? Are you cooperating with others? Are you open to your guides? Seagull can teach us many lessons of looking, living and being. It is time to listen and watch for the nuances that indicate the divine timing of action.

TANRAN REIKI SACRED SPACE INVOCATION

A powerful way of creating sacred protective healing space is through the activation of various Tanran symbols around you that represent that sacred intention of divine protection and healing. When using Tanran Reiki to create sacred space call upon the Reiki guides, healing masters, and/or Divine Elders and invite them to prepare your energy field to receive their light energy and to bless and activate the sentient life force of each symbol so that their healing energy can work within you as a universal healing force.

First, envision or draw the symbol Zee Gah Nah, once in front of you and once behind you or on either side of you. Zee Gah Nah is a spinning triple vortex that works similar to a black hole vacuuming out low frequency energies such as sorrow, anger, and confusion transmuting them into higher, lighter frequencies of wisdom, inner-standing, and gratitude for the purpose for all things. When spun counter clockwise, Zee Gah Nah suctions out and removes non-productive or toxic energy that is being release during your active meditation. When spun clockwise it works in reverse sending out energy that has been transmuted into healthy love encompassing life force which allows for the healing chi of the elements to penetrate unhindered into your chakras and/or auric field.

Next, envision Cho Ku Rei in the 8 corners surrounding you (like a cube) at the top and bottom of you auric space or the space that you inhabit, (southwest, southeast, northwest, and northeast). This helps define the space and creates a protective field around you. **Next envision Dai Ko Myo within the middle of the sacred space you are preparing.** The power and intention of this master symbol draws in the sacred energy of the infinite realms and raises the vibration as it encompasses all of the 7 elements within the universe and within nature and represents the Divine workings of all things above and below. Once done, seal the space by envisioning Doh Yah Noh around the entire area to reinforce the protection of your auric field. The following charts are a visual representation of what this may look like.

For those wanting to become attuned to activate Tanran Reiki the training process for level 1 & 2 of the Tanran system is a 2 day workshop that will cover the Origins and history of Tanran Reiki, its systems, the similarities and differences of Tanran Reiki as opposed to other systems of Reiki, a review of the Tanran symbols, their applications and functions, how they connect with the chakra system, and attune you to the energy.

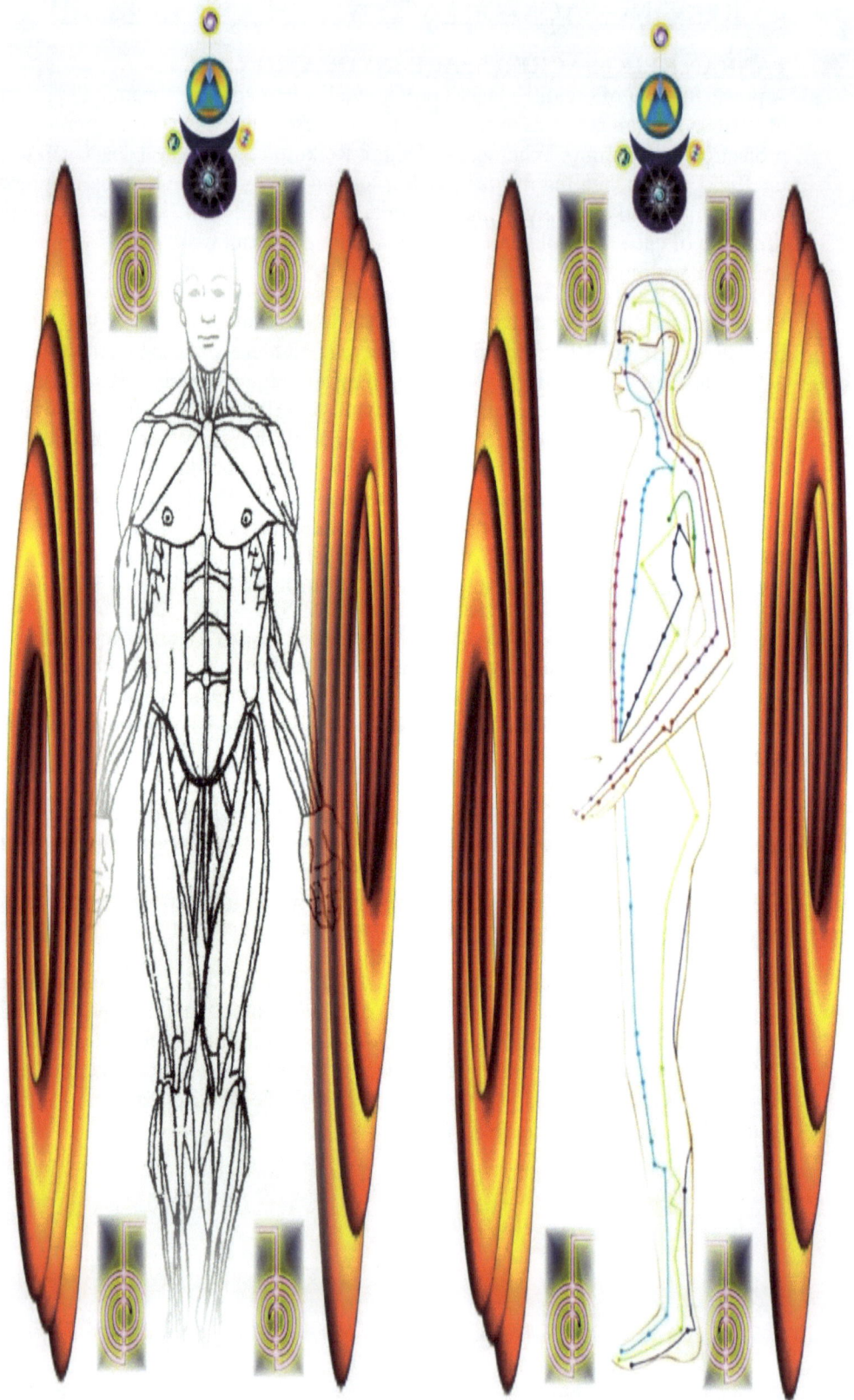

TANRAN REIKI ATUN-MENT PRAYER AND HEALING SALUTATION

BE THE UTTERANCE THAT CARRIES THE MIRACLE OF ETERNAL HEALING INTO THE UNIVERSE.

The following prayer and salutation at this stage of Kun Qi I find reactivates and attunes one to the presence of **Reiki (The Spirit of God Life Force)** and all the various sources of life force energy in a richer, deeper manner. Through affirmative prayer and focused intentional movement, the love, life, and desire that the universe contains for our greater good, becomes more evident and real.

- "Here and now I invoke the presence of the Reiki Guides, the healing and Ascended Masters, and the healing vibrations of the earthly and the universal elements to bless this space as they work in, as, and through me healing all impropriety and dis-ease within my spirit, mind, and body and that of all life forms within the universe."

- "I allow and envision the healing powers of love, life and the sentient life force of Our Creators within the Reiki symbols to enter through the "Seat of the Soul" above my head, to re-activate each symbol within each respective chakra, radiating throughout my body to awaken, cleanse, and heal my life force and to release Their healing energy into the world touching the hearts of those to whom it's being sent, as well as Mother Earth, The Elements, and all within the infinite expanse of the Universe."

- "I take in the Prana of life as my life force, visualizing, intoning, and merging the aspects of each symbol, each element, each attribute, each mudra. As I breathe in, embody, and release this healing life force to radiate throughout My entire body and the entire universe with divine unconditionally loving healing intentions, I invoke these affirmations and embrace their healing intentions within my entire being both conscious and unconscious becoming one with them." "As I move and become Kun Chi I allow it to transform my life to reflect the personification of divine health, wealth, knowledge of Self and that of creation throughout The Universe and all of Creation."

The combination of breath work, visualization and movement in this sequence are synchronized and even more powerful in their healing and transformative effects. This sequence also integrates the visioning power of the mind with the various internal/external systems of the body through the breath and the healing life force energy of Tanran Reiki deepening the healing effect multi-dimensionally.

You will again be using the 8directional movement pattern in this and the following Kun sequences however we will be slowing the movement down while intensifying the movements in order to better synchronize and internalize the sentient power of the symbols.

Stand facing south and begin circular breathing Atun -ing yourself to the Reiki Guides, your inner vision and your breath. Ask the Guides to bless and activate sacred space around you as you visualize the symbol set for sacred space from the previous page. Once you've activated sacred space bring your attention to your crown.

www.ingramcontent.com/pod-product-compliance
Lightning Source LLC
Chambersburg PA
CBHW041419290326
41932CB00042B/22